Disorder and Diagnosis

DISORDER AND DIAGNOSIS

Health and the Politics of Everyday Life in Modern Arabia

Laura Frances Goffman

STANFORD UNIVERSITY PRESS
Stanford, California

STANFORD UNIVERSITY PRESS
Stanford, California

© 2024 by Laura Frances Goffman. All rights reserved.

No part of this book may be reproduced or transmitted in any form or by any means, electronic or mechanical, including photocopying and recording, or in any information storage or retrieval system, without the prior written permission of Stanford University Press.

Printed in the United States of America on acid-free, archival-quality paper

Library of Congress Cataloging-in-Publication Data
Names: Goffman, Laura Frances, author.
Title: Disorder and diagnosis : health and the politics of everyday life in modern Arabia / Laura Frances Goffman.
Description: Stanford, California : Stanford University Press, 2024. | Includes bibliographical references and index.
Identifiers: LCCN 2024005267 (print) | LCCN 2024005268 (ebook) | ISBN 9781503638174 (cloth) | ISBN 9781503640818 (paperback) | ISBN 9781503640825 (ebook)
Subjects: LCSH: Medical policy—Arabian Peninsula—History. | Medical policy—Persian Gulf States—History. | Public health—Arabian Peninsula—History. | Public health—Persian Gulf States—History. | Diseases—Political aspects—Arabian Peninsula—History. | Diseases—Political aspects—Persian Gulf States—History. | Imperialism and science—Arabian Peninsula—History. | Imperialism and science—Persian Gulf States—History.
Classification: LCC RA395.A66 G64 2024 (print) | LCC RA395.A66 (ebook) | DDC 362.10953—dc23/eng/20240321
LC record available at https://lccn.loc.gov/2024005267
LC ebook record available at https://lccn.loc.gov/2024005268

Cover design: Katrina Noble
Cover photo: A doctor and a nurse with a patient in Abu Dhabi, 1969. Used with permission. © UAE National Library and Archives
Typeset by Newgen in 10/15 ITC Galliard Pro

To my parents,
Carolyn McCue Goffman and Daniel Goffman

CONTENTS

List of Illustrations ix
Acknowledgments xi
Note on Transliteration xv

INTRODUCTION
    Health and Power   1
1 Contagion   19
2 Hospitals   49
3 Childbirth   72
4 Experiments   96
5 Nurses   131
6 Folk Medicine   164
CONCLUSION
    The Resilient Everyday   191

Notes 197
Bibliography 247
Index 269

LIST OF ILLUSTRATIONS

Figure 0.1	View of Muscat in the early twentieth century	2
Figure 0.2	The Arabian Peninsula, Persian Gulf, and surrounding areas in the twenty-first century	5
Figure 1.1	Thomson's map of Persian Gulf ports	35
Figure 1.2	The Muscat quarantine station and an adjacent fishing village	37
Figure 1.3	Muscat quarantine station accommodations	38
Figure 1.4	Some of the structures at the Muscat quarantine station	39
Figure 1.5	View of Bushire quarantine station	40
Figure 1.6	Bushire quarantine station, first-class block with servants' quarters and kitchen on the right	41
Figure 1.7	Bushire quarantine station, third-class huts in foreground, disinfecting station behind	42
Figure 1.8	View of Basra quarantine station from the bank of the river	43
Figure 1.9	Basra quarantine station, first-class block	44
Figure 1.10	Basra quarantine station, second-class block	45
Figure 1.11	Basra quarantine station, third-class huts	46
Figure 4.1	Roger Nichols examining a child's eyes in Saudi Arabia in the 1960s	122

Figure 4.2	A townsite village in Saudi Arabia	125
Figure 4.3	An oasis village in Saudi Arabia	126
Table 5.1	Population, medical staff, and beds in Kuwait, 1965–1970	143

ACKNOWLEDGMENTS

This book represents my attempt to understand how human beings carve meaning out of a modern world that is all too often violent, frustrating, and disappointing. My intellectual and ethical conviction is that ordinary people matter, and their actions have far reaching consequences. But, because they are often lacking the power, ability, or motivation to keep their own records in ways that would make things straightforward for historians, we have a responsibility to read available archives carefully and creatively to retrieve and contextualize ordinary people's voices and experiences. These intellectual and political priorities have guided my exploration of the history of health in modern Arabia.

Any ability I have had to carry out this project is thanks to a team of wise and generous teachers, colleagues, friends, and family members who have guided me along the way. Judith Tucker, my mentor and a model of astute and ethical scholarship, patiently supported me. Life was generous to me in bringing our paths together. Fahad Bishara steered me toward invaluable sources. He provided astute questions, crucial advice, and constant encouragement. Carol Benedict's mentorship has been transformative. Osama Abi-Mershed guided me through the challenging but exhilarating ideas that forge the backbone of intellectual life. Mustafa Aksakal asked key questions at critical junctures, pushing me to consider how my work fits into the broader contours of the global Middle East.

Many colleagues during my time at Georgetown, University of Oslo, University of Arizona, University of Illinois Urbana–Champaign, and around the world provided guidance and encouragement. Georgetown's lively history cohort continues to motivate and support me, especially Jakob

Burnham, Graham H. Cornwell, Kate Dannies, Idun Hauge, Matthew Johnson, Armen Manuk-Khaloyan, Jackson Perry, Jeff Reger, Yasser Sultan, and Elizabeth Williams. Einar Wigen, Alp Eren Topal, and the rest of the Lifetimes team offered support in Oslo. In Tucson, Ben Fortna generously mentored me and commented on my entire manuscript. Also in Arizona, I benefited from the collegiality and insights of Anne Betteridge, Julia Clancy-Smith, Julie Ellison-Speight, Janelle Lamoreaux, Ute Lotz-Heumann, Maha Nassar, Yaseen Noorani, Austin O'Malley, Sébastien Roux, Brian Silverstein, Beth Stahmer, and Kamran Talattof. Jennifer Jenkins took me under her wing and offered sage advice. LouAnn Gerken hosted me for every holiday while I was in Tucson and became a valued friend and role model. Vicky Garwood offered warm friendship and Turkish breakfasts in her beautiful desert home.

I am fortunate to have found an intellectual home at the University of Illinois Urbana–Champaign. As I completed this manuscript, several colleagues shared insightful feedback at the Department of History's faculty workshop: Ikuko Asaka, Terri Barnes, Antoinette Burton, Ken Cuno, Eileen Ford, Craig Koslofsky, Marc Hertzman, Yuri Ramírez, John Randolph, Dana Rabin, and Anna Whittington. Antoinette Burton read the entire manuscript and offered invaluable suggestions.

Alex Boodrookas remains my "best colleague." So much of this book bears the imprint of his generosity and advice. Other friends, family members, teachers, and colleagues who have sustained and inspired me include Gábor Ágoston, Mahmoud Ali, Adey Almohsen, Civan Bakırgil, Abdullah Baabood, Mary Berkmen, Guy Burak, Marcia Chatelain, Omar Cheta, Amy Chidester, Salman Chowdhury, Tim Davis, Beth Derderian, Aziz Elabaseery, Rachel Engh, Crystal Ennis, Leon Fink, Lora Galabi, Lisa Goffman and Bill Saxton, Sam, Jean, Bea and Arthur, Dahlia Helmy, Elsayed Issa, Rose, Jim, Nick and Susan Jeffery, Maurice Jackson, Adrienne Kates, Rana Khoury, Allison Korinek, Ann Lesch, Reina Lewis, Rob Lewis, Jan Liverance, Zach Lockman, Meredith McKittrick, Jessie Moritz, Laila Moustafa, Shaikha Almubaraki, Tim Newfield, Leslie Peirce, Anwar Al-Saad, Mohamad Salah, Suzanne Stetkevych, Gwenn Okruhlik, Mohammed AlShakhori,

Fahed Al-Sumait, Aparna Vaidik, Kimberly Wortmann, Mohamed Youssef, Abdullah Al Zeyadi, and Ayelet Zoran-Rosen.

I am grateful for the support of a Fulbright-Hays Doctoral Dissertation Research Abroad fellowship, research sponsorship from the Gulf Studies Center at Qatar University, a postdoctoral fellowship year at the University of Oslo, and faculty research funding from the University of Arizona and the University of Illinois Urbana–Champaign.

Thank you to Kate Wahl and the editorial team at Stanford University Press for their support and professionalism. I am grateful to Katherine Faydash for her wonderful copyediting. Two anonymous readers offered feedback that was instrumental in improving this manuscript.

Much behind-the-scenes and often unacknowledged labor has gone into organizing, cataloging, digitizing, and retrieving the documents I rely on in this book. I am truly grateful to the librarians and archivists who make historical research possible. I would like to thank the kind librarians and archivists at Dar al-Kutub (particularly Mohamad Faraj and Abdul Aziz), Museum of Islamic Art Library (particularly Susan Parker-Leavy and Ahmed Al-Marzoqi), Qatar University Library, Hamad Health Sciences Library, the BP Archive (particularly Joanne Burman), Kuwait University, Qatar Digital Library, Arabian Gulf Digital Archives, the National Library and Archives of the UAE, the National Archives of India, the Zanzibar National Archives, the British Library, the British National Archives at Kew, the US National Archives, the Georgetown special collections, the University of Arizona Library, and the University of Illinois Urbana–Champaign Library. I am grateful to Maggie Lehane for designing the map. My sincere thanks also go to Abdulla Aljneibi, Mariam Matar AlKaabi, and Ahmed AlMaazmi for kindly helping me to secure permission to use the cover photograph.

Finally, I want to acknowledge that, because of the shimmer of joy in my dad's eyes when he was immersed in his research and writing, I had the privilege of growing up with a fervent (and no doubt unusual) belief that Ottoman history was the most exciting subject in the entire world. He named the family dog we got when I was six years old Bendysh, after a British diplomat to the Ottoman Empire. I'll never forget how Bendysh (the dog) would sit enraptured, his head jolting up at every mention of his name, while my dad had long phone calls with colleagues in which he buoyantly discussed the Ottoman exploits of Bendysh (the Englishman). We lost a lot when my dad had his stroke in 2006. Aphasia robbed him of his speech and writing. Now, well over a decade since I started my own formal training in Middle East history, I'm able to see that much of my academic journey has been driven by my search for the intellectual exhilaration that lit up my childhood and that I so missed after my dad got sick. It's thanks to my mother that I have been able to pursue my own academic career. Heroically, intelligently, and lovingly she has taken on the role of caring for my now disabled father. Moreover, while adjusting to life with a disabled husband, she completed her own book and developed a critical awareness of the gendered politics of caregiving even as she remained the emotional and organizational stalwart of the entire family. I dedicate this book to my parents, Carolyn McCue Goffman and Daniel Goffman, with love and gratitude.

NOTE ON TRANSLITERATION

I follow the transliteration system of the *International Journal of Middle East Studies* (*IJMES*). Personal names are transliterated without diacritics or follow the individual's preferred spelling in Roman script.

INTRODUCTION

HEALTH AND POWER

IN THE SUMMER OF 1899, the British civil surgeon Atmaram Sadashiva Grandin Jayakar knew cholera was coming to Muscat. But when he tried to alert the local authorities, no one would heed his warnings. Jayakar, stationed as a British imperial representative in the coastal city since 1873, pleaded with Sultan Faysal bin Turki (r. 1888–1913) to take precautionary measures against the cholera epidemic raging in Karachi.[1] Not only did Faysal's government fail "to wake up to the danger," but the sultan even suspended quarantine arrangements for several weeks.[2] This total absence of surveillance, Jayakar believed, allowed for infected passengers arriving by mail steamer to pass effortlessly into the local community, triggering an epidemic that progressed "gradually and insidiously."[3] Adding to Jayakar's frustration was the fact that, even as residents started developing the dreaded symptoms of diarrhea, vomiting, thirst, restlessness, and leg cramps, authorities "doubted and denied" the epidemic.[4] Local people, for their part, also proved reluctant to seek help as they and their family members fell ill. Jayakar himself learned of the epidemic only indirectly when, in September 1899, news of a twelve-year-old boy's sudden death due to "vomiting and purging" led him to "suspect the probability of the appearance of cholera."[5]

Cholera finally subsided in the twin ports of Muscat and Muttrah by January 1900, but it continued to devastate Oman, especially the interior region nestled between the Hajar mountain range and the deserts of central

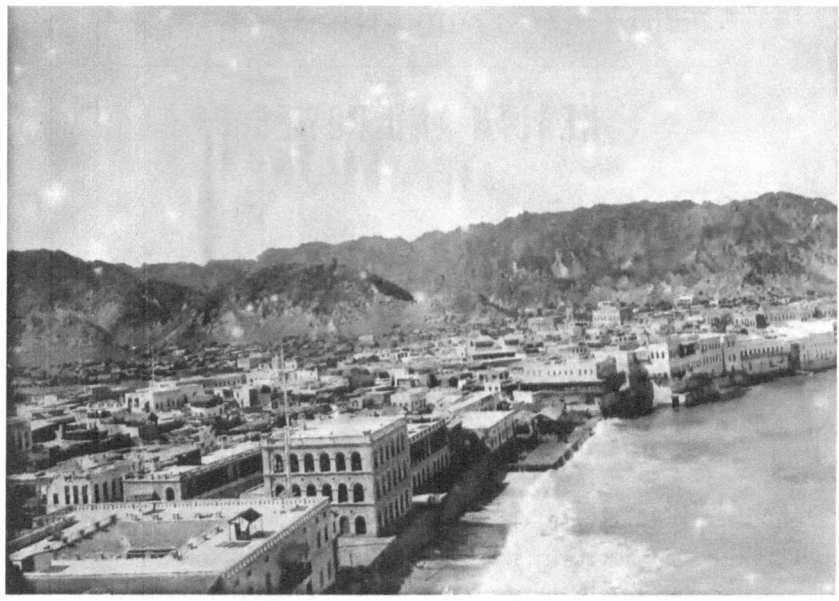

FIGURE 0.1. View of Muscat in the early twentieth century.

SOURCE: Theodore Thomson, *Report by Dr. Theodore Thomson on the Sanitary Requirements of Certain Places in or near the Persian Gulf, &c.,* Printed for the use of the Foreign Office, October 1906. London School of Hygiene & Tropical Medicine Library & Archives Service.

Arabia.[6] Local politics obstructed Jayakar's ability to surveil cholera's advancement beyond the "almost circular range of hills" that framed Muscat's "picturesque appearance from the sea" (fig. 0.1).[7] Nevertheless, from his coastal enclave, Jayakar learned that Oman suffered "enormous mortality."[8] Agricultural life in the interior region flourished thanks to an expansive network of engineered water channels, known locally as *aflāj* (sing. *falaj*), that pulled precious water down from the mountains.[9] In the time of cholera, this combination of interconnected water systems and human mobility proved deadly. The bacterium *Vibrio cholerae* that causes cholera disseminates through food or water that is contaminated with fecal matter. For people who develop severe symptoms, the course of illness is rapid and devastating. Dehydration from diarrhea and vomiting can lead within hours to kidney failure, coma, and death. The breathtaking speed at which cholera ravaged previously healthy bodies only intensified the terror of its symptoms.[10] In early October 1899, a caravan returning inland from Muttrah had introduced cholera in the village of Surur, "which lies on the highway to the Sharkiyeh or Eastern District of Oman." As Jayakar reported, "the suddenness of the invasion and the alarming rate of mortality there caused the people to be almost panic-stricken and to flee in all directions," carrying the infection with them.[11] By November, letters dispatched from Oman to the Sultan of Zanzibar, Hamud bin Mohammad, contained updates on the dire situation: "Everything is lifeless . . . The people of Oman are afflicted by the epidemic, smallpox, the famine, and the rising cost of living. Every crisis is greater than its sister!"[12]

We can imagine how in 1899 and 1900, as the water channels streamed down from the mountains, *Vibrio cholerae* also flowed through Oman's communities. Jayakar was attuned to scientific advancements that posited connections between cholera epidemics and shared water supplies. He also demonstrated a nuanced understanding of local water infrastructures. He identified patterns of "washing the dead quite close to the aqueducts" as "the determining cause" of cholera's intensity in Oman. "When a dead body is removed to one of these aqueducts for washing," he wrote, "a breach is made in the masonry of the aqueduct quite close to the place where the body is, and the water allowed to run over it, some of which evidently runs by the side of the aqueduct and eventually pollutes it. Cholera germs in abundance had thus an easy access to the water supply of most of the places and gave rise to those sudden and violent explosions."[13] Jayakar reported that cholera claimed 12,231 lives in Oman.[14] He estimated that 10,000 people lived in Muscat and 15,000 in Muttrah at the turn of the century; in other words, Jayakar calculated that the total number of deaths from cholera was comparable to the entire population of one of the main coastal cities.[15]

Reflecting British imperial classifications of the region's people, Jayakar cataloged cholera mortality and morbidity from a "racial point of view."[16] But even though he categorized the population as Baluchi, Arab, African, Persian, and Indian, Jayakar ultimately placed more emphasis on social class and wealth, rather than ethnicity, to explain how the epidemic developed.[17] He carefully documented patterns of cleanliness, medical and prophylactic practices, and the degree of willingness to seek out medical care across different communities. For example, he observed that the Baluchis suffered "the greatest incidence of attacks" because "their habitations are mostly in the filthiest localities and themselves most regardless of the commonest rules of personal hygiene." The Indian community, in contrast, enjoyed "almost absolute immunity" from cholera, Jayakar reported, thanks to the geography of their housing, the relative affluence of their living situation, and their willingness to seek out Jayakar's medical care.[18] Finally, morbidity was starkly gendered; Jayakar noted that in some communities "women were suffering more than men" at a rate of nearly double the number of cholera attacks because "the duty of nursing the sick generally devolved on the fairer sex."[19] From Jayakar's perspective, official neglect, usage of dangerous water, poor sanitation, gendered caregiving, and reluctance to seek medical help characterized the local response to Oman's cholera crisis of 1899–1900.

But, in addition to its devastating loss of life, the epidemic shifted Sultan Faysal's understanding of the relationship between health and politics. Just as cholera was retreating from the coastal cities, simultaneous outbreaks of plague and influenza struck Muscat and Muttrah.[20] Facing this renewed epidemiological onslaught, the sultan supported disinfection and inoculation, built hospital sheds, and hired a medical practitioner and assistant who had plague experience from Bombay.[21] Faysal's unprecedented willingness to take measures against plague in the aftermath of the cholera epidemic constituted a remarkable transformation. The sultan, despite persistent skepticism among residents and subjects, had recognized public health as a responsibility of sovereignty and an instrument of governance.

* * *

Jayakar's description of the devastating cholera epidemic in Oman at the turn of the twentieth century opens a door to the questions that this book seeks to examine. Jayakar, an official British doctor, begged the sultan to take measures that would allay the spread of epidemic by placing restrictions on the movement of people. Local people, in turn, resisted or ignored

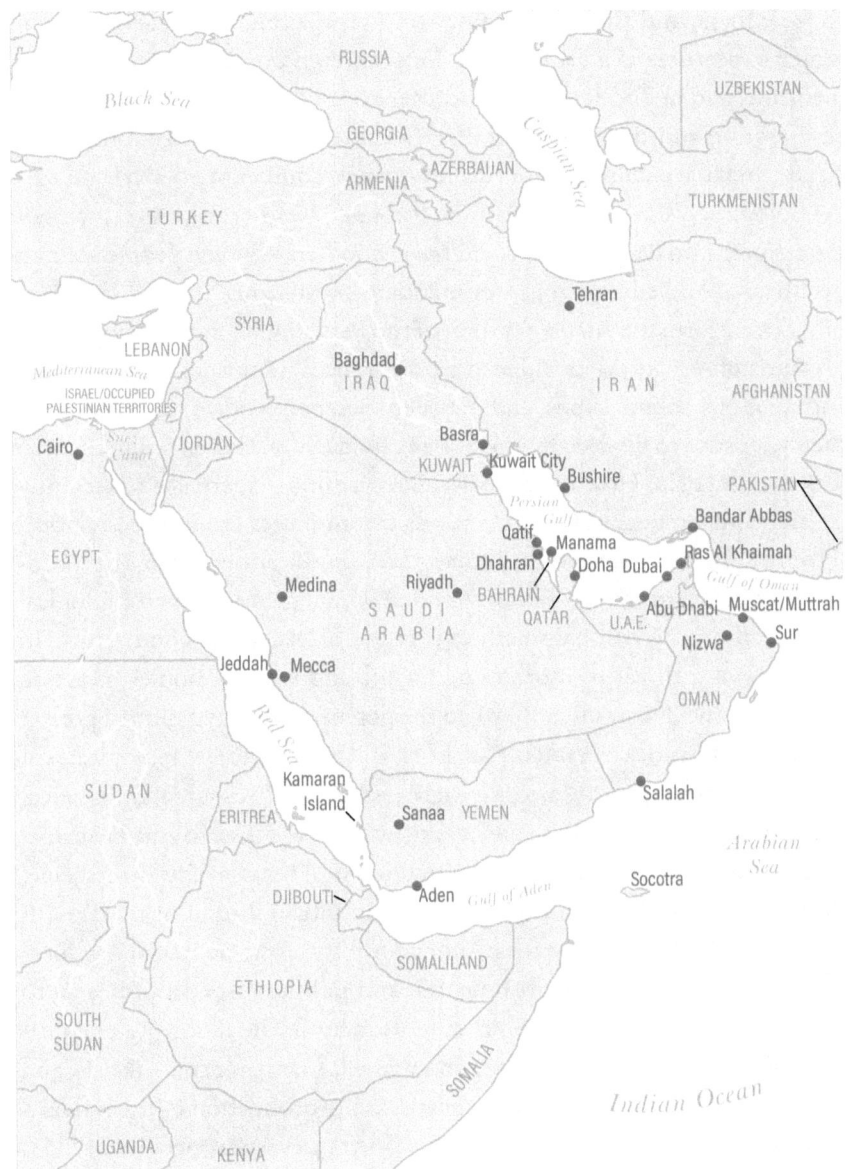

FIGURE 0.2. The Arabian Peninsula, Persian Gulf, and surrounding areas in the twenty-first century. Map by Maggie Lehane, University of Wisconsin Cartography Lab.

those efforts, and the sultan came to interpret refusal to participate in sanitary measures as a challenge to his sovereign power. State formation, medicine, and public health became interwoven during this age of imperial competition and the consolidation of local rulers in nascent monarchical states. Imperial and local actors diagnosed new sources of political and epidemiological disorder in Arabia and responded by inserting novel forms of state power into daily life. How did the encounters between people seeking health and people bestowing—or inflicting—public health practices upon others transform the Arabian littoral of the Persian Gulf in the modern era? Jayakar's observations included stark differences in mortality across racial and religious communities, and between men and women, depending on their exposure to disease, their labor as caregivers, and their willingness to seek medical help. How were medical interventions experienced differently by men and women and by the various communities around the region?

From the late nineteenth century, the intensification of the British imperial presence in the Gulf corresponded with a growing microbiological understanding of contagion among the global scientific community. In emerging as a threat to more valued white and wealthy bodies, nonelite people and the diseases that they had the potential to carry assumed greater visibility in historical records. Thanks to this confluence of biological, social, and political factors, astonishingly resilient and resourceful historical characters emerge out of the crevices of accounts of disease and medicine.

Disorder and Diagnosis is a social and political history of how medicine, disease, and public health transformed the Arabian littoral of the Persian Gulf from the late nineteenth century until the 1973 oil boom. By integrating the biological, environmental, and political aspects of health to highlight the role of nonelites in state formation, the following chapters challenge the predominant assumption that oil, Islam, imperial officials, and autocratic monarchies were most central to the production of the modern Gulf. Rather, this was a transformation shaped by everyday people. In 1862, steamships linked Gulf ports to Bombay and Karachi, and thus initiated a new era of accelerated connectivity and British imperial integration. In the late nineteenth and early twentieth centuries, quarantine stations and hospitals incorporated the bodies of Gulf residents into an unprecedented medical infrastructure that was built on existing networks of transregional mobilities. The search for oil in the first half of the twentieth century and its aggressive exploitation in the aftermath of World War II expanded the focus of colonial medical interventions from the coast into the hinterland, and from white and elite bodies to indigenous and itinerant laborers. And, in the 1960s and 1970s, the transition of the Gulf's Arabian littoral from British spheres of influence to formally sovereign states accelerated the transformation of peripatetic populations into increasingly rigid categories of citizens and noncitizens.

Over this *longue durée*, an array of medical projects—quarantines, hospitals, childbirth, vaccinations, nursing, and folk medicine—illustrates how the Gulf and its Arabian hinterland served as a buffer zone between "diseased" Asia, the Ottoman Empire, and white Europe; as an object of development; and as a space of scientific translation. Mobile, multiethnic, and multiconfessional residents of regions that would become Kuwait, Saudi Arabia, Bahrain, Qatar, the United Arab Emirates, and Oman accepted, modified, or rebelled against top-down medical institutions. From the mid-nineteenth century, the relationship between ideas of contagion and contamination and racial and spatial segregation were institutionalized on a global scale. In the Gulf, the paradigm of health as a colonial and civilizing mission and, consequently, as a method of cultural erasure mediated interactions between local populations and doctors as well as imperial and state officials. From this increasing entanglement of public health, governance, and everyday life, new venues of interaction and negotiation between states and populations emerged.

Beyond National Borders and Chronologies

This book places overlooked historical actors at the center of the development of the modern Gulf and Arabia. It also positions the Arabian littoral of the Persian Gulf as a nexus of global circulations of people and pathogens. Along with urban spaces, illicit and licit trade, and fluid legal systems, modern public health and medicine emerged through the intersecting behaviors and beliefs of a range of actors. *Disorder and Diagnosis* explores the tension between the Gulf and its Arabian hinterland as a coherent epidemiological and medical space and as a disorderly crossroads of imperial and local political projects and imaginaries.[22] Previous scholarship has constructed histories around ways that the flows of pathogens transcend state and national borders and shape emerging political frontiers.[23] Building on such insights, this book emphasizes movement to demonstrate the importance of considering the Persian Gulf and Arabian Peninsula as an epidemiological region in the prenational period, and even well into the twentieth century. The modern state, with its claims to control space and time as part of a presumed natural and logical ordering, aims to deprive individuals of the ability to imagine alternatives by removing, or making unthinkable, any space not tied to a single temporal and spatial national identity.[24] By privileging mobility and connectivities, *Disorder and Diagnosis* moves beyond the stark spatial and conceptual limitations of the national frame and locates alternative historical imaginaries amid the fluctuating contours of regional configurations.

As well as insisting on the permeability of national borders, this book also overturns predominant chronologies of Gulf development. Emphasizing how Gulf societies steered their own course as they navigated their way into oil-funded modernity challenges the long-standing assumption that this region's history has moved in a separate, stagnant time scale.[25] In the late nineteenth and early twentieth centuries, British imperial officials and American missionaries fostered the belief that the people of this region existed outside of prevailing definitions of modern progress. In the context of health and disease, they expressed such sentiments by describing local medicine as mired in unscientific traditions and resistant to, or incapable of, change or development in conversation with other medical systems. A second assertion of regional inertia occurred when the post–World War II oil state (echoed by its ideological interlocuters) declared itself the exclusive provisioner of progress, modernity, and social welfare. Centralized state medicine planned by foreign experts and staffed by noncitizen workers was projected to supersede the demand for local curative practices.

Resulting from such extensive erasure and denial of the dynamism of bottom-up local histories, discussions of the Gulf and the Arabian Peninsula have been subjected to a persistent exceptionalism.[26] Narratives of the region produced by contemporary states and social scientists alike have embraced deterministic paradigms positing that oil wealth resulted in authoritarian regimes and passive citizens, privileging global economic forces over local politics.[27] Meanwhile, specialists in other areas of the Middle East and Arab world have overlooked the mutually constitutive connectivities and shared experiences between the modern Gulf and the wider region. National accounts wholeheartedly promote a narrative in which the predominantly Arab states of the modern Gulf are supposed to have leaped from a period of darkness and relative isolation before the discovery of oil and arrived with dazzling speed in well-financed and tightly controlled global cities characterized by commoditized affluence.

Much Gulf historiography, spanning nineteenth-century British dominance and the current age of American hegemony, focuses on describing a series of skirmishes, treaties, and agreements and locates the driving force of historical change in negotiations between regional elites and global superpowers. More recently, however, scholars have explored local archives and read sources "against the grain" with the important aim of recovering historical voices that have been left out of this elite and imperial-centered political narrative by focusing on urban histories and the lasting effects of imperialism.[28] A related body of scholarship seeks to integrate the Gulf into the Indian Ocean world, looking at how individuals, institutions, and economies operated under the imperial radar and complicating assumptions regarding the omnipresence of British authority.[29]

While oceanic history is central to the Gulf experience, much of the extant scholarship depicts this world of trade and mobility largely (though not exclusively) as the purview of men.[30] Until we consider how women fit into this milieu of fluid connectivity between land and water, we risk erasing a large part of the region's history. The intersections of the politics of health, childbirth, motherhood, and gendered medical labor particularly show women to be productive and creative agents. Moreover, while trailblazing work has considered the interplay of religion, politics, women, and gender in the region, the lens of health allows us to shift our focus toward questions of reproduction and political economy.[31] While there is a real methodological challenge in uncovering women's contributions, histories of health reveal dense archival discussions of women's lives and thus offer an opportunity to fill this void. The chapters on hospitals, childbirth, experiments, and nurses emphasize women's experiences as patients, mothers, and workers in the framework of a politics of health. Working beyond and between national frames of time and space allows such stories to shift toward the foreground of Gulf modernity.

Between Politics of Health and Theories of Power

The devastation of epidemic makes visible the politics of everyday life. Histories of the Gulf and Arabia have focused on the political and economic dynamics between local elites, transregional merchant communities, British officials, and tribal challengers. But, as Jayakar's estimates on cholera mortality in the 1899–1900 epidemic poignantly illustrate, disease was the overwhelmingly predominant cause of daily hardship and loss of life for local communities of the pre-oil period. Indeed, British imperial officials believed that the Gulf climate was so dangerous that the Government of India was reluctant to appoint significant numbers of Europeans as local agents in the Gulf until the twentieth century; as a British Indian, Jayakar's own lengthy tenure in Muscat from 1873 to 1900 exemplifies that trend.[32] Such fears were not unfounded. Disease took a hefty toll on European and local communities alike. Between 1800 and 1810, four British agents in Muscat died from climate-related causes.[33]

Disorder and Diagnosis intersects with a range of historical studies seeking to make sense of the relationship between disease, state, and population. One way of taking stock of current trends in the history of medicine is to ask how different scholars have grappled with Michel Foucault's assemblage of territory, security, discipline, and population.[34] Historians long have struggled to reconcile the inescapable reality of Foucault's influence with disciplinary vexation over his methods. As Allan Megill put it: "The main complaint is perspectival and methodological. Foucault leaves unanswered, even unasked, questions that historians find essential; his generalizations are usually supported by insufficient warrants."[35] Nevertheless, scholars productively have crafted sharp research questions in response to Foucault's broad strokes. David Scott, for example, encourages researchers working on the colonial state to identify "the point or points of power's application, the object or objects it aims at, and the means and instrumentalities it deploys in search of these targets, points and objects."[36] In approaching health as a lens onto the politics of everyday life, this book pursues a series of related questions: Which political rationalities and methods do state actors employ to manage a population and individuals simultaneously? How does the state apply power over territories and populations both conceptually and materially? Which mechanisms enable sovereigns to define the people and geographies they claim to govern? Which conditions of possibility prompted corporate agents to turn to epidemiological studies and medical experiments to render populations legible and more productive? How do institutions like quarantine stations, clinics, and hospitals encourage individuals to self-regulate or to find ways around such disciplining interventions? Finally, and most crucially for this study, how do the everyday practices of a range of people nuance or overturn doctrinaire categories of biological, social, and political personhood?

We can trace Foucault's influence across recent studies of medicine in the modern Middle East in which scholars continue to interact with and push back against his claims in creative and innovative ways.[37] In her study of madness, modernity, and war in Lebanon, for example, Joelle M. Abi-Rached critically synthesizes how histories of mental health have interacted with Foucault's framework. She notes the shift from a triumphalist postwar position on the continual progress and improvement of medicine to Foucault's famous critique that "moral and hence psychological treatment was more insidious and perverse than the physical shackles used to restrain the insane, for it trained and turned the will against itself."[38] The current historiographical wave aspires to a middle ground, managing, as Abi-Rached puts it, "to display through contextual specificities the multiple functions of asylums and the porousness of the institutional politics of mental illness that together involve different actors with diverse resources and interests."[39] Similar trends may be observed in the history of medicine more broadly, in which concerns with overarching institutional power are mediated by the activities and choices of individuals as reconstructed by historians through close and critical readings of available archives.

Without claiming to have escaped the long shadow of the Foucauldian corpus, this book builds on such approaches to the history of medicine by offering a commitment to historical methodology as something of a restraining check on totalizing theories. It is unhelpful to elide the fact that institutions, often with the support of debilitating state violence and astonishing influxes of wealth, have transformed the lives of people in the Gulf and the Arabian Peninsula on a massive scale from the mid-nineteenth century to the present. But, as often as not, grandiose theory crumbles when we work to construct meaning from quotidian choices and actions rather than from sweeping generalizations. "States and municipalities," as Helen Tilley writes, "have never had a monopoly over cultures of care."[40] Individuals—and even entire categories of people—who have been expunged from master narratives emerge as creative and active historical figures when they choose, as we will see, to abscond from quarantine, give birth at home, or seek hospital treatment.

Empire, state building, and modern medicine are projects that share an impulse to diagnose disorders and prescribe solutions. Such dynamics of health and power—and their remarkable limitations—are the central concern of this book. The idea of health systems, medical imaginaries, and scientific practice in this region that existed "before" the introduction of biomedicine is integrated into the chapters as appropriate; however, my narrative rejects the rigidness of a before-and-after timeline.[41] First, the assumption of indigenous medicine as it was practiced "before" and "after" external influence presumes a homogeneous and unchanging medical system, depriving the region of its own vibrant health histories. Second, the convergence of the state, public health, and medical institutions as an experience of modernity constitutes a key venue through which the Gulf and Arabian Peninsula were integrated into global processes. Third, the nature of my sources shapes the content of my discussion. I integrate British imperial records, American missionary writings, Islamic scholarly opinions, scientific studies of the health conditions of local people, local newspapers, and Arabic-language histories of health and *al-ṭibb al-shaʿbī* (folk medicine). This interweaving of a wide range of archival genres allows this book to foreground the influence and experiences of populations who might otherwise remain absent from the historical record.

The Chapters Ahead

Quarantine stations and hospitals demonstrate two distinct examples of how British imperial visions of modern medicine and local imaginaries of health and mobility intersected. In the late nineteenth century, quarantine stations materialized Britain's efforts to fend off its Gulf rivals. Chapter 1, "Contagion," positions the Gulf in the global networks of disease, empire, accelerated communications, and scrutinized contagions of the late nineteenth and early twentieth centuries. Quarantine stations allowed state actors to wield sovereignty and to construct new classifications of the population in the name of sanitation. The chapter turns to the scale of local life to reconstruct experiences of disease and notions of contagion leading up to the imposition of imperial quarantines. Then, a tour of the quarantine stations that knitted Gulf ports together reveals how this imperial infrastructure's unprecedented claims over Gulf bodies integrated categories of race, class, and gender into a sprawling sanitary infrastructure. But the limitations of the imperial sanitary imaginary were evident in the persistent disorder that the lens of social history exposes. Even as imperial intermediaries at the local level embraced quarantine, the reluctance of travelers to interrupt their journeys rendered the stations so porous that they proved ineffective as a means of blocking the spread of disease.

From quarantine stations that forcibly fixed travelers in space and time, I turn to medical institutions that drew in health-seeking patients from around the region. Chapter 2, "Hospitals," reconstructs how communities in Manama, Muscat, and Kuwait made use of American missionary and British Agency hospitals in the early twentieth century. It traces how hospitals produced new forms of gendered personhood, in which medical care was delineated between spaces for men and women, and between male and female medical professionals. An emergent competitive medical marketplace created pressure on local elites to integrate health services into their broader projects of governance. In stark contrast to the quarantine stations, hospitals emerged as a top-down medical infrastructure that eventually enjoyed popular local buy-in. The nascent hospital infrastructure prompted local rulers, American missionaries, and imperial officials to scramble to meet the evolving medical expectations of everyday people.

The British Empire, operating on the cheap, depended on intermediary actors such as American missionaries and Indian doctors, like Jayakar, to invest time, money, and concern in the ailments of local people. At the same time, hospital projects would have failed had they not achieved bottom-up popularity. Local people expressed their enthusiasm with their feet, traveling far to access hospital care.

Yet local people's embrace of hospitals remained strategic and selective. Their behavior did not align neatly with doctors' normative vision of patients who obediently accepted scientific diagnosis. Despite the growing popularity of hospitals, childbirth, a critical event in women's lives, remained beyond the control of women missionary doctors throughout the early twentieth century. Chapter 3, "Childbirth," counterbalances the focus on the rise of institutionalized medicine and public health as driven by male elites and missionary doctors. In defiance of women missionaries' efforts, local women resisted the medicalization of childbirth and persisted in giving birth at home under the care of midwives and women relatives. This chapter makes women's worlds visible in the face of a historiography that has overwhelmingly characterized the rhythms of oceanic mobility and national development as masculine experiences. Taken together, quarantines, hospitals, and childbirth remind us of the nuance and contingency of empire and state building in everyday life by revealing how local people could alternately resist and tactically make use of medical infrastructures.

Motherhood as a category of health and an act of politics is also an important theme in Chapter 4, "Experiments." In the post–World War II period, a new imperial structure achieved hegemony in the Gulf in the form of the oil industry's corporate colonialism. To unpack how this emergent geopolitical alignment intersected with local experiences of health, I examine medical experiments carried out in eastern Arabia under the auspices of the Arabian American Oil Company (Aramco). Rather than assuming local passivity in the face of the postwar corporate onslaught, my intention is to stress that the emergence of health care as a central demand of popular movements in Arabia is just as important as the goals of company officials and university scientists for understanding how medicine developed. The racial segregation and extractive exploitation of the oil industry coincided with global decolonization and regional Arab solidarities. Popular and labor movements envisioned health care as a universal right that people could demand from their employer and their state. From the 1950s to the 1970s, amid these broader changes in the popular politics of health, Aramco funded a Harvard project to use the people of the region as a population on which to test experimental trachoma vaccines. In Aramco's capitalist frame, the goal of medicine was to produce healthy bodies of laborers and sanitized environments for work. As a result of oil exploitation and state consolidation, public health expanded from the Gulf coasts into Arabia's interior. The partnership between Harvard and Aramco constructed eastern Arabia as a space of medical experimentation contingent on the desire of local parents to seek care for their children's infected eyes.

Chapter 5, "Nurses," shifts the focus from women as health-seeking parents to women as noncitizen workers. In the 1960s, migrant Arab women nurses in Kuwait drew on pan-Arab solidarities to attempt to advance their professional claims. Over the course of postwar state building, noncitizen women performed the labor of birthing Kuwait's medical system, a hallmark of the country's welfare project. Interviews with nurses in the Kuwaiti press from this period show that these women actively positioned themselves as vanguard Arab modernizers. They drew on the discourses of Arab unity and modernist development to push back against patriarchal norms that constrained their professional and personal lives. Noncitizen Arab women nurses struggled to convince the Ministry of Health and the Kuwaiti public that they were essential professionals who deserved fair pay and decent working conditions. The chapter concludes with the post-1973 pivot away from the Arab world and toward South Asia as a source of health-care workers as the Ministry of Health, in step with other agencies, prioritized cheaper labor.

Finally, in chapter 6, the narrative springs forward to the late twentieth and early twenty-first centuries to explore how more than a century of imperial, corporate, and state Gulf medical modernization never fully supplanted local esteem for folk medicine. Instead, the demographic anxieties produced by autochthonous citizenship and exploitative labor practices created conditions that fostered nostalgia for the folk medicine of pre-oil Arabia. This chapter shifts methodologically to a socially situated textual analysis. It examines how two Arabic-language accounts of *al-ṭibb al-shaʿbī* (folk medicine) construct health history as a space of nostalgia for a pre-oil, nativist past. The resurgence of *al-ṭibb al-shaʿbī* overturns the idea of a teleological progression of medicine. This counternarrative of medicine is made possible by a resurgent interest in folk medicine that frames certain health practices as indigenous to the region's Arab Muslim population. In this conceptualization, *al-ṭibb al-shaʿbī* is an immutable cultural artifact, a tool for delineating national inclusion, and a foil to biomedicine as an alienating and overly institutionalized experience.

The accelerated globalization of disease and the subsequent elaboration of medical knowledge and institutions transformed the relationship between imperial and local political elites and everyday people in the modern Gulf and Arabia. The periodization of the first five chapters of this book ends in a dynamic moment of transition from public health as a poorly funded and sporadically implemented manifestation of British imperialism and American missionary work to top-down development projects that targeted the bodies of oil workers and emerging citizen and noncitizen populations. Chapter 6, however, examines an alternative reading of the stories I unravel in the preceding case studies. Looking back from ideological narratives of medicine constructed by citizens in the late twentieth and early twenty-first centuries, these politicized accounts express nostalgia for pre-oil society in their attempt to reconstruct folk medicine as a yardstick of national belonging. By fashioning the history of folk medicine as a site of heritage, such narratives contribute to broader patterns of demarcating inclusions and exclusions among local populations in modern Arabia and the Gulf.

Across these chapters, my method has been to focus on striking and surprising archival fragments, encircling them with thick contextualization to reconstruct their social, political, and medical worlds. I identify the pursuit of health as an assemblage of motivations that guided collective, but largely uncoordinated, action.[42] While the theme of health seeking as a form of politics unifies the narrative, I am attentive to how the concept of health itself is historically fluid. That is, I locate the politics of collective, uncoordinated action in changing medical infrastructures and social dynamics. People in Arabia adjusted their expectations of what constituted health in dialogue with state projects, missionary hospitals, and globalizing science. I seek to shift the focus of this region's modern history away from the actions and schemes of ruling elites and corporate executives and toward the ambitions and activities of middling intermediaries and ordinary people. As the following chapters show, even when powerful actors, be they local, imperial, missionary, or corporate, aspired to use medical and health institutions as tools for demarcating and disciplining populations, the nimble creativity of everyday people complicated or even undermined those top-down visions. Rather than chronicling a teleological march toward modernity, I attempt to find a balance between aspirations of totalizing power and resurgent moments of unanticipated consequences, persistent disorder, and even chaos.

CHAPTER I

CONTAGION

IN THE DEAD OF NIGHT ON APRIL 9, 1903, under a luminous moon, five men from the Omani coastal town of Sur clambered over the low rocks encircling the coast to escape Muscat's quarantine station. Their travel companion, Abdulla bin Khamis, was waiting for them in a small boat, and together they fled into the night.[1] The next morning, Sultan Faysal bin Turki (r. 1888–1913) was furious. He dispatched his quarantine superintendent, Ali Salman, to the British Agency to request that the HMS *Perseus*, at anchor in Muscat harbor, chase down the truants. The British were eager to acquiesce to his request. They associated Sur with the slave trade, and this city's merchants had long frustrated British officials by evading their attempts to curb the Gulf's persistently robust traffic in enslaved people.[2] The steamship took off down the coast, carrying the quarantine official so that he could identify the missing men. Scanning the coastline with his field glasses, Ali Salman was relieved to find that the fugitives could not escape inland, as "the place where we came up with them was overhung by the steep sides of a cliff and they could get nowhere."[3] He recalled the moment of recapture: "I called out the name of each and said we had come for them and they came without further trouble seeing we were armed."[4]

In the late nineteenth and early twentieth centuries, British officials had established a network of quarantine stations around the Gulf. A powerful technology, the quarantine system manifested an imperial aspiration to systematize space and mobility in a region British officials imagined as a disorderly crossroads of contagious diseases and unruly travelers. Following their initial aversion to yet another demonstration of imperial encroachment, local rulers came to embrace sanitary measures as a means of bolstering their own sovereign claims over contested territories and itinerant populations. Yet, as imperial and local elites made these initial forays into public health, they rarely attempted to communicate the interlocking relationship between contagion, epidemics, and mobility to the region's people. Even as the global scientific community painstakingly moved toward general acceptance of direct person-to-person contagion or indirect infection through the transmission of water, air, or other contaminated particles as the driving forces of pandemics, around the world imperial governments predominantly relied on compulsion rather than communication to enforce the expanding tentacles of the global sanitary regime. For his part, the sultan's enthusiasm for quarantine in the wake of the Suris' escape appears to have stemmed from his eagerness to quell domestic opposition more than from his fear of disease.

Indeed, this particular evasion of quarantine in 1903 surfaces in the imperial archives only because it was recorded in the context of an international legal dispute over the status of ships that transported enslaved people in defiance of the British and the sultan. These ships displayed the French flag to avoid having to submit to British maritime inspections. Abdulla bin Khamis, the man who helped his companions escape from quarantine, captained dhows carrying French flags and registration papers and claimed to be a French subject.[5] Such strategic French flagging posed a significant challenge both to the sultan's sovereignty and to British claims that they "protected" him from external interference.[6] By drawing on a legal-medical framework in which the Suris' bodies were potential vectors of disease, the sultan seized the escape from quarantine as an opportunity to assert his authority over individuals who were passing through the territories he claimed to rule. As for the British, the quarantine investigation offered a chance to record the lawlessness of French-flag wavers. The logic of contagion as it was materialized in the quarantine station offered legal and political cover for the sultan to tame domestic insurgency and for the political agent to curtail an imperial rival. Moreover, the comparative archival silence on other escapes from or avoidance of quarantine suggests that evading sanitary measures was not typically worth the effort of enforcement, let alone official comment.

As the events following the Suris' escape from quarantine make clear, Sultan Faysal's sovereign claims over Oman's residents depended on British support.[7] For their part, in leaping to implement the sultan's jurisdiction through quarantine enforcement, the British sought to streamline their influence by maintaining a local sovereign. After forcibly returning the captured men to quarantine in the spring of 1903, the sultan framed the incident in terms of a sanitary violation that threatened the well-being of the population. He stated that the five men "most flagrantly and lawlessly violated the whole of the quarantine regulations which I had introduced . . . in the interests of public health and safety."[8] As for the Suris, their testimonies do not indicate that they had any knowledge of the sultan's claim that quarantine could protect their communities from disease. Instead, from their perspective, quarantine restrictions simply differentiated travelers according to the class of steamship ticket they had been able to afford. While deck passengers remained confined to quarantine for a week, second-class passengers only had to report to the British Agency hospital. As one of the escaped men, Khalfan bin Hamad bin Mahomed, testified, "I came from Bombay last mail, and travelled second class to avoid going to the quarantine station."[9] In contrast to the general uncertainty regarding the precise mechanisms of disease transmission, everyone involved in the case—from state sanitary officials to steamship deck passengers—had a clear understanding of the relationship between ticket class and quarantine restrictions.

The 1903 escape from quarantine and the punitive response of the sultan and the British offer a view of the politics of contagion on the threshold of public health. How was the Gulf positioned, spatially and politically, in globalizing concerns of disease transmission and imperial rivalries? How did local people understand contagion and disease? Which political and epidemiological messages did quarantine stations convey to Gulf travelers and international observers? The architecture and social composition of Gulf quarantines reveal that erratically enforced quarantine regulations proved more effective at conveying distinctions of class and race than they did at communicating bacteriological notions of contagion to Gulf travelers. Rather than educating and protecting a populace, Gulf quarantines evolved as a justification for British empire and a mechanism of monarchical power.

The Gulf and the Globalization of Disease

In the nineteenth century, a global sanitary hierarchy, as materialized in imperial quarantines, increasingly represented the world according to the flow of disease through the movement of people and goods. This spatial imaginary positioned the Middle East as a buffer zone between pathogens moving from the east toward Europe.[10] Framed as a middle passageway for disease to travel from Asia to Europe in the bodies of Muslim pilgrims, European and Ottoman sanitationists and government officials targeted the Red Sea for experimental sanitation and quarantine measures. They believed that human movement to and from the hajj represented a dangerous connection between India, seen as a source of cholera, and Europe.[11] Persian Gulf quarantine measures received less attention than those of the Red Sea region as it was a route away from Europe for returning pilgrims. Yet with its centrality to trade from India and the flows of movement from the Persian Gulf along the Tigris and Euphrates and into Persia, the region was also a focal point of international rivalries. Global powers including the British, French, Germans, and Russians cultivated complex relationships with local rulers while negotiating Ottoman and Qajar claims. The Persian Gulf quarantine infrastructure emerged as a field of competition for the territorial and economic ambitions of rival empires.

Differences in the management of quarantine in the Red Sea and the Persian Gulf highlight how tensions over commercial profits, the demands of the annual hajj, and international quarantine regulations shaped sanitary practices in the Persian Gulf region. Following its opening in 1869, the Suez Canal connected the Mediterranean to India—a navigational and environmental transformation that enforced the imperial metaphor of the Middle East as a "natural highway" for disease into Europe.[12] In addition to its commercial centrality, the Red Sea region was the annual destination for Muslim pilgrims, many of whom were subjects of European empires. The 1865 cholera epidemic in the Hijaz spread to Europe and the United

States, resulting in heightened international attention on sanitation and Muslim pilgrims.[13] Until the British occupation of Egypt in 1882, international sanitary organizations monitored ships passing through the Suez Canal and occasionally quarantined and detained British-owned steamships, passengers, and cargo.[14] These detentions cut into the profit margins of the rapid double-piston steamships that carried goods from India, foreshadowing tensions between imperial powers, sanitary discourses, and debates over the means of transmission of disease.

Sanitary outposts at Kamaran Island (an Ottoman-run quarantine station off the coast of Yemen in the southern Red Sea) and El Tor (on the southern coast of the Sinai Peninsula) illustrate how the interplay of politics, science, and architecture forged state of the art quarantine stations. The Kamaran quarantine station opened in 1882. In the initial years of Kamaran's "medico-penal regime," the thousands of pilgrims who disembarked at Kamaran experienced the poorly equipped quarantine station as a space of incarceration.[15] After arriving, the pilgrims and their luggage were taken off ship and disinfected while the ship was washed and scoured with carbolic acid and sulfur.[16] In the late 1890s, when the plague pandemic was underway, inspection and fumigation for rats and other rodents were added to the agenda. The unsanitary conditions in the quarantine facilities only exacerbated a discourse in which "'starving and importunate' pilgrim clusters began to be termed a 'public nuisance' and a microbe-generating hazard."[17]

While Kamaran guarded the entry to the Red Sea from the Indian Ocean, the quarantine camp at El Tor, in the southern Sinai Peninsula, sought to prevent disease that had already infiltrated the Red Sea region from entering Europe through the Mediterranean.[18] At El Tor, according to a 1902 report, "the pilgrims are conducted into a spacious dressing room. Here they receive each a sterilized gallabieh with which to cover their nakedness. Then they pass on to the bathroom, where, according to the choice of each, the pilgrim may have a cold or hot douche or a cold or hot sea-water bath. The washing over, they proceed to another room where their disinfected goods are handed back to them. While dressing themselves in their disinfected garments in this room they receive a visit from the quarantine doctor, and the list of their names is taken by the passport authorities."[19] Responding to the annual flood of pilgrims and growing geopolitical concerns with contagion, the quarantine stations in the Red Sea partitioned and managed human movement on an enormous scale. In the decades following the opening of the Suez Canal in 1869, El Tor and Kamaran received much international scrutiny as two of the most important guard posts preventing the spread of disease from the annual pilgrimage into Egypt, the Mediterranean, and Europe.

While order, discipline, and science seem to have been the themes of the age, the smaller quarantine stations in the Persian Gulf took on a more idiosyncratic character than spaces that enjoyed (or suffered from) greater international scrutiny. Shifting allegiances of political sovereignty and imperial influence converged in the porous, unevenly regulated, and starkly classed and racialized Gulf quarantine stations (as I discuss in the final section of this chapter). The Ottoman state implemented empirewide sanitary regulations from the 1830s.[20] Ottoman quarantine stations represented the first imperial public health initiatives in the Gulf region, starting with the Basra quarantine that the Ottoman government established in 1865 to inspect ships from India.[21] The Qajar state claimed jurisdiction over the eastern coastal ports, but it struggled to enforce maritime quarantine in a manner that satisfied increasing international scrutiny. Moreover, as a result of tensions over the treatment of Shi'i pilgrims traveling to holy sites at Karbala and Najaf, the Qajars resented the stringency of some Ottoman sanitary measures in the Gulf, particularly at Basra, and even enacted retaliatory quarantines in the 1870s.[22]

Such frictions between the Qajars and the Ottomans put the British in an awkward position. While the British were reluctant to take on the cost of sanitary conditions in the region, they were in the process of cultivating their influence in Persia while carefully maintaining trade relations with the Ottomans in the Gulf. In 1862 the British India Steam Navigation Company had initiated regular steamship service from Bombay to Basra, with stops at Muscat, Bandar Abbas, Bushire, Basra, Lingah, and Bahrain. At Basra, it connected with Euphrates and Tigris Steam Navigation Company's river steamers.[23] British involvement in the Persian Gulf intensified at the turn of the twentieth century, propelled by Lord George Curzon's (Viceroy of India, 1899–1905) belief that any encroachment by rival imperial powers in the Gulf represented a direct threat to India. Nevertheless, ultimate responsibility for the region's sanitation provisions remained uncertain. Under an 1864 agreement, British medical officers recruited from the Indian Medical Service (IMS) managed quarantine measures in the Gulf. In 1896, the Qajar government assumed financial responsibility for quarantine provisions at Lingah, Bandar Abbas, Muhammarah, Bushire, and Jask, but British doctors continued to staff the stations.[24] IMS doctors managed the quarantines, but they were not responsible for the general public health of the town, and they had no authority to stop residents from fleeing across the Gulf during periods of epidemic.[25] All IMS doctors in charge of quarantine stations in the Gulf were under the orders of the Residency surgeon at Bushire, a hierarchy that ran parallel to the subordination of the political agents stationed at Gulf port cities to the Political Resident at Bushire.

Debates over appropriate quarantine measures reflected geopolitical competitions. In the early twentieth century, officials of rival empires publicly challenged British sanitary measures as insufficient in terms of both the length of quarantine duration and the provision of quarantine stations. For example, Frédéric Borel, a French doctor with experience as an Ottoman medical official, including a post as sanitary officer at Basra, argued that the Persian Gulf was a dangerously weak thread in the global net of prophylactic sanitary measures.[26] In 1904, Borel wrote that the sanitary protections for the Persian Gulf were woefully behind those provided for pilgrims returning north from the Hijaz.[27] Moroccans, Syrians, Turks (Ottoman Muslims), and Russians had designated last-stop quarantine stations, but in comparison, the Persian Gulf "is in no way protected against the return of pilgrims," and "nothing is done against the caravans."[28] Borel observed that "cholera in the Hijaz is followed shortly by cholera in Yemen and the Persian Gulf."[29] Indeed, unlike in Europe, quarantine stations that guarded major overland transportation routes were not commonplace in Arabia.[30] Borel also feared that the ill-defined borders of the region (at least by European standards) would lead to epidemiological disorder. He warned, "There is, I think, a great danger here: the sanitary service of the two Gulfs [of Persia and Oman] would soon degenerate into a political organism, and hence would become harmful rather than useful."[31] Borel recognized the political nature of a sanitary regime that required cooperation among states, and he feared that such concerns would result in a weak "political organism" that would fall short of the scientific needs of a sanitary cordon in the epidemiologically critical but politically unstable region. Such epidemiological observations were themselves politicized critiques of inadequate British sanitary measures, articulated at the height of interimperial rivalries.

Contagion in Gulf Communities

As they jostled for dominance in the global sanitary competition, imperial statesmen and ambitious scientists generally did not consider the perceptions of local Gulf communities relevant to their debates. But in fact there is evidence that people in the region engaged with the idea of contagion before the introduction of bacteriology.[32] Given the mobility of traders, pearl divers, enslaved peoples, pilgrims, and others in the Gulf, Arabian Peninsula, and Indian Ocean world, residents of the region had long suffered from epidemic diseases. Indeed, both imperial and local accounts of nineteenth-century epidemics attest to the region's integration into the disease zone of the Indian Ocean world.[33] Scattered descriptions of how Gulf populations experienced disease appear in local scholarship, community lore, British records, and American missionary writings. Taken together, these vignettes offer evidence of how Gulf populations engaged in observation-based prevention and treatment and interacted with corpses before the introduction of imperial medicine and sanitation.

Local historians report, for example, that in 1773, residents of Basra fleeing plague carried the disease to Kuwait, Qatif, Bahrain, and other Gulf coastal areas. Plague had purportedly spread to Basra from Baghdad.[34] The nineteenth-century Iraqi historian 'Abd al-Rahman bin 'Abd Allah al-Suwaydi mentioned the spread of plague to Kuwait but claimed that it did not have a great impact there.[35] Ahmad Mustafa Abu-Hakima argues that plague mortality along the Gulf coast was low because "they had taken adequate precautions to prevent the movement of any individual from the infected regions to their territories," but it is unclear how widespread such measures could have been in the eighteenth-century Gulf.[36] His assertion that ports along the Gulf's western littoral made economic gains as a result of merchants abandoning plague-stricken Basra seems to contradict the idea that the ports were effective in preventing movement from Basra.[37]

Contagion, of course, is not limited to humans, and local people also took measures to protect their livestock. An 1880 British report on the Persian mule listed two epidemic diseases that regularly threatened the valuable animal, "'Ranj' or 'Koft' and 'Mashmashi.'" Both were "considered very contagious." Muleteers identified *ranj* by the symptoms of stomach rumbling, whiteness in the gums or eyes, and red urine and dung. Once the disease was recognized, "animals attacked are placed apart." The symptoms of *mashmashi* included yellow discharge from the mule's nose, enlarged glands, and loss of appetite. The sick mule was "simply separated from the others and allowed to die."[38] On the Arabian side of the Gulf, the missionary Paul Harrison described a local method of vaccinating sheep against anthrax. After herders recognized the first animal to die of the disease, they would cut out the lungs and place "a bit of the juicy and slightly putrescent lung" into a scratch they made in the ears of the remainder of the flock.[39] "The Arabs tell me," Harrison reported, "that of a flock so treated only one or two will die, whereas in an untreated flock hardly more than that number will be left alive."[40] Such practices of identifying symptoms among livestock and taking preventive measures of isolation and inoculation offer evidence that local people acted on their observations of contagion.

Documented responses to other diseases also reveal some notion of person-to-person contagion. Many enslaved Africans contracted diseases and died en route to the Persian Gulf.[41] One reference offers some sense of how local people who were engaged in the slave trade understood the risk of disease spreading between passengers on crowded vessels. An 1872 account of particularly brutal efforts to curb contagion reports that "at the first discovery of smallpox among [enslaved people] by the Arabs, all the affected slaves were at once thrown overboard, and this was continued day by day until . . . 40 had perished in this manner."[42] Not only do these drastic actions suggest a sense of person-to-person contagion, but they also underscore the unequal value that local, as well as colonial, actors placed on the lives of different categories of passengers.

In ʿAbd Allah al-Tabur's 1998 history of folk medicine in the Emirates (see chapter 6), his informants describe isolating patients with diseases like smallpox and leprosy.[43] He uses the word *ʿazala*, which can mean "removal," "dissociation," or "isolation," and reports that the designated isolation site was called *maʿzil*, or "place of isolation."[44] Al-Tabur explains how the people of Ras Al Khaimah would take the person inflicted with leprosy or smallpox to a small cluster of islands where he or she would remain for forty days. On the islands, "one person is employed in caring for the infected one. This person must have immunity against this disease, by virtue of having been exposed to it before, and having recovered from it."[45] Another historian reports that communities along the Gulf coast would shield children from measles by isolating them in a dark enclosure with no sun.[46] While these references are based on oral accounts taken after the introduction of biomedicine to the Gulf and may be projecting a modern understanding of contagion onto the past, the fact that these methods are situated so specifically in local geography and practice suggests some accuracy in reporting.

At the beginning of the 1820s, cholera first disseminated across the Persian Gulf region after British troops from Bombay introduced the disease at Bushire.[47] Capturing local people's sense of the origins and movement of this disease, Arabic-language histories refer to the cholera epidemic of AH 1236 (1820) as "India's gift" (*hadiyyat al-hind*), describing how it arrived in Bahrain and then spread throughout the region.[48] The nineteenth-century Najdi scholar ʿUthman bin Bashr recounted the onset of the epidemic and its symptoms in Arabia:

> In this year (AH 1236) a great epidemic [*al-wabāʾ*] occurred that spread universally and exterminated all living creatures as far as the eye could see [in all the horizons]. It was a pain that struck in the stomach causing it to empty and severe vomiting. And a person dies on the same day or after two or three days, and I have never known of anything like this in this world. The epidemic first occurred in the region of India, and moved from India in this year to Bahrain and Qatif, and a great many people were exterminated by it, then it fell upon al-Hasa, Basra, Iraq, Persia, and so on.[49]

In 1831, an epidemic of plague devastated the region. Signifying the scale of its impact, Kuwaiti historians refer to the period as "the year of the plague."[50] James Raymond Wellsted, an officer in the Indian navy who surveyed Arabia's coast in 1833–1834, described with flair the plague's arrival in Baghdad: "It stalked its awful march of death from village to village, withering, like the lava flood, all life that came under its baleful flow."[51] The 1831 plague was believed to have spread from Basra to Zubayr and Kuwait and its surroundings.[52] According to ʿUthman bin Bashr, the plague of 1831 "was unlike any epidemics that had come before it . . . houses were emptied of their families. If a man entered a house he would not leave it again . . . people were struck down in their homes and they found no one to bury them."[53]

In Kuwait, the plague of 1831 reportedly killed three-quarters of the population.[54] Stories from the time of plague demonstrate that people in Kuwait sought to physically isolate themselves from disease, a common reaction around the world.[55] In one account, a local shaykh called on his community to abandon the plague-infested town center and to relocate to huts in Shuwaikh, an outlying district. Another story relates that one family in the eastern part of the city "closed the door to their home, hoarding sufficient food and drink. They didn't allow anyone to enter out of fear that the plague would infect them." They permitted one woman who sought news of her family to leave the house by lowering her from a window by rope, but when she returned, "they didn't allow her to enter, and she perished."[56] In a third account, a thief received his due when temptation carried him into the path of plague. In one household, where no one was left except for a plague-inflicted woman, the thief entered and "took a goat in the house, but the woman was unable to cry out." While the thief was trying to leave with the stolen goods, he too was struck by the plague and died in his place; the woman recovered to reclaim her belongings.[57]

The Kuwaiti historian and author ʿAbd Allah Khalid al-Hatim, born in 1916, recounted that Kuwait was so inundated with corpses that the entire port town became a gravesite as cemeteries overflowed into homes and public squares.[58] Because the plague was most virulent in Kuwait during pearl-diving season, most of the male population would have been away. One scholar has even suggested that the men's avoidance of the epidemic and subsequent return prevented the annihilation of Kuwait's community.[59] Nevertheless, it must have been devastating for the sailors and divers to arrive home to find their houses empty and their communities turned into graveyards. ʿAbd al-ʿAziz al-Rashid vividly describes men returning in the aftermath of the plague only to discover that their wives had perished. He claims that they were forced to seek out women from surrounding areas like Zubayr and Najd, "and thus they saved the country from nothingness and extinction" (*al-ʿadam wa-l-fanāʾ*).[60] While plague narratives written several decades after the event are likely a mix of fact and hyperbole, the persistence of such stories in local histories and collective memory attests to the severity of these epidemics in Gulf port cities.

What can we know of how local communities experienced epidemics and the accelerated rate of death that accompanied their onslaught? To superimpose modern hygiene and bacteriological etiology onto religious legal opinions is to fall into the trap of "medical materialism," that is, to reduce symbolic systems to modern medical explanations or to confuse ritual and hygienic notions of cleanliness.[61] But the questions people posed to the late nineteenth- and early twentieth-century blind Ibadi jurist ʿAbdullah bin Humayd al-Salimi (d. 1914) offer local perspectives on experiences of death and burials in Oman in the era of cholera.[62] In writing to the jurist, Muslims who submitted questions to al-Salimi left traces of their handling of corpses during the critical stage between death and burial.[63] One individual, for example, asked al-Salimi if a corpse's ritual purity was voided if tears came out of the eyes. Al-Salimi offered two possible interpretations, with the usual caveat that God knows best. First, that moist bodily emissions rendered the ritually cleansed corpse impure; second, that the ritual purity remained intact because the Muslim believer is always pure, either in life or in death.[64] In a particularly poignant inquiry from "the days of plague" (*ayyām al-ṭaʿn*),[65] a man named Ahmad wrote to al-Salimi "by his own hand" because he remained troubled by an encounter with a corpse from several years earlier. A Baluchi servant was found dead in a dried-out *falaj*, or water channel.[66] It took two days for Ahmad and his men to learn of the incident. By the time they arrived, "we found him gravely damaged from the swelling and the pus," they said, and they were confronted with the decaying body's foul smell. But the body was wedged into the *falaj* at such an angle that they were unable to remove it from its place. The people of the area were terrified by the event and the decaying body, so, out of desperation, Ahmad and his men threw stones and pebbles over the corpse to cover it in its place. At the time, he had asked the prominent Omani jurist Saʿid bin Khalfan al-Khalili (1811–1871) if his actions had been acceptable. Al-Khalili replied that he could not see that Ahmad had another option, and he had done well not to leave the corpse "exposed amongst the Muslims for the beasts to eat it." Yet years later, Ahmad revisited the event and his memories of the Baluchi servant, dead but out of reach in the *falaj*, this time addressing al-Salimi. Unsurprisingly, al-Salimi supported al-Khalili's ruling, answering Ahmad with a pithy reassurance that al-Khalili's opinion had been correct, and God knows best.[67]

In the mid-nineteenth century, al-Khalili (the same jurist who ruled on the Baluchi corpse) also addressed questions relating to cauterization (*al-kayy*), providing us with some sense of the professional and social milieu of this medical practice. One questioner asked if he could seek out cauterization and medication from a stranger who might be a non-Muslim, with the intention of seeking healing, and then compensate the healer for his services with a generous payment. Al-Khalili assured the questioner that it is permitted to seek out healing, as well as to offer payment. Another questioner wanted to know if he could cauterize his wife and his slave even if they did not consent, so long as he believed it would benefit them. Al-Khalili replied that it was permissible for him to cauterize his wife "with her consent for the purpose of remedy"; without specifying whether the slave also needed to consent, he suggested that it was permissible to cauterize a slave so long as the purpose was to bring "remedy and benefit" (*al-dawāʾ wa al-maṣlaḥa*).[68] Of course, "remedy and benefit" was subjective; according to Matthew Hopper, "the branding of enslaved men appears to have been used to 'cure' insubordination or their inability to dive for pearls."[69] In the early twentieth century, the missionary doctor Paul Harrison discussed cauterization in the Gulf as a "counter irritation," or a method "to bring infection to a head and facilitate its discharge externally as a pus," and he believed that the procedure could be "very beneficial."[70] Missionaries also observed that women often performed cauterization, citing a hadith establishing that "in case of necessity it is legitimate for one sex to medically treat the other."[71]

Long experienced in the ravages of epidemics crisscrossing the region, Gulf communities labored to reconcile the demands of health with religious and cultural norms. As we will see in the next section, what was novel about quarantine for local populations was the reality of state-mandated and enforced public health measures that imposed categories of race, class, and gender onto people long accustomed to freedom of movement between sea and land. Rather than parents, neighbors, and religious scholars guiding health decisions, quarantine offered imperial officials and local rulers unprecedented claims over Gulf bodies and territories.

Quarantine

Quarantines, in all their epidemiologically fluid interpretations and socially unequal implementations, represented one of the heaviest imperial footprints in the Gulf from the late nineteenth century until World War I. The Gulf quarantine stations, established by imperial decree and eventually embraced by local rulers, introduced local communities to state-driven public health. In Europe, "railways effectively invented social classes in their modern form, by naming and classifying different levels of comfort, facility and service."[72] In the Gulf's ocean-oriented port towns, steamships and quarantine stations performed a similar role. Quarantine restructured travel, trade, and social life by sorting people into categories of class, race, nationality, and gender. As a legal framework, quarantine also mapped onto a local notion of territorialism that encompassed both land and water. Coastal rulers, for example, claimed jurisdiction over itinerant divers.[73] Unsettled and fluctuating understandings of the nature of contagious diseases and their means of transmission granted significant room to imperial officials and local rulers to construct claims of public interest while protecting profits, surveilling travelers, and undermining political rivals. Global configurations of imperial competition and sanitary discourse created opportunities for local rulers in the Persian Gulf to escalate their claims over subjects and territories by manipulating porous quarantine policies. Travelers, in turn, experienced these infrastructures of mobility as a sorting process that differentiated people according to their race and the income they could expend on travel.

Initially, Gulf rulers resisted "British interference in matters of internal government."[74] But a clear transition occurred in the early twentieth century. As local rulers came to understand the symbolic significance and political utility of quarantine, they began actively to enforce and even to fund quarantine arrangements in their ports. Even though he had refused "the adoption of any precautionary measures against plague" until 1897 and suspended quarantine arrangements while cholera raged in Karachi in the summer of 1899, in the 1903 incident described at the beginning of this chapter, Sultan Faysal chased down, imprisoned, and fined some of his subjects who had broken quarantine.[75] In 1897, Shaykh Isa bin Ali Al Khalifa of Bahrain refused British assistance with sanitary protections "founded ostensibly on the repugnance of his subjects to scientific plague precautions, and in support of his statement the Shaikh submitted a petition to which a number of signatures were attached."[76] In 1910, however, the same shaykh of Bahrain sought permission from the British Agency to appoint his own quarantine doctor and fee-collecting agents.[77] In short, by the second decade of the twentieth century, local rulers had come to embrace quarantine as a mechanism of control over their subjects and a means of legitimizing power in their territories, albeit under the protective surveillance of British agents and ships of war.[78]

Quarantine and the vision of contagion it invoked remained a top-down endeavor, whether mandated by Ottomans, British, Qajars, or local rulers. A crucial distinction emerged between imperial officials and local elites, however, in the driving motivations of the sanitary agenda. For the British, the primary audience for the quarantine stations was the international community. British officials sought to prove that they took their great-power status in the Gulf seriously enough to prevent the movement of disease from India into Europe while safeguarding the commercial interests of the shipping industry. Local rulers, in contrast, approached quarantine as an opportunity to incorporate individual travelers into an emerging articulation of their sovereign populations. Quarantine stations provided an apparatus for the surveillance and classification of individuals within a biomedical ideology that enjoyed the endorsement of an increasingly globalized scientific discourse.

Quarantine asserted an innovative connection between coercive state regulations and the management of life and death. British officials kept records estimating epidemic mortalities. While the official death counts are imprecise and even impressionistic, they serve as a measurement of how disease moved through the region and affected wider imperial political and economic concerns. British records indicate that death rates remained high during years of epidemic well into the twentieth century. In Bahrain, also without a quarantine station through the first decade of the twentieth century, an estimated 301 people died of plague in 1903, and 2,000 were reported to have died of cholera in 1904.[79] Around 2,000 people in Bahrain died of plague in 1907.[80] In an outbreak of plague on the Trucial Coast in 1911, an estimated 2,000 people died at Dubai and 500 at Sharjah.[81] As late as 1924 an outbreak of plague thought to have been imported from Dubai caused 4,000 deaths in Bahrain.[82] As debates over the means of disease transmission raged across the globe among imperial bureaucrats and scientists, the actual deaths were far from theoretical.

At the turn of the century, the confluence of political rivalries and emergent understandings of disease transmission fostered a politics of contagion that reinforced Gulf quarantine arrangements. The Government of India was wary of the sanitary-related critiques of rival empires that "continue[d] to be increasingly jealous of the British Administration of the quarantine."[83] In 1906, the Foreign Office arranged for Dr. Theodore Thomson, a medical inspector, to undertake a tour of Gulf quarantine stations. Notably, Thomson's visit was prompted by a sanitary tour of the Persian Gulf by a French doctor that had occurred a year earlier, underlining the competitive nature of the Gulf sanitary infrastructure. The geopolitical context of Thomson's tour led to paradoxical conclusions. On the one hand, Thomson framed epidemiological arguments to justify ongoing British predominance in Gulf quarantine. On the other hand, he sought to protect British shipping interests from the stringent sanitary measures of rival powers. The diversity of the quarantine stations' designs reflected different levels of imperial interest, which in turn corresponded to the political and economic significance of each city. The chosen locales of steamship routes and quarantine stations (or their absence) and their architectural characteristics articulated the relative importance of ports to global trade and European travelers and devalued indigenous trade routes. In his map of Persian Gulf ports, he included ports of call for steamships passing through the region while leaving out ports that primarily served internal markets; for example, he gives no mention to Doha or towns along the Trucial Coast (fig. 1.1). The organizations of the ships and quarantine buildings inserted Gulf bodies into a classed and racialized infrastructure.[84] Recalling her 1921 voyage

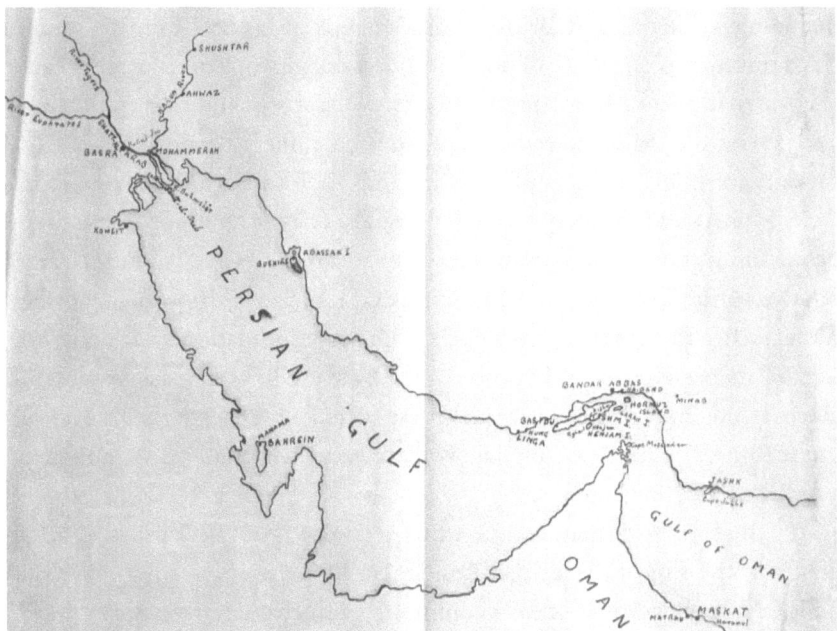

FIGURE 1.1. Thomson's map of Persian Gulf ports.
SOURCE: Theodore Thomson, *Report by Dr. Theodore Thomson on the Sanitary Requirements of Certain Places in or near the Persian Gulf, &.*, Printed for the use of the Foreign Office, October 1906. London School of Hygiene & Tropical Medicine Library & Archives Service.

from Bombay, the American missionary Cornelia Dalenberg illustrated this reality: "The four of us [missionary women] were the only first class passengers on the Gulf steamer. A few Indians were in second class and the Arabs traveled 'deck.' This meant they remained out in the open with their goats, sheep, camels, donkeys, parrots and chickens."[85]

From the early twentieth century, the Government of India oversaw Muscat's foreign affairs with every state except for France and the United States, which enjoyed preexisting treaty relations with Muscat.[86] Muscat was a chief emporium for pearls, dates, textiles, foodstuffs, and horses in transit between Gulf waters and Indian markets, but the steamship routes of the 1860s and 1870s that traversed the Gulf upended Muscat's mercantile preeminence.[87] The globalization of the date trade in the late nineteenth and early twentieth centuries offered Muscat some economic relief to its diminished status. In 1906, Muscat enjoyed considerable steamship traffic, including weekly calls by British India Steam Navigation Company steamships traversing Persian Gulf ports and occasional stops from other steamships arriving from Bombay or Europe. Muscat's quarantine station was in a bay on the mainland at Haramul, located a mile and a half from Muscat and accessible by sea and footpath (figs. 1.2–1.4). Muttrah, two miles from Muscat and similarly located along the coast, was a port for indigenous sailing craft but not steamships. The location of the quarantine camp relative to the two ports emphasized its targeting of European steamship traffic rather than indigenous vessels. The accommodations were only for third-class passengers, and "no provision is made for first-class or second-class passengers." The quarantined passengers had to "ease themselves on the seashore," water was supplied from a nearby well, and provisions came from Muscat.[88]

By the early twentieth century, Bushire was Qajar Iran's principal Gulf port and the site of the British Residency, which oversaw the other Gulf political agencies. Difficulties in communication characterized the relationship between the coast and the Persian interior. In the 1890s, it took five or six days to travel the 182 miles from Bushire to Shiraz; with good winds, it was possible to navigate the 170 miles from Bushire to Kuwait in just twenty-two hours.[89] Even as Britain's Gulf interests shifted toward pacifying

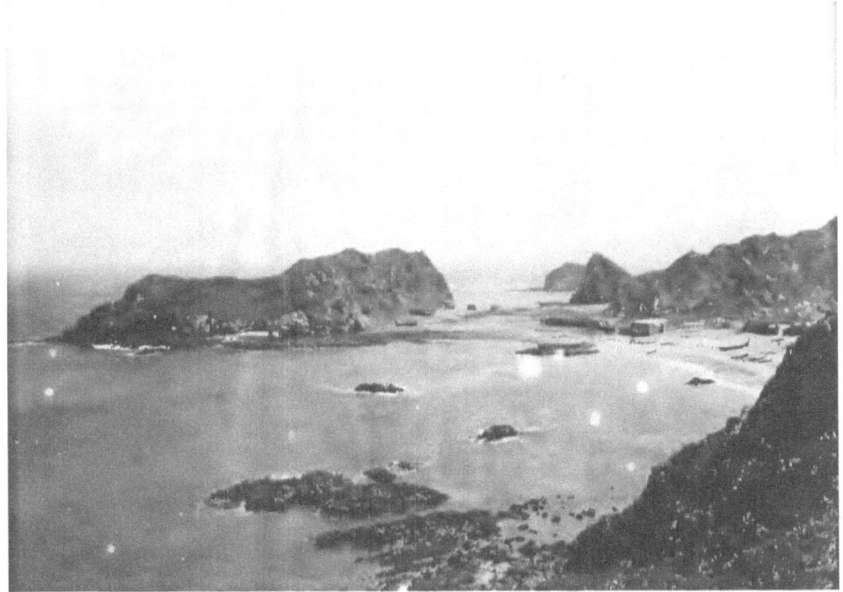

FIGURE 1.2. The Muscat quarantine station and an adjacent fishing village.

SOURCE: Theodore Thomson, *Report by Dr. Theodore Thomson on the Sanitary Requirements of Certain Places in or near the Persian Gulf, &*. Printed for the use of the Foreign Office, October 1906. London School of Hygiene & Tropical Medicine Library & Archives Service.

the Arabian coast in the nineteenth century, the British maintained the Residency in Bushire until 1946, when the headquarters were moved to Bahrain.[90] By the outbreak of World War I, a mail steamer reached Bushire from Bombay in just seven or eight days.

Bushire's political and economic importance also placed it on the front lines of recurrent waves of epidemic disease. Sanitary control of Iran's Persian Gulf port cities emerged as an important field for great-power politics and local expressions of resentment for outside interventions. With their Russian rivals controlling quarantines along the eastern Iranian frontiers, Britain jealously guarded its sanitary authority over the Persian Gulf, but in practice its sanitary policies were consistently lax. Iranian resentment of European-run sanitary measures also reflected underlying tensions over the growing interference of foreign powers in domestic affairs. In 1898, the population of Bushire was so hostile to British sanitary measures that

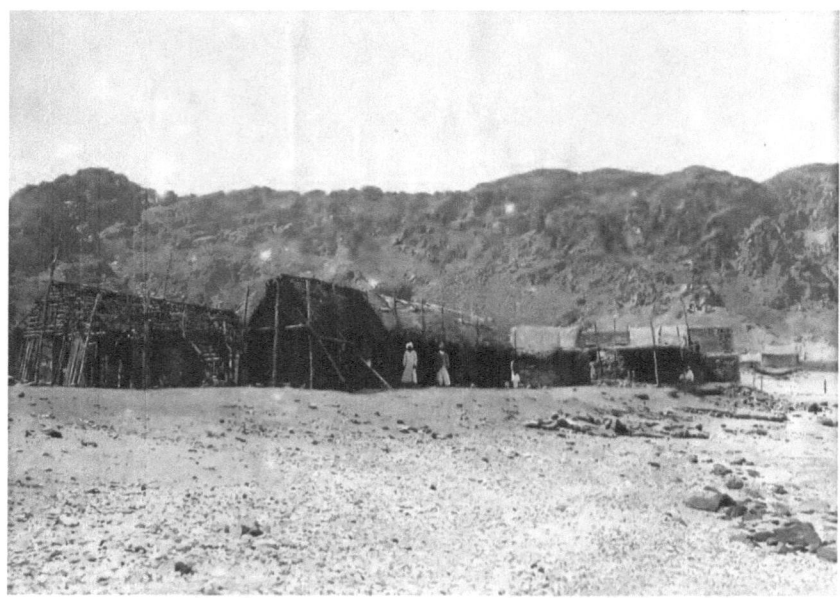

FIGURE 1.3. Muscat quarantine station accommodations. Hut on the left shown in the process of construction.

SOURCE: Theodore Thomson, *Report by Dr. Theodore Thomson on the Sanitary Requirements of Certain Places in or near the Persian Gulf, &*. Printed for the use of the Foreign Office, October 1906. London School of Hygiene & Tropical Medicine Library & Archives Service.

riots and strikes broke out, with demonstrators throwing stones through the windows of the Indo-European Telegraph Department and the British consulate.[91] The British and the Iranian government reacted by dispatching troops. In 1904, on a wave of Iranian nationalism that foreshadowed the constitutional revolution, the Iranian government attempted to wrest sanitary control away from the British. British reconciliations with the French and the Russians, however, undermined Iranian efforts and solidified British control over Persian Gulf quarantines.[92]

When Dr. Thomson, the sanitation inspector, visited in 1906, it was in the wake of a period of increasing British control over Persian Gulf sanitation despite Iranian resistance. In 1906, Bushire enjoyed weekly calls from British India steamers as they stopped on the way up and down the Persian Gulf. Due to its status as the region's major port of call, Bushire

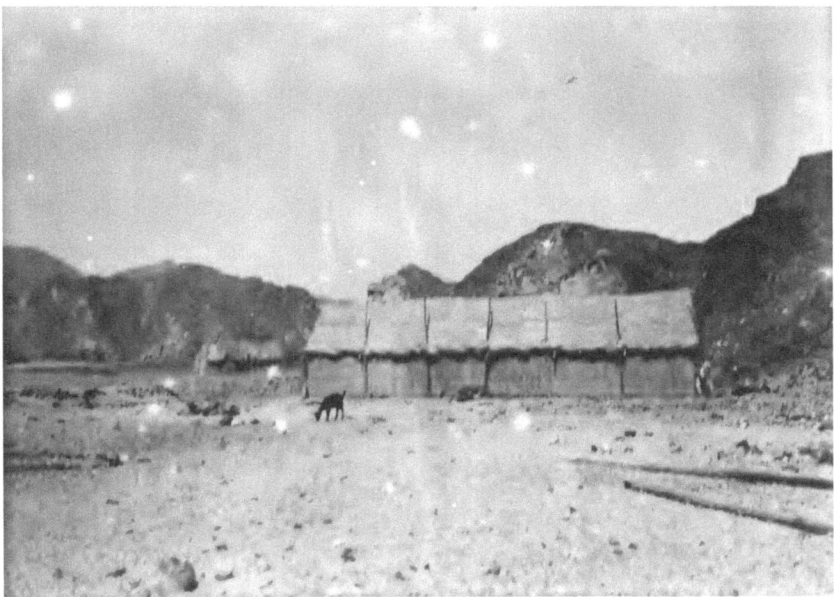

FIGURE 1.4. Some of the structures at the Muscat quarantine station.

SOURCE: Theodore Thomson, *Report by Dr. Theodore Thomson on the Sanitary Requirements of Certain Places in or near the Persian Gulf, &*. Printed for the use of the Foreign Office, October 1906. London School of Hygiene & Tropical Medicine Library & Archives Service.

had quarantine accommodation for first-, second-, and third-class passengers (figs. 1.5–1.7). But the Residency surgeon's "biased practices," such as "giving clean bills of health to British ships while impounding Russian vessels from the same point of origin," created tensions over jurisdiction and sovereignty with the government in Tehran.[93] In his report on his tour of Gulf quarantines, Thomson commented on the "substitution of surveillance for observation in the case of first-class passengers on vessels from other ports."[94] That is, some passengers were allowed to reside outside of the quarantine stations under surveillance rather than physically remaining alongside the lower-class passengers in the stations. Moreover, "a date-stick hut is not suitable . . . if the occupant should happen to be a European, who is not likely to be accustomed to accommodation of this kind."[95]

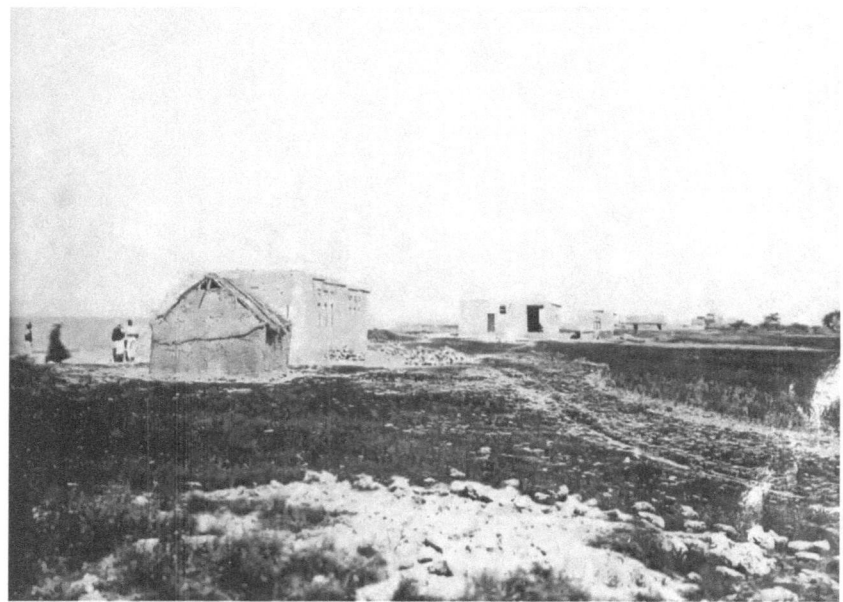

FIGURE 1.5. View of Bushire quarantine station. The second-class block is in the foreground on the left, the first-class block in the center, and the third-class huts and disinfecting station are behind on the right.

SOURCE: Theodore Thomson, *Report by Dr. Theodore Thomson on the Sanitary Requirements of Certain Places in or near the Persian Gulf, &*. Printed for the use of the Foreign Office, October 1906. London School of Hygiene & Tropical Medicine Library & Archives Service.

In Basra, the Ottomans had embraced quarantine measures to combat both the epidemiological threats of cholera and plague and the geopolitical hazards of economic and political Gulf rivals. Following its military conquest in the sixteenth century, Basra provided Ottoman access to the Persian Gulf and integrated this region into networks of communication that facilitated the diffusion of disease across the empire.[96] An outbreak of plague and a Persian siege in Basra in the 1770s weakened the city's regional position, resulting in increased trade traffic to smaller Gulf ports.[97] The Ottomans sought to bolster their presence in the Gulf and Arabia from Basra, and the cholera and plague pandemics of the nineteenth and early twentieth centuries placed sanitation efforts at the center of Ottoman expansionism

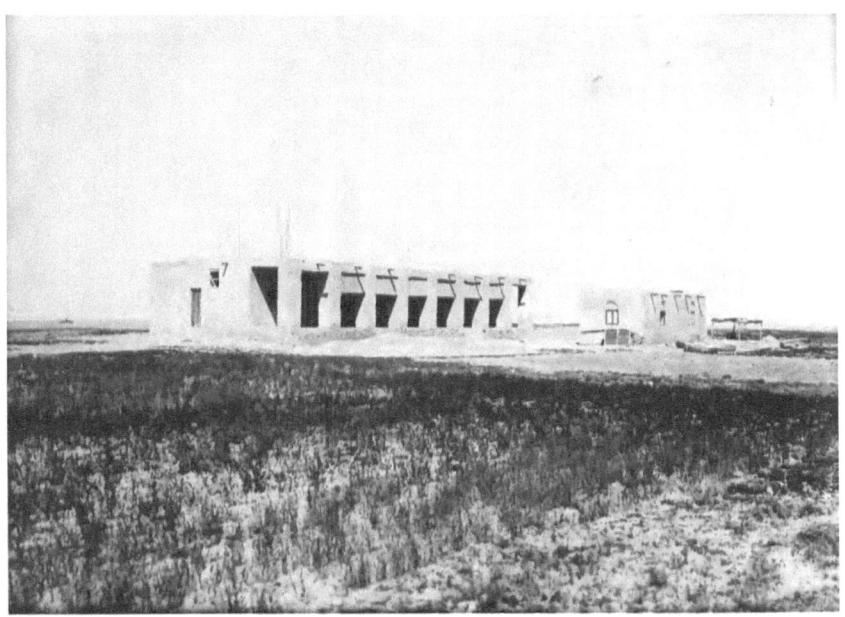

FIGURE 1.6. Bushire quarantine station, first-class block with servants' quarters and kitchen on the right.

SOURCE: Theodore Thomson, *Report by Dr. Theodore Thomson on the Sanitary Requirements of Certain Places in or near the Persian Gulf, &*. Printed for the use of the Foreign Office, October 1906. London School of Hygiene & Tropical Medicine Library & Archives Service.

in the region. Basra also was an important destination for Shi'i pilgrims arriving from British India and Qajar Persia, prompting the Ottomans to address the possibility that Qajar and British subjects were spreading cholera and plague.[98]

The Ottomans had sought to revive their military and administrative interests in the Gulf from the 1870s. The threat of global pandemics in this period further heightened Basra's importance as a bulwark against the admission of epidemics into Ottoman territories. In this context of renewed Ottoman efforts in the Gulf and the global threat of disease, the Ottomans relied on their quarantine stations for epidemiological and political ends. Two medical officers who had been appointed by the Constantinople

42   CHAPTER ONE

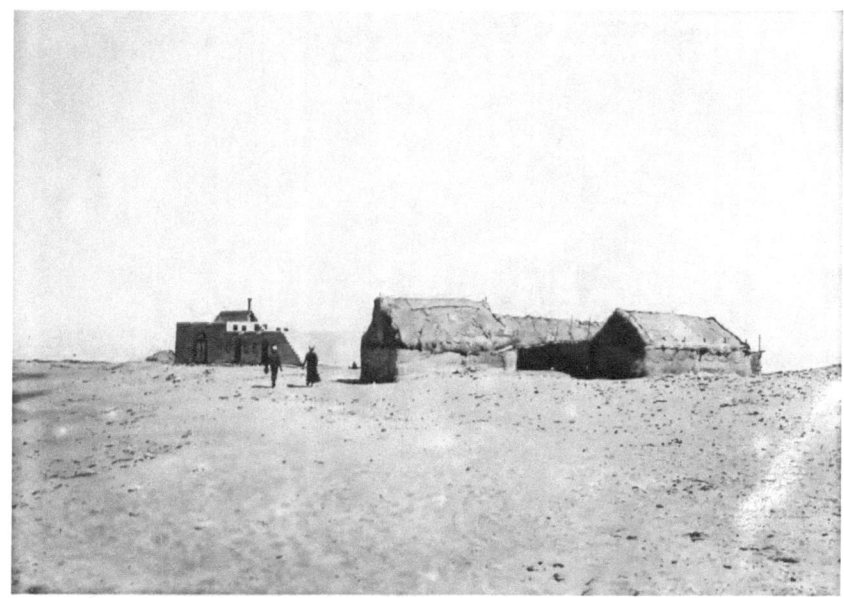

FIGURE 1.7. Bushire quarantine station, third-class huts in foreground, disinfecting station behind.

SOURCE: Theodore Thomson, *Report by Dr. Theodore Thomson on the Sanitary Requirements of Certain Places in or near the Persian Gulf, &*. Printed for the use of the Foreign Office, October 1906. London School of Hygiene & Tropical Medicine Library & Archives Service.

Board of Health ran Basra's quarantine (figs. 1.8–1.11). In his 1906 report, Thomson expressed the belief that Ottoman severity was due to economic or political malice rather than scientific reasoning: "The measures applied to incoming shipping, based upon Regulations that have been made by that Board from time to time, are in several respects unduly stringent."[99] While Thomson (somewhat ironically) was allowed to bypass quarantine requirements at British-run quarantine stations during his tour, at Basra, he reported, "My information as to the circumstances of this station comes mainly from personal observation during a short period of quarantine which I underwent there."[100] Thomson would, of course, have stayed in first-class accommodation during his time in quarantine.

South of Basra in Kuwait, political intrigue and great-power rivalries formed the backdrop to the port city's first experiences of modern

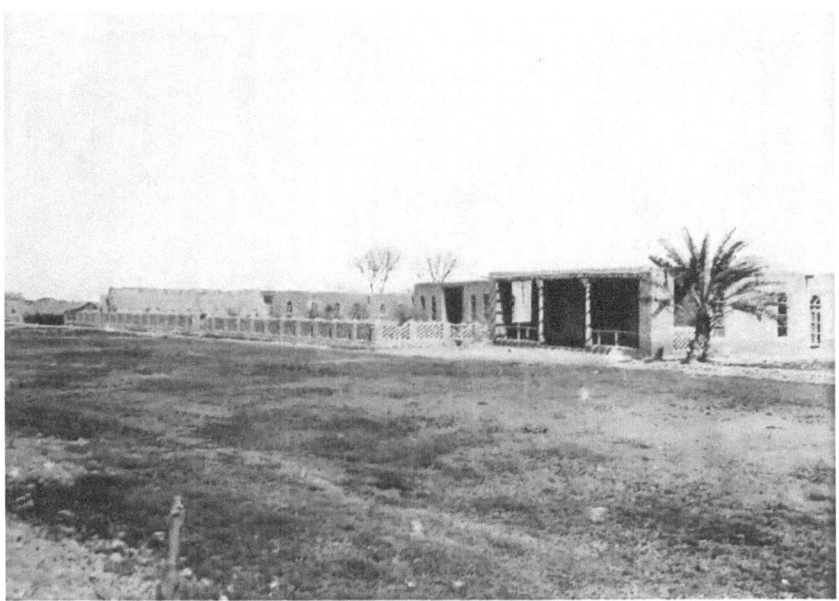

FIGURE 1.8. View of Basra quarantine station from the bank of the river. First-class quarters in the center and on right, second- and third-class quarters on left.

SOURCE: Theodore Thomson, *Report by Dr. Theodore Thomson on the Sanitary Requirements of Certain Places in or near the Persian Gulf, &.* Printed for the use of the Foreign Office, October 1906. London School of Hygiene & Tropical Medicine Library & Archives Service.

sanitation in the late nineteenth and early twentieth centuries. Istanbul remained confident in Ottoman claims over Kuwait at the beginning of the 1890s. In May 1896, Shaykh Mubarak Al-Sabah (r. 1896–1915) came to power after assassinating his brothers, prompting the Ottoman governor in Basra to call for military occupation. The Porte was sluggish to respond to the coup, allowing an opening for discussions that would result in the secret 1899 agreement between Britain and Mubarak granting Kuwait protected status.[101] Mubarak also owned extensive lands along the Shatt al-Arab around Basra, and periodic dispatching of armed forces to the area posed a threat to Ottoman sovereignty.[102] The Ottoman state appointed Ibrahim Bey quarantine officer from 1897 to 1901, but Shaykh Mubarak resented this expression of Ottoman influence, especially the taxes collected to cover quarantine expenses and staff salaries.[103] Talal

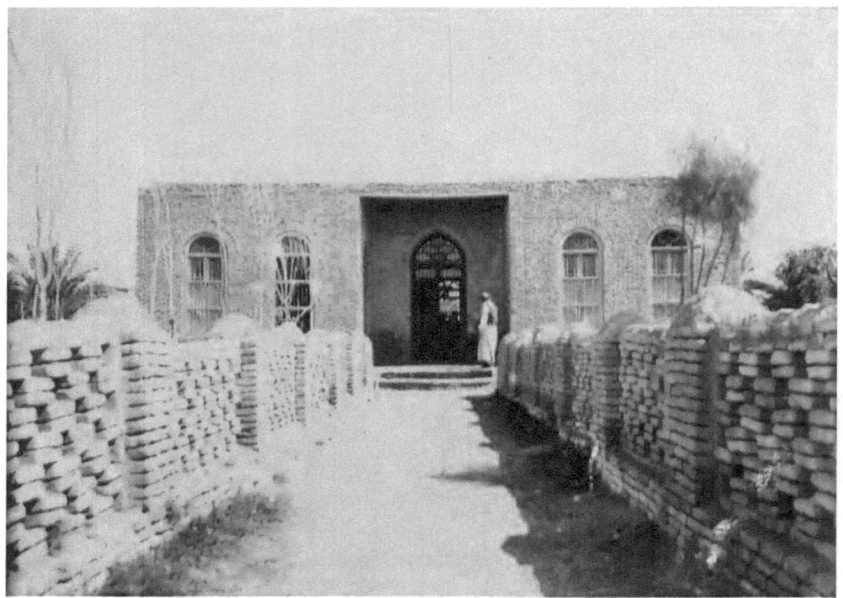

FIGURE 1.9. Basra quarantine station, first-class block.

SOURCE: Theodore Thomson, *Report by Dr. Theodore Thomson on the Sanitary Requirements of Certain Places in or near the Persian Gulf, &.* Printed for the use of the Foreign Office, October 1906. London School of Hygiene & Tropical Medicine Library & Archives Service.

Saʿd al-Rumaydi recounts an incident in which Mubarak used the quarantine regulations against incoming Ottoman ships that were arriving in Kuwait's port. He relates that Shaykh Mubarak Al-Sabah did not welcome them and instructed Ibrahim Bey not to allow the Ottomans entry unless they quarantined for fifteen days. They reluctantly agreed but later decided to leave Kuwait after Shaykh Mubarak addressed them from the coast.[104]

Despite the political tumult of the period, the Ottoman state did manage to establish sanitary authority over Kuwait's port. Indeed, the first state medical professionals in Kuwait were the Ottoman quarantine officer and his assistants, who were posted in Kuwait from 1897 to 1901.[105] News of the third global plague pandemic emerged during the same period that saw Mubarak dispose of his brothers.[106] The 1896 outbreak of plague in India

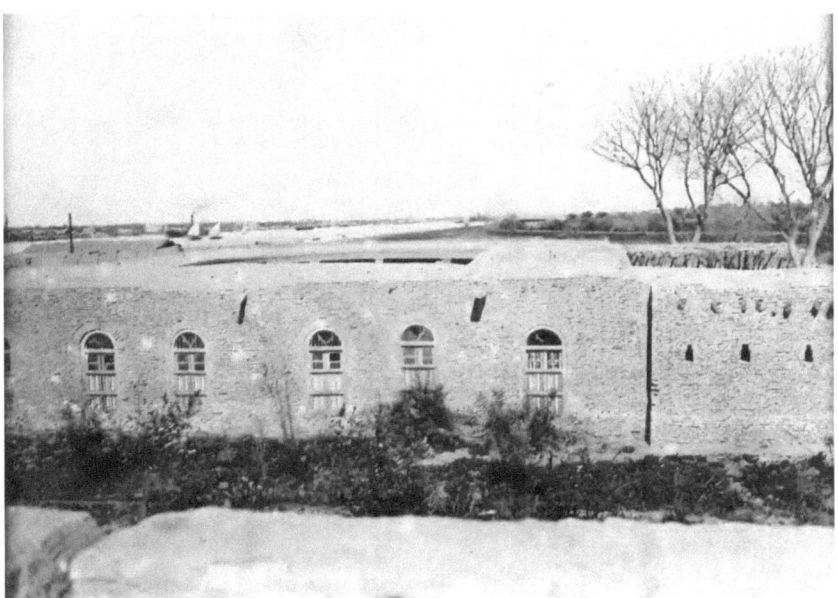

FIGURE 1.10. Basra quarantine station, second-class block.

SOURCE: Theodore Thomson, *Report by Dr. Theodore Thomson on the Sanitary Requirements of Certain Places in or near the Persian Gulf, &*. Printed for the use of the Foreign Office, October 1906. London School of Hygiene & Tropical Medicine Library & Archives Service.

and the 1897 international sanitary conference prompted the Ottomans to initiate quarantine in Kuwait. The station charged quarantined passengers a fee to cover expenses, including salaries of the employees. The quarantine station at Kuwait, and Mubarak's resistance to the Ottoman sanitary presence, were emblematic of wider Ottoman efforts to demonstrate the Sublime Porte's ongoing claims over Gulf territories in the 1890s through public health measures. But even in sanitary matters, Ottoman influence was waning. While the Ottomans had succeeded in establishing quarantines at Kuwait and Qatif in 1897, the British blocked Ottoman efforts to open stations at Bahrain and Qatar.[107]

There was a gap of three years at Kuwait between the closing of the Ottoman station in 1901 and the British establishment of their own doctor in 1904. Two factors converged to prompt the British to send a doctor.

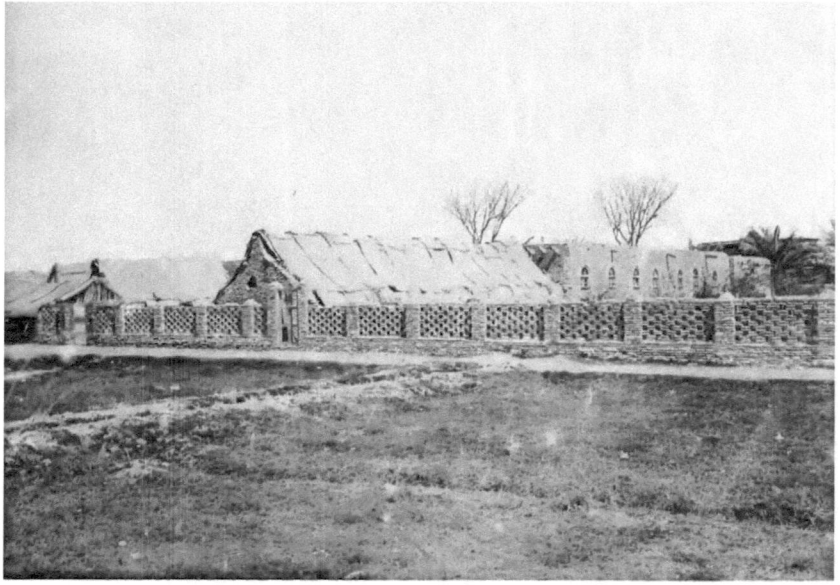

FIGURE 1.11. Basra quarantine station, third-class huts.

SOURCE: Theodore Thomson, *Report by Dr. Theodore Thomson on the Sanitary Requirements of Certain Places in or near the Persian Gulf, &*. Printed for the use of the Foreign Office, October 1906. London School of Hygiene & Tropical Medicine Library & Archives Service.

First, the Ottoman governor at Basra wanted to restore the Porte's sanitary presence in Kuwait, and both the British and Mubarak desired to prevent this renewal of Ottoman authority. Second, Mubarak was eager to initiate medical services without allowing Christian missionaries into Kuwait (the missionaries' role as catalysts of medical institutions is the subject of chapter 2).[108] Trade with Ottoman Gulf ports also remained a paramount concern, and the British sought to appoint a doctor who would have sufficient qualifications so that the clean bills of health he issued to ships would satisfy the health authorities in Istanbul.[109] But when Thomson undertook his tour, he found "no quarantine station or isolation accommodation for cases of infectious disease, nor any disinfecting apparatus" at Kuwait.[110] He noted that, other than the fortnightly British India boats, "there is little other steam communication."[111] When Thomson visited Kuwait, Shaykh Mubarak was in the process of transitioning from an Ottoman quarantine regime that he regarded as a hostile intervention to wresting control of British sanitary policy in order to advance his own sovereign claims.

Public Health as Coercion

The global and regional demands for and debates over quarantine contributed to territorial and sovereign consolidation in the Persian Gulf region in the early twentieth century. At the same time, the integration of these institutions into port communities embedded spatial and social hierarchies in the lived experiences of an emergent public health regime. By the end of the first decade of the twentieth century, rulers along the Arabian coast of the Persian Gulf acknowledged that quarantine was a critical institution for their port cities. The social class differences inscribed in the quarantine stations indicate that the emerging predominance of this view depended more on imperial categories and political rivalries than on sanitary concerns. Indigenous rulers understood that their prophylactic measures were the by-product of imperial politics, but they came to embrace the institutions and their scientific ideologies as mechanisms for the consolidation of their sovereign power over the circulation of Gulf populations.

In the Persian Gulf, quarantines emphatically did not create separate social spaces in which all were equal before the onslaught of sickness. Instead, quarantine stations served as physical structures for the compulsory isolation of different populations, and, as such, they materialized hierarchies of class and race. As in other parts of the world, poor and nonwhite travelers were disproportionately treated as likely sources of contagion and targeted for quarantine measures. Sanitary experts and imperial officials blamed any resistance to top-down prophylactic measures on superstition and ignorance while justifying increasingly invasive measures in the name of scientific progress. Such experiences were certainly not unique to the Middle East, or even to imperial settings. In as distant a port as New York Harbor, higher-class cabin passengers escaped quarantine while immigrants were sent to Ellis Island for prolonged medical inspection.[112] During the Great Manchurian Plague of 1910–1911, lower-class Chinese migrant workers were treated with contempt by Western-trained Chinese and Russian doctors alike "for their senseless refusal to comply with regulations issued for their own protection, their superstition and their desperate attempts to seek relief in traditional medicine."[113] Moreover, the "construction of 'coolies' as an epidemiological Other" in need of active and interventionist sanitary reform in Chinese state medical discourse prompted transformations in sanitary governmentality.[114]

In the early twentieth century, little effort was made to convince indigenous Gulf populations that this increasingly prevalent public health measure would benefit local people. As a result, quarantine stations emerged as a public health infrastructure that expressed the coercive powers of elites rather than conveying the potential health benefits to the target populations themselves. Quarantine represented the frontline materialization of imperial intervention, a central concern of interimperial political debates, and the initial point of contact between local populations and an emerging idea of state-driven public health.

The next chapter follows evolving health paradigms as they pivot from top-down quarantine measures to the individualized medicine offered by missionaries and hospitals. Imperial officials and local rulers imposed quarantine on reluctant passengers and forced travelers to pause in space and time. Hospitals, in contrast, actively attracted Gulf patients who journeyed considerable distances for the purpose of addressing particular ailments. The popular demand for hospitals reveals how even as quarantine measures represented state coercion, another modern medical project was unfolding across Gulf cities as a result of the emerging health imaginaries of everyday people.

CHAPTER 2

HOSPITALS

ON FEBRUARY 6, 1909, six years after he had called on a British steamer to chase down the passengers who had slipped out of quarantine, Sultan Faysal of Muscat held a town meeting. In his appeal to "natives of this place as well as others who are settled in my territory," his goal was to collect donations for the construction of a new hospital.[1] The diverse audience for the sultan's fundraising efforts included representatives of Muscat's Bhatia (Hindu Indian merchants), Agha Khani (Nizari Isma'ilis), Memon (Sunni Indian merchants), Khoja (Shi'i Indian merchants), Arab, and British communities. The medical situation was urgent. Four years earlier, in 1905, the Government of India had refused to provide a new hospital building "until satisfactory evidence had been adduced that the Sultan desired a new hospital and would support it, and that the local community, Arabs and Indians, were prepared both to found and maintain the institution."[2] Then, in 1907, the "filthy and insanitary" room the British Agency borrowed from Sultan Faysal for use as a dispensary "fell down with a deafening crash," prompting a visiting Public Works Department official to condemn the building as "dangerous and uninhabitable."[3] Yet even as the Government of India withheld funds from medical development and Muscat's British-run dispensary literally collapsed, hospitals, alongside sanitary regulations, were emerging as sites of fierce competition around the Gulf. Alarmingly for the sultan, at the time of his meeting, American Christian missionaries had already established medical stations in other Gulf communities. It was only a matter of time before they would attempt to expand into Muscat and Muttrah.

Taking matters into their own hands, early in 1909 the sultan and the political agent set about gathering funds for a new hospital from the local community. In January the political agent wrote a letter "to all British subjects in Muscat to ask them to subscribe generously" to the fundraising effort.[4] The sultan then took "an unprecedented step in convening a meeting for a charitable purpose" when he gathered his constituents on February 6.[5] His speech and his success in garnering financial support for a hospital suggests, first, that residents were willing to view themselves as an integrated population, united by their shared health concerns. Second, they demonstrate that local people were coming to see medical institutions as an essential component of political leadership. Faysal declared to the assembled community members:

> You all know that the existence of a Hospital in the town is for the safety of health and beneficent to all rich and poor. The object for assembling you in this meeting is to request help for the erection and finishing [of the hospital] because this work is profitable for the residents of this place as well as for others who come from other parts, and it is a kind of charity. It is therefore incumbent on all whether present in this meeting or absent, to give help in this according to their means because it is necessary and every one is profited by [the hospital]. Today is the day for giving your donations, and I have hopes of the assembly. It is my wish that no body should leave this meeting till I see the foundation of this work before my presence, and I expect help from God regarding the settlement of this affair.[6]

The availability of individualized medical care required collective political and financial participation for a state-provisioned hospital that would support a multireligious, multilingual community. The sultan suggested that contributing constituted an act of charity on the part of all residents to care for the poor and the sick. He concluded with an expansive vision of the stakeholders in his hospital project: "I am obliged to all the natives of the place, British, Arab and Foreign subjects that they have joined me in this great work."[7]

While soliciting funds from local people for public works projects was not an atypical example of the British Empire operating on the cheap, the public meeting and the attempt to gather contributions from the community was much more than a reaction to British stinginess. Surrounding the hospital discussions was a sense of genuine frustration in the exchanges between the agents on the spot (including both doctors who took pride in their professional standards and political agents who saw the Persian Gulf as integral to British India), and the Government of India, which resisted financial entanglements. More significantly, the sultan included multiple Muscat communities in constructing an institution that would, he argued, represent their own best interests as a collective.

Many Muscat residents and communities appear to have been convinced by the combined appeals from the political agent and the sultan. Letters that accompanied donations demonstrate how people living in Muscat envisioned and sought to influence the new hospital through their contributions. But the new unity did not abolish long-standing distinctions; in fact, the hospital project reinforced social boundaries. The Bhatias donated Rs. 10,000 to the new hospital, on the condition that it include a separate ward called the Bhatia Mahajan Ward. In that ward, they demanded a "separate room for Bhatias, who come to take medicine in the Hospital"; it had to include "two separate rooms in the ward for male and female patients, who wish to remain in the Hospital," and "there must be one separate cooking room, bath room and latrines." They also reserved the right to send an elected representative to serve on the hospital management committee. Finally, they stipulated that "no patient should be allowed to stay in the Bhatia Mahajan Ward, unless he produces written permission from the B.M. representative of the Hospital Committee."[8] Even while contributing to an institution aimed to serve multiple communities, this relatively wealthy group was careful to preserve its distinction through separate hospital spaces and institutionalized communal representation.

Those with the means to contribute significant funds exhibited a sense of entitlement over hospital space and patient treatment, whereas more modest pledges came with no such demands. The Agha Khani residents of Muscat and Muttrah wrote to the political agent on February 5, 1909: "A few days back we held a meeting and have been able to collect Rs. 500 only. We are very sorry that it is a very small sum, but it could not be helped, as we are few in number and are poor people. We request you to excuse us for giving such a small sum."[9] Memon Abdul Latif Isani Kutchi, representative of the Memon community of Muscat and Muttrah, stated in his letter, "With due deference and proud reverence I beg to approach with this application that your honour ordered of for charity of Hospital; there are three Memon Kachi only in Mutrah and Muscat, two are in poor condition only Abdul Latif Isani willing to pay Rs. 400."[10] While the archives preserve only the letters from British subjects answering the call of the political agent, the list of names of fifty-three donors represented the diversity of Muscat's and Muttrah's merchant communities.[11]

Following long-standing patterns of cooperation between the ruler and the various merchant communities, the construction of a new hospital in Muscat at the end of the first decade of the twentieth century resulted from a joint effort between Sultan Faysal, the British Political Agency, and members of the ethnically and religiously heterogeneous population who donated funds. This act of collaborative medical institutionalization was not unique to Muscat. In fact, the British Empire relied on the cooperation of local elites to advance imperial projects across the Gulf. The sultan placed himself in an intermediary position between the British hospital project and the health needs of Muscat's residents. He thus extended his claims over the people of Muscat beyond collecting port customs and enforcing quarantine to include the targeted care of individual bodies. The combined appeals from the political agent and the sultan appear to have persuaded Muscat's various ethnic and religious groups. They responded to the town meeting with promises of donations accompanied by letters that sought to influence the hospital's organization.

Hospital projects also demonstrate how dynamics of imperial competition in the early twentieth-century Gulf produced new forms of gendered personhood. Besides the fact that the previous building had collapsed and the hospital was occupying makeshift lodgings, the lack of suitable accommodations for women patients was one of the principal grievances of the British Agency surgeon Norman Scott with Muscat's medical facilities in 1908, the year before the sultan's public meeting. Local women, Scott suggested, were eager to come to the hospital, but the lack of proper facilities disproportionately affected their care. He opined, "Had there been more and better accommodation to offer especially for women many more of the inhabitants would have sought relief as indoor patients."[12] The Bhatia Mahajan community also accompanied their hefty donation for the new hospital with the caveat that "there must be two separate rooms for male and female patients."[13] For the British doctor and the local community members alike, a modern hospital entailed the partition of medical space and the categorization of patients along gendered lines.

The timing of the public concern of the British and the sultan for medical care in Muscat, as I indicated earlier, was not coincidental. It was the American missionaries of the Reformed Church in America who were, like missionary organizations in Bombay, the "ideological and organizational catalysts" of medical institutional change in the early twentieth-century Gulf.[14] This competitive medical marketplace motivated early hospital projects in Muscat, Bahrain, and Kuwait at the beginning of the twentieth century. Competition among British agents, local elites, and American missionaries drove the emergence of hospitals; what one British official represented in 1909 as the "recent aggressive endeavours of the American Mission," for example, spurred British officials and local elites to action in Muscat.[15] Notions of contagion and the movement of disease intersected with environmental, social, and economic factors. For British officials, the driving objectives of quarantine were to facilitate free-flowing international trade by forcibly confining travelers in space and time and to forestall rival imperial encroachments in the Gulf. Both quarantines and hospitals emerged out of a convergence of foreign and indigenous investment in medical institutions. These institutions reified the claims of local elites over residents and increased the influence of imperial officers and Christian missionaries on the ground.

Hospitals differed from the quarantine system in important ways: hospitals represented a more intimate framework of individualized medical care. Hospitals targeted a group of patients who were defined spatially by residential (if, in many cases, transient) proximity to the hospital. But most significantly, while top-down measures to prevent epidemics, like the quarantine stations, were intrusive and likely to encounter resistance, people *chose* to make use of a hospital. The fact that residents of the Arabian side of the Persian Gulf came to desire and even seek out hospital care in the early twentieth century triggered a greater level of engagement among communities on the ground than did the quarantine stations. The expansion of hospital care, as documented by rising numbers of men and women patients, entailed a bottom-up social process driven by local people crafting new roles as consumers of medicine through their interactions with foreign doctors and nurses. Ordinary people thus played a powerful role in institutionalizing modern health services. By demanding formalized medical treatment and then making their desires felt by attending hospitals and clinics in large numbers, patients forged a new realm of political contestation out of emerging health services.

Competing Hospitals Emerge

Over the first two decades of the twentieth century, hospitals emerged across several Gulf port cities as spaces of political jostling in a competitive medical marketplace. Inside these hospitals, the focus was, first, on diagnosing specific illnesses and, second, on treating individual patients. The mobility of local populations and the instrumental use of medicine for evangelical and political ends shaped experiences of personalized medicine. As hospitals became an accepted part of the landscapes of port cities, some patients traveled far for medical care, having heard of missionary and British health services from transient Bedouins, pearl divers, and merchants.

From the end of the nineteenth century, missionaries fanned out across the Gulf, hoping that their medical skills would win them access to Muslim constituencies. The missionaries believed that their medical and educational humanitarian work would inspire people to convert to Christianity.[16] For the missionaries, medicine was a means to the end of evangelism.[17] They understood that doctors could gain access to privileged spaces.[18] The different legal arrangements and political alliances also played a role in shaping the emergence of hospitals across the Gulf. In Bahrain, the British claimed a protectorate. In Kuwait, the Ottomans maintained tenuous rights which the British and Shaykh Mubarak sought to weaken by preventing the reestablishment of Ottoman sanitary authority. In Muscat, the United States had a direct treaty with the sultan dating to 1833.

The missionaries' relationship with the British agencies was one of wary codependence. Similar to Christian missionaries in Egypt, "they could come because the British made it possible, protecting missionaries at the same time that they watched them."[19] In the 1880s, a group of young American men formed the Arabian Mission while they were students at the New Brunswick Theological Seminary of the Reformed Church in New Jersey. The mission's founding fathers chose to focus their efforts on "Arabia" because they viewed it as the "homeland of Islam," which they saw as "the main rival of Christianity."[20] Following a successful fundraising tour of midwestern churches, the missionaries rapidly established a foothold across multiple Gulf communities. Members of the mission opened a station in Basra in 1889, where they identified medical services as a way to gain access to local people.[21] As the Arabian Mission established outposts around the Gulf, it developed a complex relationship with the British agencies. While British imperial officials recognized the usefulness of the missionaries' medical skills and generally appreciated the addition of white Christians to their social circles, they were also leery of the presence of a group of American outsiders whose agenda in the region did not always correspond to the goals of the Raj. Moreover, British representatives were concerned that the local population would not differentiate between American proselytizers and British administrators, fueling additional resentment against and resistance to the imperial presence.

The missionaries established a Bible shop in Bahrain in 1893.[22] Attuned to Manama's status as a regional entrepôt, they opened the Mason Memorial Hospital in Bahrain in 1903. Architecturally and institutionally, the hospital—built on land purchased in 1901, constructed in 1902 and opened in 1903—transformed Gulf medical care. The Mason Memorial Hospital was the first hospital in the Gulf that focused on caring for local people.[23] The missionaries emphasized the symbolic effect of the building as elevating local health care from the primitive to the civilized. "Where a year ago were mat huts," John Van Ess proclaimed, "now stands that magnificent building. . . . Like the Saviour's arms, its doors are always open to receive the sick in body, and like the Saviour too, those in charge try to give healing for the body, and, best of all, healing for the soul as well."[24] The mission's doctor Sharon Thoms described the design: "With the twelve foot verandahs entirely surrounding the building, and the sun shades to be put up at the east and west ends, the sun will at no time during the day touch the walls of the building proper."[25] The building itself not only showcased the mission's ability to conquer disease but also demonstrated the power of modern architecture over the local climate.

Local communities were hostile to Christian evangelism, but they also observed the benefits of targeted medicine. Some residents responded by seeking alternative avenues of care. Over the same period that the missionaries were establishing their medical services, other actors were demanding that local elites and British representatives provide the administrative scaffolding for parallel health institutions. For example, when a leading Hindu merchant in Bahrain offered to donate Rs. 5,000 toward establishing a British hospital in Bahrain in 1901, the assistant political agent's enthusiastic support stemmed from his suspicion of the missionaries. He noted that many locals sought treatment at the mission dispensary, but "there are large numbers of poor people who refrain from doing so on account of religious scruples and persons of this class will greatly appreciate a hospital which they can visit without compunction."[26] After more local merchants offered generous sums, the Government of India finally agreed to sponsor the hospital. In July 1905, an assistant surgeon arrived to work in the Victoria Memorial Hospital.[27] As a medical outpost of British Empire, Victoria Memorial Hospital existed because Bahrain-based merchants had clamored for an institution that offered a viable alternative to the Christian missionary hospital.

Even in this competitive medical marketplace of the turn-of-the-century Gulf, the American health services enjoyed a steady stream of patients. After constructing their hospital in Bahrain, the missionaries set out to establish similar institutions in other Gulf cities. Initially, local rulers around the region proved resistant to their presence. In August 1904, Shaykh Mubarak of Kuwait (r. 1896–1915) abruptly forced a small outpost of the Arabian Mission to close its Bible and book shop.[28] But while Mubarak's antagonism toward the missionaries and their evangelism was typical of local elites, news of missionary medical services had reached Kuwait. The port city's residents also started to call for institutionalized health services.[29] Recognizing this unprecedented pressure to provide medical care to the people of his port city, Mubarak wrote to the political agent at Kuwait in September 1904: "An English doctor is needed in our town of Koweit . . . and this doctor should be skillful in his art, wounds, and diseases. That will be beneficial to us and all our subjects."[30] As had the local merchants in Bahrain, at the beginning of the twentieth century Mubarak turned to the British Empire to provide an alternative medical infrastructure that would stymie the encroaching missionary influence.

Mubarak's interests also aligned with British fears that the Ottomans would post a doctor in Kuwait to supervise sanitation and quarantine. The presence of a British doctor on the ground in Kuwait would allow the British to rebuff renewed Ottoman sanitary claims (see chapter 1). In October 1904, the British Agency opened a charitable dispensary at Kuwait. It offered medical advice and treatment free of charge from morning until 1 p.m. every day except Friday.[31] Mubarak hoped that the British clinic would satisfy his subjects' demands for medical services and hold the missionaries at bay, while the political agent believed that a doctor would strengthen Britain's local presence in that "Sheikh Mubarak will be impressed by the advantage to him and his people of a resident English medical man."[32] Poor patients received free treatment, and those who had the means were expected to pay a fee.[33] The first "resident English medical man" in the dispensary was the Indian assistant surgeon Daudur Rahman. Rahman recorded high attendance between October 1904 and March 1905 (3,976 patients treated; 2,316 men, 1,127 women, and 533 children).[34] But the British doctor, whose duties were split between the dispensary, caring for the employees of the Political Agency, and sanitary supervision, could not keep up with the high volume of local demand for medical care.[35]

A positive encounter with a mission doctor who successfully operated on his daughter's eyes in the nearby town of Muhammarah apparently lessened Shaykh Mubarak's hostility to the American Christians.[36] After several years of being turned away from Kuwait, the missionaries opened a dispensary in 1910, a school in 1911, and a hospital in 1914.[37] When the American missionaries first opened their medical services to the public in Kuwait, people remained hesitant to embrace their treatments. According to one account, many of the locals initially "mocked and avoided" them.[38] To test the mission doctor's abilities, Mubarak sent his horse, suffering from a large abscess in his leg, to the hospital for treatment. Although the doctor was not trained to treat animals, he realized the symbolic importance of the situation, and so the first operation performed in the Kuwait mission hospital was on the shaykh's horse. Fortuitously for the longevity of mission medical services in Kuwait, several days later the animal recovered.[39] The horse's revival, the story goes, prompted the shaykh and other locals to trust the missionaries' medical abilities.

The British Agency's Doctor Rahman used local categorizations that differentiated between townsfolk and itinerant Bedouin populations, which also revealed the interplay between indigenous and imperial delineations of the population. Bedouins appeared to make up a significant proportion of patients, as "attendance fell off" in the winter when "the Bedouins went out of the town."[40] In the spring, "as the severity of the winter abated and caravans of Bedouins from the interior began to visit the town, the attendance began to rise again."[41] Rahman's clear delineation between Bedouin and settled patients foreshadowed other public health discourses and practices. After completing their hospital in 1914, the American missionaries placed a wire fence around the building to maintain some distance between the hospital and the tents of the Bedouins who had traveled to the hospital for medical care.[42]

The missionaries and British also might have picked up on local contempt for Bedouin practices. For example, Rasim Rushdi's 1955 study pointed out differentiations in Bedouin health practices, claiming that Bedouins believed that some odors, such as the smell of menstruating women, caused disease.[43] When he entered the city, the Bedouin "stuffed his nose with a rag" soaked in foul-smelling liquid to negate potentially harmful odors.[44] In a separate account, the mission doctor Stanley Mylrea wrote in 1921, "Now among the people of Kuwait the belief is strongly held that certain aromatic odors are fatal to the healing of a wound and it is an everyday sight to see people going about with the nostrils plugged up with cotton and asafetida to keep themselves from inhaling these dangerous smells."[45] Unlike the Kuwaiti authors, the mission doctor did not distinguish between Bedouins and townspeople in his description of this medical belief. Such contempt for Bedouin hygiene, however, permeated foreign and local urban discourse alike well into the twentieth century, offering a glimpse of class differentiation through cultures of health. In a 1965 article, the Egyptian doctor Kamal Fahmy also remarked on local responses to smells associated with women. "In some tribes in Arabia," he wrote, "the local women put a perfumed substance resembling chewing gum high up in the vagina immediately after normal labour, to prevent bad odour of the lochia."[46]

In Muscat, the competitive dynamics of hospital creation unfolded along parallel lines as they had in Kuwait. The sultan used the fact that he—with the support of local communities—had already planned for a hospital (as described at the beginning of this chapter) as an excuse to fend off missionary advances. But Sultan Faysal's objections also demonstrated his awareness of the politicized medical situations unfolding in other Gulf cities. The missionaries proved adept at drawing on Muscat's 1833 treaty with the United States to strengthen their case for establishing medical services. In early March 1909, just a month after Sultan Faysal held his meeting to solicit funds for a hospital, he faced unwanted advances from the Arabian Mission. The sultan learned that the missionaries were planning to rent a house in Muttrah for a hospital "without obtaining his sanction."[47] Missionaries had been practicing medicine in Oman since the 1890s and had established a clinic in 1904, but a hospital represented a clear escalation of their activities.[48] Faced with this slight to his sovereignty, he turned to the British for assistance.

Unlike in Bahrain and Kuwait, in Muscat the mission's determination to open a hospital resulted in a legal debate that involved the sultan, the British political agent, and the American consul. The issue highlighted the ambiguity of Muscat's relationship to the British Empire and challenged the strength of its long-standing treaty with the United States. Legally, the heart of the matter was whether or not Christian missionaries could be categorized as "traders." According to an 1833 treaty of amity and commerce between the United States and the sultanate, "The citizens of the United States resorting to the ports of the Sultan for the purpose of trade shall have leave to land and reside in the said ports without paying any tax on importation whatever for such liberty other than the general duties on imports which the most-favoured nation shall pay."[49] This argument depended on an interpretation of missionaries as traders akin to merchants. Holland, the British agent in Muscat, found this assertion dubious. He contended, "To the layman it seems at least questionable whether a missionary, whose actions are not ordinarily governed by commercial considerations, can be regarded as a trader."[50] For his part, the sultan feared for his local political standing. He worried that "the doctor's successes will result in the conversion of patients."[51] The sultan also was concerned that "local disturbances may arise from the missionaries' interference with their patients' religion."[52] But because of the existing treaty between the Sultan of Oman and the United States, the political agent was not empowered to stop the missionaries through direct intervention. The missionaries, with the support of the American consul, persisted, and in April 1909, the mission doctor Sharon Thoms moved into a house and opened a dispensary. Underlying the missionaries' claims of benevolence was an understanding that the American consul would offer political support to their right to practice medicine in Oman.

Gulf Patients and Gendered Medicine

From initial planning stages through the establishment of medical routines, Gulf hospitals produced new forms of gendered personhood. Missionary and British doctors alike assumed that medical institutions in the Arabian Peninsula needed to maintain completely separate areas for men and women. This practice gave the American missionaries a distinct advantage over the British in providing hospital care. In contrast to the British outposts—where the political agents struggled to attain the salary for a single male assistant surgeon from the Government of India—the Arabian Mission aggressively recruited women doctors and nurses. Their goal was to spread the Gospel to local women, whom the missionaries assumed were inaccessible to foreign men. Women missionaries also provided a highly marketable narrative for their magazine *Neglected Arabia*, which operated largely as a fundraising publication. Missionary writings portrayed Arabian women "as experiencing intellectual deprivation, domestic oppression and sexual degradation."[53] The female missionaries' claim that their access to Muslim women allowed them to "lift the veil and show you things as they are" would have been especially enticing to their American audience.[54]

The missionaries made a strong case that they were successful at drawing patients into their clinics and hospitals. *Neglected Arabia* regularly mentioned specific numbers of patients seeking treatment. Such empirical data demonstrated to American audiences the popularity of medical work among local people, as well as the missionaries' success at spreading the Gospel. The religious aims of medical care were unambiguous. In the early twentieth-century Gulf, the treatment experience entailed first listening to a Christian sermon and then receiving medical care. Dr. Sharon Thoms described the setup in Bahrain's dispensary (before the hospital had opened) in 1901:

> The medical work has been most wonderfully blessed. We are treating, on an average, about fifty patients a day, and doing three or four operations. Some of the most satisfactory operations are those for cataracts, of which we have performed seven, for they come here blind and go away seeing—but what is this compared to that privilege of giving them the Light of the World, Jesus. During the last four weeks we have treated over twelve hundred patients and done a goodly number of operations. As we have no assistance, except an uneducated native, you will understand how busy we are. When the men leave for the pearl fields we will probably get a breathing-spell. We are improving this glorious opportunity of presenting the Gospel to the people who assemble here for treatment each day, as best we can. As most patients bring with them a friend or two, you see the Gospel is preached to a great many more than are treated.[55]

Like medical care, preaching was gender segregated. As Amy Zwemer recounted the scene in 1902: "These summer mornings men and women gather early at the dispensary, the women in their little room and the men on seats in the porch and outside. Every morning, with few exceptions, a preaching and prayer service is held for the two gatherings, men and women."[56] More challenging to measure, of course, was whether or not the waiting patients chose to listen. Mrs. Zwemer expressed some frustration following her visits to women in their homes: "It is difficult to read to them for any length of time because they comment on the book or the words to each other, and I have to read at the top of my voice so as to be heard above the tumult."[57]

The architecture of the new hospitals also inscribed gender difference into medical spaces. In Bahrain, the missionaries segregated their hospital by men's and women's sections. The women's quarters included "a chapel or waiting room and a treatment room down stairs, besides a ward large enough for eight beds up stairs."[58] Women patients, like their male counterparts, were subjected to "our Gospel reading and 'lay preaching'" in the waiting room before receiving treatment.[59] The mission doctor Eleanor Calverley chose the rooms for her first women's clinic in Kuwait based on the fact that "women patients could enter, be treated, and leave without danger of having their faces seen by men."[60] When the Kuwait women's hospital opened in 1919, she said, "To shield our patients from the view of men while they were waiting outside the doctor's office, a wooden lattice screen was built into the end of the veranda nearest the Men's Hospital."[61]

For their part, the British hospital in Muscat partitioned space by European and "native" as well as by men and women. After the new British hospital opened in October 1910, the Political Agency's surgeon Captain N. N. G. C. McVean noted how the building provided "separate accommodation for the different classes of patients and special accommodation for females."[62] In contrast to the missionary institutions, the primary goal of the British hospital was to care for Europeans. The fact, however, that the British hospital in Muscat enlisted an interpreter who spoke Arabic, Persian, Baluchi, Swahili, Hindustani, and English, "all of which languages are daily in use at the hospital," attests to its wide use by non-European patients.⁶³

It also is evident that many of the injured and the ill, both men and women, who found their way to the foreign doctors first had attempted their own methods of treatment. In 1900, for example, the mission doctor Sharon Thoms reported that "a pearl diver was brought in from the pearl banks with one arm very badly mangled and the other bitten entirely off just below the elbow by a shark while diving for pearls."⁶⁴ Despite the severity of the wound, the dispensary had not been the man's first stop upon returning to shore. The "accident had occurred the day before and the wounds had been covered with burned dates and pitch."⁶⁵ This initial treatment had "stopped the bleeding," but "one bone of the arm was gone entirely, and the splintered end of the other projected some distance beyond the torn flesh of the elbow."⁶⁶ The operation was serious, as Thoms had to "amputate some distance above the elbow," but as soon as the man had regained consciousness, "he insisted upon walking some distance to a boat in which he went to his home."⁶⁷ The missionary's efforts to save the man did not go unappreciated. When the patient's father and brothers returned from the pearl banks several days later, they accompanied the injured man back to the dispensary. Thoms reported, "The whole family showed signs of gratitude, but the father weeping covered my hands with kisses and my head with blessings."⁶⁸ This incident demonstrates how a patient first turned to local supplies (burned dates) before visiting the mission clinic out of desperation. The man apparently was from another area, one reached by boat, and he and his male relatives accessed the mission dispensary en route between their home and the pearl banks. Although it is quite possible that Thoms exaggerated the family's gratitude, a pattern of such life-saving operations would have gone a long way toward converting local people into hospital patients.

Women missionaries frequently referred to their exceptional access to local women, but some accounts of actual interactions undermine the missionaries' assertions of gendered solidarity. Misunderstandings prevailed on all sides as soon as the first woman inpatient was admitted to the mission hospital in Manama in November 1902. Marion Thoms (a woman doctor, and the wife of Sharon Thoms) recounted:

> She was very dirty and ragged, and we wanted to give her a bath and put on a clean garment before taking her into the operating room. She was perfectly docile and apparently ready both for the bath and the clean dress, but she took a sudden fright at some movement of mine and rushed out half-dressed upon the verandah. I could not restrain her without exerting force, which I did not want to exert unless it proved to be necessary. She kept going from pillar to pillar down past the men's wards, and even the warning that there were men there had no effect upon her. Usually that is all that is needed to cause any woman to retreat. She was all the time calling out quite loudly, and the people in the huts nearby came out to see the cause of the commotion. All I could understand was "I am an old woman." Finally when we were just half-way round the hospital she tried to climb over the railing of the verandah and a mason came to the rescue. He spoke to her in Persian and she told him she was afraid she was going to be killed. He reassured her and I led her back to the bath-room.[69]

Marion Thoms's description of this woman's first hours at the hospital reveals how strange the experience could be for patients in Bahrain. Procedures that seemed natural and sanitary to the missionaries terrified the woman, who later revealed that she was afraid the doctor was going to "take her eye out, cut it, and put it back again."[70] This patient's alarm at the prospect of cataract surgery contrasted sharply with the contemporary missionary claim that "the restoring to sight of those who have long been blind is regarded as a miracle, and is helping to break down the prejudice toward our work."[71] The missionaries, moreover, incorrectly assumed that local proclivities for gender segregation were so strong as to prevent the woman from running away if men were present.

Marion Thoms also portrayed the patient through a particularly American racialized lens. The first woman patient was "an old black woman, a slave I think," but it is unclear whether Thoms had any reason to assume she was a slave other than her dark skin.⁷² Marion Thoms discursively resolved the unsettling experience for her American readership by presenting the patient in typical American Black caricature: "When dressed in a clean pink garment, with a pink handkerchief tied over her head, she looked not unlike one of our southern 'mammies.'"⁷³ When the missionaries encountered resistance to their hospital practices, they assumed that such reactions resulted from religious "intolerance," racial inferiority, or cultural ignorance. Marion Thoms consoled herself: "It is hard not to feel impatient with such ignorance and not to feel depressed at being so misunderstood, but we must take lessons from the 'patience of Christ' and learn to 'have compassion upon the ignorant.'"⁷⁴ In drawing from a distinctly American cultural canon to categorize the people they encountered, Marion Thoms rendered her experience legible to a predominantly white American Christian readership. Once the patient accepted the missionaries' medical services, they transformed her into a familiar racialized stereotype.

The 1903 arrival of the third global plague pandemic to Bahrain, just months after the American mission had opened its hospital, further tested the missionaries' claims to have special access to local women. Amy Zwemer recalled the height of the plague epidemic: "As soon as the disease was well established and panic had taken possession of the people the dispensary patients dropped in numbers very suddenly, and in the Women's dispensary almost entirely; just an odd one would venture to come."⁷⁵ Zwemer reported on an alarming rumor that blamed the missionaries for bringing plague to the island. She wrote, "The story noised abroad was that the doctor had taken the poison serum which he had sent for to Bombay and had scattered it about the town and so infected the people; some of them said that he had done this in order to kill off all the Moslems and have a Christian island!"⁷⁶ The idea that the Christian missionaries were trying to poison Muslims was not an entirely unbelievable interpretation of the missionaries' vision of evangelizing Arabia by saving (or eliminating through conversion) Muslim souls. In Amy Zwemer's response to the rumors, she stressed both the importance of their work with Muslim women and their complete unity with the male missionaries, who were in many cases their husbands. Zwemer wrote from the "female" perspective of the mission when she asserted that her access to women hospital patients and her admission to the harem section of people's homes granted her a particular understanding of local culture.

Amy Zwemer described what it was like to treat patients at home during the plague outbreak when hospital attendance had plummeted. Her discussion of the unsanitary, crowded, and poorly provisioned situation of patients she visited provided a stark contrast to the new mission hospital's modern and permanent appearance. She explained that, in contrast to what her American audience might have expected, there was no segregation camp or government aid in response to the plague outbreak, and "each patient remained in the place where he was and so we had to go from house to house each morning with dressing-trays, stimulants and tonics."[77] Initially, three women died even after receiving treatment from the Americans. Amy Zwemer attributed the fatalities to preexisting conditions and an unfavorable environment, writing, "It was difficult to treat both symptoms [a previous illness and the plague] at once, especially in the dirty, close, stifling-hot huts on the desert-plain where we found the patients."[78] The missionaries were also frustrated that, as before the plague outbreak, they were only a last resort for patients who "always treated new symptoms with their own remedies first."[79] Amy Zwemer described the local treatments in detail: "The native specific for the buboes was fried horse-manure and the internal treatment worse still; the patient's diet, to *cool* the fever, was often raw cucumbers."[80] Another young girl had covered her bubo with "a black sticky mixture like cobbler's wax."[81] For the missionaries, such details emphasized the backwardness of local medicine and the desperate need for the mission hospital.

Fortunately for the residents of Bahrain and the missionary enterprise, not even the bubonic plague could maintain its virulence in the scorching temperatures of a Gulf summer. Amy Zwemer reported that "after the intense heat began the plague germs died out and the death rate rapidly decreased, while patients began to come again to the Hospital."[82] Hospital attendance increased by the middle of June, approximately six weeks after the first reported case of plague. The missionaries had opened their hospital to gain a footing in the local community that would facilitate their proselytizing by carrying out their humanitarian goals. Indeed, local attendance demonstrates that there *was* a need for and appreciation of these medical services, if not for the accompanying Christian message. The missionaries reported 807 cases in their dispensary between July 1 and September 11, 1900. Samuel Zwemer took pride in the fact that they were attracting their target demographic, stating that "nearly all of them were very poor people and with the exception of a dozen Jews and Jewesses they were Moslems."[83] In 1904, "on an average there were sixty cases being treated every morning at the dispensaries, to say nothing of the calls attended in the homes of the people."[84]

The missionaries and their hospital weathered the plague and emerged with a stronger presence on the island. They combated suspicion by adapting to local needs and expectations and providing home treatments for those who refused to come to the hospital. Yet, as some residents increasingly turned to the mission hospitals, other local actors with access to capital responded to this bottom-up demand for health care by funding and organizing alternative and non-Christian institutionalized medical services.[85] While local women continued to provide care and oversee childbirth in domestic spaces (see chapter 3), male elites founded institutions to rival the missionary presence. In 1910, a group of Kuwaiti merchants and educated men, motivated by transregional discussions of Islamic reform, as well as by their own travels to places like Egypt, Iraq, and Mecca in pursuit of education, joined together to start a local school that would, they hoped, obstruct missionary influence.[86] The Kuwaiti merchant class enjoyed close ties to cities like Bombay and Basra and also "espoused Islamic modernist ideology" during this period.[87] Enthusiastic readers of Muhammad Rashid Rida's magazine *al-Manar* (The lighthouse), Kuwait's modernists were consummate reformers who "would lovingly nurture their community with spiritual rather than materialistic values, even when they needed money to realize their aims."[88] In 1911, a group of Kuwaiti merchants and educated men joined together to open a local school (which would welcome students starting in 1912) intended to stymie missionary influence by offering history, geography, arithmetic, English, and Arabic.[89] The missionary Edwin Calverley referred to Rida as "the editor of an influential Moslem journal in Cairo, who knew the methods and universal tendencies of Christian missions." Calverley described Rida's dramatic 1912 visit to Kuwait: "In daily lectures in the principal mosque of the town, he urged them to avoid association with us and to make it unnecessary for the people to come to us by themselves providing medical and school facilities along progressive lines. The whole town agreed with him as regards the advisability of avoiding the Christians, and sermons to that effect were preached in the other mosque."[90]

In 1913, following Rida's rousing visit to Kuwait, a group of reformist merchants formed the Arab Charitable Association.[91] They recruited a Muslim doctor from Ottoman Basra to staff their new dispensary, which provided free health services to the poor.[92] The project was short-lived; the doctor resigned the same year, forcing the dispensary to close. According to one Kuwaiti historian, however, the clinic represented a momentous change in Kuwait's medical landscape, as "despite the short time the clinic operated, the experience was the beginning of effective national participation for institutional health work, and following it a number of civic pharmacies were established."[93] Writing in 1915, Calverley admitted that the American missionaries' "school, Bible shop and medical work have all been seriously affected."[94] Sadly, Farhan al-Khal, the charitable organization's founder, was not able to witness these developments in the local health establishment. He died on a ship while he was returning to Kuwait from Bombay in 1914.[95]

World War I altered the dynamics between missionary and British medical services on the ground in the Gulf, as the British were willing to accept any available medical help from allies. In the wake of the Great War, local elites and nonelites alike came to see medical institutions as desirable components of the urban landscape. In Kuwait, for example, even as local merchants and religious leaders pursued rival medical projects, residents continued to turn to the mission hospital at key moments. When the Ikhwan attacked Kuwait at Al Jahra village in 1920, the mission hospital treated 120 injured Kuwaitis.[96] The mission doctor Stanley Mylrea described the incident: "Most of [the wounded] arrived on October 11th but the worst cases were brought by water and did not reach us till the following day. Nearly all of them came to the American Hospital and I am glad to say that we lost only four of them." Mylrea went so far as to complain of the extent to which the community was depending on the mission hospital. When "the twentieth prominent man had told me how God would reward us," Mylrea "boiled over" and retorted:

> That's all very fine, talk is the cheapest thing in the world. You people pile all this work on me, but it never occurs to one of you to do anything or to help either financially or in kind. In my country, the rulers would be the first to visit the wounded and to do all in their power to see the sufferers have every attention. Here the Sheikh's slaves dump helpless men on the hospital verandah and that is all there is to it—no thought of how my small staff is to cope with all this extra work.

Mylrea claimed that his outburst paid off, when the next day "a man who has been a bitter enemy of the American Mission in the past" came to the hospital and "handed me a bag containing Rs. 500."[97]

Nevertheless, the desire to provide a local, Islamic version of institutional medicine persisted. In the early 1920s, an assembly of merchants convened in the majlis of Hamad 'Abd Allah al-Saqr to pursue the idea of opening a Kuwaiti hospital that followed the model of the American hospital.[98] Although this plan was not realized due to the failure of the committee to reach a consensus, its efforts do reveal the growing sense of the importance of wresting responsibility for the community's medicine away from the Americans and British. In 1924, Shaykh Hamad ibn Isa Al Khalifa of Bahrain even proposed "start[ing] a hospital Dhow to tour round the pearl banks," thus envisioning hospital care as an act of the ruler's patronage as integral to pearl diving, the island's main economic activity.[99] By suggesting the insertion of hospital services into the pearl-diving industry, Shaykh Hamad signaled his responsibility to provide health care to a population that he conceptualized according to their status as productive (if itinerant) residents of Bahrain.

Over the course of these local innovations, practices of gender segregation that the Americans and British built into their hospitals continued to cast a long shadow over modern medicine in the Gulf. By the 1960s, local observers of the momentous changes underfoot in their society were embracing medical gender segregation as a natural arrangement. For example, the Kuwaiti scholar ʿAbd Allah Khalid al-Hatim wrote that the missionaries had opened the first women's hospital because they saw that "the Kuwaiti woman was living at that time in a position in which she was not permitted to receive treatment in the men's hospital at the hands of male doctors."[100] Such narratives of absolute gender separation in the pre-oil period simultaneously picked up colonial discourses of women's segregation as evidence of backwardness and emphasized the modernizing and civilizing role of the post-oil development state as a rupture from past practices.

Hospitals and Patients

American missionaries working in the Arabian Peninsula associated the care of bodies with the saving of souls. They promoted medicine as a means to entice people to hear their religious message. British doctors argued that hospitals and dispensaries offered an opportunity to demonstrate the benefits of empire to local people. As hospitals emerged around the region, rulers and merchants also recognized health care as an assertion of their leadership. Residents of Gulf port cities initially were suspicious of and hostile to the new medical institutions, particularly the Christian missionary projects. Local elites sought to prevent missionary efforts to set up medical facilities, fearing religious tensions and a new source of foreign influence. By the second decade of the twentieth century, however, people across the region were demanding and utilizing these new medical institutions. Hospital architecture and divisions of medical labor naturalized gender segregation, constructing novel forms of personhood for men and women patients.

The mission hospitals reached diverse elements of Arabian and Gulf society. In one notable example from the 1930s, the Bahrain hospital played a central role in an enslaved man's manumission. The formerly enslaved pearl diver Suwailim bin Faraj recalled, "During May 1934 I fell sick at Qatar and my master sent me to the Hospital at Bahrain for treatment." The man seems to have seized on his hospital visit as a chance to claim his freedom. When his master came to collect him from the hospital, he said: "I refused to accompany him as he was not kind towards me. As there was no hope of his getting me to go with him to Qatar he left me and went away."[101]

The mission hospitals continued to receive a steady flow of local patients until state public health services finally outpaced their facilities after World War II. Yet even as local people increasingly sought out hospital care, the biomedicalization of a critical event in women's lives proved elusive. In the next chapter I explore how folk medicine remained important in childbirth throughout the twentieth century as first missionary and then state doctors struggled to infiltrate women's reproductive worlds.

CHAPTER 3

CHILDBIRTH

IN THE EARLY TWENTY-FIRST CENTURY, Hussa Ahmad bin Sayf, a Bahraini woman, recounted to her daughter her experiences of childbirth in the late 1940s. Looking back from decades later, she recalled her unusual refusal to pack her vagina with salt in the days following childbirth. Hussa explained:

> When I was about to give birth to my first baby, I asked my husband's sister, who preceded me in childbearing, about the pain of childbirth. She told me that the true pain is not the one that accompanies labor, but rather [the real pain is] that which comes after childbirth, when pieces of salt are placed daily inside the vagina. This makes the woman who has just given birth feel that there are burning embers in her abdomen, and the pain doubles when the postpartum woman is deprived of drinking water, which she desperately needs. Based on what I heard from my husband's sister, I adamantly refused to put salt [in my vagina] or to abstain from drinking water, even though my mother was angry and reprimanded me. I did not accept this [practice] in any subsequent births.[1]

What was this postpartum practice that Hussa Ahmad bin Sayf refused? Why did the women of her family expect her to partake in something that she understood would entail great pain and trauma? And how had childbirth, as a social and biological event, changed in such a way as to prompt her to articulate these intimate memories of the 1940s in the early twenty-first century?

Rather than tracing a linear teleology in which women, obediently following the directives of male-dominated institutions, move from the home to the hospital to have their babies, this chapter unpacks how three constellations of Gulf childbirth across the twentieth century reveal the vibrancy of women's social worlds. First, even as American missionaries popularized hospital care in the early twentieth century, they failed to infiltrate childbirth because women persistently relied on midwives from their own communities. Second, as state hospital projects expanded in the post–World War II period, a new cohort of foreign doctors flocked to the region. In a series of scientific articles aimed at an international audience of medical colleagues, these doctors documented how their women patients in Arabia suffered from vaginal atresia, or abnormal narrowing or closure of the vagina. Identifying acquired, as opposed to congenital—that is, a condition present from birth—vaginal atresia as exceptionally common in Arabia, they determined that the medical condition stemmed from local practices of packing postpartum women's vaginas with salt.[2] Local women met the doctors' attempts to surgically correct vaginal atresia and to culturally alter postpartum practices with a variety of responses, demonstrating how a complex field of interactions, rather than top-down social engineering, characterized postwar medical modernization. Third, this chapter's final section considers an Egyptian anthropologist's late twentieth-century study of Gulf folk medicine. Oral histories featured in his discussions of women's health reveal how local women continued to practice and find value in folk medicine decades after the proliferation of state medical services.

Importantly, the late twentieth-century interviews I explore do not contradict or correct earlier doctors' discussions of postpartum uses of salt. Indeed, as in Hussa Ahmad bin Sayf's account, memories of salt's pain reverberated over decades. Yet in contrast to the writings of doctors who encountered pregnancies and the aftermath of childbirth as medical problems to be solved, local women emphasized how childbirth was central to the maintenance and reproduction of women's social worlds. In tracing the three distinct discussions of childbirth across a range of genres of sources with the goal of rendering women's experiences historically visible, I counterbalance the previous chapter's focus on the rise of institutionalized medicine as driven by local elites, imperial agents, and American missionaries. Even as foreign doctors and state agents worked to bring Gulf health care in line with what they imagined to be universal standards of modernization, the ways that local women collectively navigated the critical event of childbirth over the course of the twentieth century profoundly shaped medical practice.

Women Missionaries, Male Authority, and Medical Conversion

As demonstrated in the previous chapter, missionary medical services enjoyed a regular stream of local patients starting in the early twentieth century. But even as the missionaries drew women into their hospitals and clinics, they struggled to access the world of childbirth. Part of their challenge was that, in contrast to exceptional ailments that ruptured ordinary life, most people in Arabia conceived of childbirth as a "natural process that required no outside interference" rather than a medicalized event.[3] Midwives remained a "source of opposition" to missionary doctors, because the midwives "resented their competence being questioned and also feared the threat Western medicine posed to their livelihood."[4] Avner Giladi's description of childbirth as a distinct domain of women's subculture in the premodern Middle East is also relevant here. Childbirth, he writes, was an event that "sharply split the community along gendered lines. Men were usually excluded . . . whereas the women of the family and the neighborhood rushed in not only to help and support the woman in labor but also to take part in an event in which the midwife was a key figure."[5]

Nevertheless, eager to sell their successes to their audience of potential donors back in the United States, missionaries recorded several exceptional instances of intervention in childbirth. Through a close reading of these encounters, I show that missionary women relied on male authority to bypass local midwives and to penetrate the birthing space.[6] Further, I build on Catherine S. Woodward's observation that, as the twentieth century wore on and the Arabian mission failed to convert more than a handful of people, they turned to their medical work as evidence that they were still achieving results for Christ, and for donors in the United States. As Woodward summarizes the situation in Bahrain in 1939, the missionaries "could point to 67,000 or more dispensary treatments, but only five converts."[7] As the failure to evangelize was increasingly evident, missionaries instead represented local people's transition from reluctance to willingness to go to the hospital as a conversion to a missionary-driven medical modernity.

The missionaries depicted local midwives as elderly and dangerously ignorant, and the typical birth room as dirty and disorderly. In her memoir, Eleanor Calverley described her arrival at one birthing scene in Kuwait: "We found Faheema on the floor of a room dimly lighted by a lantern. She was squatting on a pile of sand and two old midwives sat by to support her, one in front and the other behind. Nearby was a pile of sacking and discarded clothing. I heard the old women muttering, 'Why did you call the *Englaiziya*? Leave us alone, and the child will soon be born!'" As the "night wore on," Calverley grew concerned because "the child's heartbeat with the stethoscope sounded a little less strong" while "Faheema was growing weary." When she felt she could wait no longer, Calverley informed Faheema that the time had come to "use instruments [forceps]. . . . The nurse will help you to inhale some medicine which will put you to sleep. When you wake up, if Allah wills, we will show you your living child." Faheema, exhausted, was amenable to the suggestion, but her mother and aunt cried out, "No! No!" and the "two old midwives were more bold now, in their mutterings," sending Calverley and her nurse "black looks" as they complained, "If we had been allowed to have our way, the baby would have been here long ago."

In response to the midwives, Calverley turned to Faheema and asked, "Is your husband in the house?" As Sulimaan, Faheema's husband, arrived, "all the onlookers pulled their veils over their faces." Ignoring the crowd of women, Calverley "stepped over to speak with him," declaring: "We have waited long enough. . . . I want to use instruments in order to bring the baby quickly while its heart is still beating strongly. Will you, please, give the order, so that I can proceed?" Calverley achieved the desired effect in calling Sulimaan. He issued the order to "let the *hakeema* do as she wishes," speaking "in a clear strong voice. Then he disappeared."[8] The recalcitrant women fell back at the husband's words, and Faheema gave birth to a healthy boy. In contrast to the irrational local women, blinded by their fear of the missionary and her medical tools, Calverley depicted her own actions as rational and calculated. It is also notable that, instead of attempting to explain or reason with the women, she bypassed them by summoning the husband into the birthing room. The women's quick veiling and the husband's immediate disappearance after issuing his command emphasize the exceptional nature of inviting a man to interfere in childbirth.

Other missionaries similarly reported turning to the household's men, usually excluded from the childbirth room, to assert their authority over local women. In Bahrain in 1930, Dr. M. N. Tiffany described arriving to a courtyard to assist a woman with her first birth. The woman in labor was attended by "four or five women" who were "fearful and not disposed to trust us too much." To make matters worse, when it started to rain, "the courtyard became a mudpuddle." After a baby girl was delivered, "the patient had severe hemorrhage and retained after-birth." When Tiffany instructed her nurse to give the mother anesthetic, "the women pushed us away." The newly delivered mother's "old father stood outside and exhorted the women on no account to let me give anaesthetic." When "the girl's condition became critical," Tiffany "went out into the rain and mud to talk to the father. The poor old man wailed, 'My girl, my girl,' and began to cry. So I cried a little, too, and begged him to give me permission to do what was necessary to save her life." Tiffany, like Calverley, achieved the desired result by appealing to male authority: "Suddenly he said, 'I believe you all right. Do what you like.' And he shouted to the women to hinder me no more. We went to work quickly and in the nick of time. It was all over in a jiffy and the patient recovered nicely."[9]

Calverley and Tiffany both introduced men to the childbirth event to leverage authority over local women. Moreover, when, in the missionaries' writings, women were the ones who embraced missionary medical expertise, they did so in language that was reminiscent of religious conversion. In 1949, Cornelia Dalenberg described a conversation with Zainab, a woman in Bahrain who had called on Dalenberg to help a mother in labor. After saving the mother's life, Zainab explained to Dalenberg why she had sought out the missionary's help: "I have been in the hospital, and my eyes have been opened."[10] In 1951, Dalenberg wrote another article of medical conversion, this time assuming the voice of a fictionalized village woman. In the first person, she described her terror of going to the hospital even after several painful days of prolonged labor. Finally she consented, and as she recovered in the hospital, she watched from the window as another woman arrived by car, but this time too late for her life to be saved. When the imagined narrator returned home, she told the other village women: "I have lost all my fear. I want to kiss the feet of the Doctor and Doctoria and the nurses every time I see them. Why was I so fearful before? We are animals. No one ever told us that at the hospital everyone would be so kind to us." Suggesting that successful medical procedures helped local people to appreciate other aspects of missionary work, Dalenberg continued her narrative in the local woman's voice: "I see now. I see why the teacher Sarah and the Doctoria and Um Bushra come and read to us and pray for us." Not only has the imaginary woman accepted hospital care, but she also embraced the pairing of medicine and proselytizing. Dalenberg concluded, still assuming her fictional role-play, "May Allah bless [the medical missionaries] and keep them always for the *Muslimeen*!"[11]

Dalenberg's use of an imaginary village woman's perspective to sell to audiences back home the idea that medical work helped local people to "see" takes on a tone of desperation if we consider that, in the 1950s, "the mission's optimism about being needed in the Gulf began to fade."[12] As the mission's 1952 annual report admitted, "In Bahrain it is beginning to become more apparent . . . that we are facing a competitive medical set-up with the Government."[13] Similarly in Kuwait, one visitor in the early 1950s declared, "It appeared that the Mission Medical Service had lost favour among the population due, no doubt, to the total absence of religion at the New State Hospital, and to the greatly improved facilities there."[14] In contrast to Dalenberg's suggestion that the mission hospital continued to introduce locals to medical salvation, the report indicated dissatisfaction with the facilities: "The people are demanding better and better service such as airconditioned rooms, cleaner sheets, even though they may never have used sheets before, better bathrooms and better nursing. They expect more and more attention."[15] By 1955 one missionary wrote, pleading for money, "There was a day when the mission hospital in Bahrain had the respect of the whole island, but lately we have been told that unless we improve our buildings and equipment we will lose that respect and the government may be rather hard on us."[16]

By the 1960s, as state health care proliferated across booming Gulf cities, the missionaries found themselves superfluous.[17] The postwar dynamic between underfunded Christian missionaries and dramatically improved state services offers a revealing contrast to the situation Beth Baron describes in Egypt in the early twentieth century, when Egyptian elites and British colonial officials alike preferred to subcontract social welfare services on the cheap to foreign missionaries.[18] Reflecting on the closure of Kuwait's mission hospital, a 1967 report explained that "the state's medical services had developed to a level comparable with most western countries, with hospitals and equipment better in many respects than that of the mission. Had the board of the mission decided to continue their medical work, they would have been obliged to undertake expensive modernisation: instead, they came to the conclusion that the mission hospital had fulfilled its purpose."[19] It closed on March 31, 1967, and the premises were leased to the Kuwaiti government as an isolation hospital for children. As the post–World War II development states supplanted the mission hospitals with their own medical institutions, they also replaced an ideology of Christian salvation with one of national realization, thus superseding the missionaries' role as competitive catalysts of medical modernity.

The Vaginal Atresia of Arabia

Between 1957 and 1965, several foreign doctors working in the new state hospitals in Qatar, Saudi Arabia, Bahrain, and Kuwait published articles in international obstetrics and gynecology journals in which they described an alarming pattern, albeit one the missionaries had long been familiar with.[20] Their shared medical concern was the prevalence of vaginal atresia, or obstruction or closure of the vagina, among local women patients. What made Arabian vaginas worthy of scholarly consideration in international medical journals was the unusual cause of local women's anatomical blockage. "Most cases of vaginal atresia," Ismail El Guindi wrote in 1962, "are congenital" (present from birth), whereas "acquired vaginal atresia, especially the traumatic obstetrical and the chemical types, are rare."[21] But in his two years of medical practice in Saudi Arabia, he had found that "the ratio between acquired and congenital cases . . . is reversed."[22] For these doctors and their scholarly audience, vaginal atresia in Arabia was distinct from similar cases found elsewhere in the world—and thus worthy of comment in scientific writing for the global medical community—in that among Arabian women, it was an acquired condition rather than a birth defect.

Why was acquired vaginal atresia so common in Arabia as to generate a flurry of scientific articles? In the days following childbirth, the doctors learned, it was common for midwives or women relatives to place salt in the new mother's vagina, as recounted by Hussa Ahmad bin Sayf at the beginning of this chapter. Given how mothers and their midwives avoided the medicalization of childbirth, foreign health professionals most likely encountered salt-packed vaginas only when the procedure had gone terribly wrong. Salt served as a powerful disinfectant and could prevent puerperal sepsis (infection of the genital tract following childbirth).[23] But to the foreign doctors' dismay packing the vagina with salt could also cause searing pain and potentially debilitating long-term effects such as vaginal atresia, the closing or narrowing of the vaginal passage due to scarring, in response to the salt. The atresia could make sexual intercourse painful and childbirth difficult, dangerous, or even impossible. The missionary Ida Paterson Storm described the impact of atresia on childbirth: "One of two things happens. The baby cannot push through and the mother, weak from a long hopeless labor, dies; or the baby forces itself out, tearing everything in the effort. Sometimes the injury is so great that the mother dies."[24] Some local women sought the missionaries' help with this condition; during a five-month medical tour to Najd in 1935, for example, they performed seven operations to correct vaginal atresia.[25]

Packing the postpartum vagina with salt was a widespread practice around the Gulf, although techniques varied. 'Ali al-Sayyid Baqir al-'Awwami described the technique in his posthumously published memoirs: "A portion of salt was placed on a clean, thin cloth. Then it was inserted in the woman's vagina to absorb the liquid substances and to help heal the wound."[26] Al-ʿAwwami was critical of local midwives, explaining that the "method was dangerous, for often the midwife miscalculated the amount [of salt] she placed [on the cloth], or the length of time that [the salt-soaked cloth] remains [in the vagina]." Finally, he mourned local women's loss of the ability to have sex: "[The salt] would cause the vagina to become dry, or [the vagina] to become blocked, such that sexual intercourse becomes painful for the woman, or even impossible, sometimes. And thus the woman loses her femininity in the beginning of her youth."[27] Al-ʿAwwami's recollection of the midwives' use of a salt-covered rag reveals a different technique from Hussa Ahmad bin Sayf's description of the pieces of salt recounted at the beginning of this chapter. Kamal Fahmy, an Egyptian doctor working at Kuwait's Al-Sabah state hospital in 1965 (and with previous experience in Dammam, Saudi Arabia), provided further detail of regional variations:

> The technique varies in different countries, and even in different places in the same country. In Saudi-Arabia, predominantly of Bedouin population, a piece of rock salt the size of an almond or bigger is inserted high up in the vagina morning and night for 4 days after labor. Sometimes, larger pieces of salt are used initially with progressive decrease in size until the eighth day post partum. In Qatar . . . a ball of rock salt the size of an egg is put in the vagina from the fifth to the twelfth day after delivery by the patient's female relatives or the local handy women [midwives]. In Kuwait . . . balls of rock salt are packed in the vagina from the second day after delivery, and are changed twice daily for 11 days. In Bahrain . . . a piece of salt roughly the size and shape of an egg is pushed into the vagina daily for 2–15 days after delivery.[28]

Why did women in Arabia agree to pack their vaginas with salt after childbirth? As mentioned, salt is a powerful disinfectant. Moreover, discussions of this question by foreign observers must be read cautiously, as the authors frequently looked down on local society, especially women, and were not immune to viewing postpartum women through a sexualized gaze.[29] They also reproduced explanations of their patients' medical conditions that drew on both Orientalist assumptions of Arab depravity and contemporary medical cultures that sexualized the doctor's voyeuristic gaze on women's bodies. In the medical articles on Arabian patients, these observations apply to male and female doctors alike.

Notably, one source cited in the medical articles is the memoir of Charles Belgrave, political and financial adviser to the ruler of Bahrain from 1926 to 1957, demonstrating how interest in local reproductive health practices and sexuality circulated among a range of foreign hired experts. Infamously absolutist, Belgrave represented British colonial interests in Bahrain and enjoyed thirty years as "the executive in chief and effectively the country's first prime minister" until Arab nationalism and anti-British popular feelings rendered his position untenable.[30] In his memoir, Belgrave referred to midwives' "dangerous and disgusting practices."[31] "Often after childbirth," he wrote, "the unfortunate mother was packed, internally, with salt in order to tighten up her muscles, to provide the husband with more sexual satisfaction."[32] This notion of salt packing for male sexual pleasure also appeared in the medical studies. In his 1957 article "The Vaginal Atresia of Arabia," the British doctor A. E. Kingston (formerly of the Indian Medical Service) cast the practice as a timeless tradition and connected it to Islamic culture. "For hundreds of years," he wrote, "it has been the custom to insert salt into the lower genital tract after parturition. . . . Traditionally, this application is thought to restore the parts to the desirable nulliparous condition." He continued: "Bizarre symptoms suggesting frustration are often noted. Islamic custom permits four wives and the victim may have been rejected for another spouse."[33] Kingston seems to have set the tone for subsequent scientific discussions of the practice. Kathleen Frith, for example, offered the following explanation: "In parts of the Persian Gulf it has been the custom for Arab women to pack the vagina with rock salt during the puerperium to shrink it back to the nulliparous state. The Arab men feel that the parous and relaxed vagina offers less sexual stimulation than the nulliparous vagina."[34] In 1964, Betty Underhill wrote, closely following Kingston: "For hundreds of years it has been the custom of Arab women to pack the vagina with salt for the first week after delivery. This is popularly supposed to restore the vagina to its nulliparous state and to add to the husband's sexual pleasure."[35]

Probably better able to converse with his local patients than were his British colleagues, the Egyptian doctor Kamal Fahmy offered a more nuanced explanation as to why women used salt after childbirth. "The women," he wrote, "use this regimen of salt packing to diminish bleeding after labour, and to act as an antiseptic. Some use it as a contraceptive measure."[36] Indeed, as a contraceptive, the practice may have drawn on Islamic medical tradition. The tenth-century Persian physician ʻAli ibn ʻAbbas Majusi wrote in his well-known medical encyclopedia that "conception will be prevented if women insert rock salt [in the vagina] during coitus, or induce the man to anoint his penis with the same material."[37] Yet Fahmy, echoing the other doctors, also concluded that salt's "main use is to constrict the vagina after labour, thereby preserving sexual pleasure for men. Men may divorce their wives, or marry other women if sexual pleasure is diminished by a patulous vagina resulting from parturition."[38] In short, as far as these doctors could determine, women's reasons for inserting salt into the vagina after birth included the desire to heal the lacerations of childbirth, to avoid infection, to prevent another pregnancy, and to ensure their husbands' sexual pleasure.

Because the general pattern was that only exceptional medical cases made their way to the hospitals, the doctors' accounts capture a mere fragment of the larger story of Arabian childbirth during this period. Nevertheless, because the medical articles are based on the doctors' clinical interactions with women patients in Arabia in the 1950s and 1960s, they offer an invaluable window into how local women and their doctors negotiated childbirth on the cusp of state-driven medical modernization. Two recurring themes through the articles illustrate this dynamic. First, even while suffering serious symptoms, some women proved reluctant to visit the hospital and sometimes were even coerced by state agents. Second, after receiving hospital care, local women's beliefs about the healing process and the meaning of reproductive health influenced how medicine was practiced. Their behavior sometimes baffled or frustrated foreign doctors, who saw themselves as offering vital care, and even forced the hospitals to alter their treatment programs in response to women's choices.

Local women interacted with the foreign doctors in a variety of ways. Although some women arrived at the hospital voluntarily, others were conveyed by force. Describing specific cases that she treated between November 1957 and March 1958 while working in Qatar's state medical service, the British doctor Kathleen Frith noted a variety of responses to her medical work among her patients. Her first case, "Ruma bint S——," was twenty years old and had been "brought unwillingly from her desert village by a visiting medical officer." We are not told exactly what information prompted the medical officer to convey Ruma from her village or which means of force the state medical officer employed. Frith wrote that Ruma had suffered from amenorrhea (the absence of menstruation) for three years, leading to lower abdominal pain. "Her 4 confinements," Frith stated, presumably after obtaining a patient history, "had been followed by the salt treatment and she had no living child." Once at the hospital, Ruma underwent "examination under anaesthesia in the theatre" and was found to have "complete vaginal atresia 1 inch from the vulva and the uterus enlarged to the size of a 20-weeks' pregnancy." An operation released "twenty ounces or more of retained menses."

After the bladder healed from the first operation, Frith planned for a second procedure in which she would place a graft "in the recanalized part of the vagina." But Ruma had other views. According to Frith, "the patient refused a second operation, being convinced that she was cured as she had seen a flow of menstrual blood." Frith also wrote that Ruma "was afraid that her husband would take another wife if she stayed away longer." Ruma left the hospital after just one operation, and the medical officer visited her again two months later only to find that "she had no further loss of blood"; in other words, her symptoms had returned. But at this point "vaginal examination was refused." In the end, for Frith, Ruma's case was "most disheartening as I had hoped that with adequate grafting she would have had her normal menstruation restored."[39] We do not know Ruma's thought process over the course of these events or why exactly she refused the second operation. Frith may have been correct in her belief that Ruma feared what her husband might do if she stayed away longer. Or she may not have understood, or have had it adequately explained to her, that the surgery was a two-part process. Or it may be that the sequence of being forced to attend the hospital, placed under anesthesia, and operated on at the hands of a foreign doctor was simply unbearable, even if she gained some relief of her symptoms.

Frith's next example, "Nadiah bint A——," presented a remarkably different set of behaviors from those of Ruma. Nadiah "came voluntarily to hospital." What prompted her to seek medical care were two months without menstruation followed by "abdominal pain and slight bleeding." Frith wrote that "her second delivery 8 months before and her first 12 years before had been followed by the salt treatment." Dilating her narrowed vagina revealed a small blood clot. Frith operated through lateral incisions in the dilated vagina, and reported that after a "pack of paraflavine gauze was left in for 5 days" Nadiah's vagina was "virtually normal." Unlike Ruma, Nadiah sought out hospital treatment. As with Ruma bint S——, Frith again commented on her beliefs about her patient's sexual life in the context of medically anticipating her future reproductive activities: "this patient had separated from her husband and had no wish for a new one."[40]

The fact that her patients repeatedly refused to follow prescriptive or postoperative recommendations also prompted Frith to adjust her treatment programs in response to local women's actions. When she treated "Ghariba bint F——," suffering from atresia and two years without menstruation as a result of the application of salt in her vagina after childbirth, Frith recalled lessons she had learned from Ruma. She wrote, "From my experience in the first case I felt it unlikely that the patient would stay in hospital for a second operation."[41] Betty M. L. Underhill had a similar experience in Bahrain, where she complained that "the virtual impossibility of following up cases makes it very difficult to assess the efficacy of any treatment. The patients can seldom be persuaded to come to hospital unless they are ill. Attempts to find them in their villages are regarded with great suspicion and they refused examination."[42] In response to her former patients' actions, Frith attempted a different operating strategy. Although Frith believed that Ghariba "should have a good functional result" following treatment, she could not verify those hopes because the patient "returned to her family and could not be traced."[43] We do not know the long-term results for Ghariba's health, but the fact that Frith altered her surgical work in response to patients' behaviors suggests that local women's actions influenced the quotidian procedures of medical professionals.

These case studies also emphasize that the notion of choice is not nuanced enough to explain women's arrivals at the hospitals and the methods and strategies they employed in the pursuit of health. As in the rare instances when local people asked the missionaries for help with childbirth, many women arrived at the hospital out of desperation. Kamal Fahmy explained in reference to his work in Dammam, "In most cases in which there was marked vaginal or cervical fibrosis and atresia or obstruction, the progress of labor was interfered with and there was prolongation of labor with subsequent danger of rupture of the uterus." In other words, the atresia often prolonged the period of labor, pushing women to seek outside assistance. As a result, "Some patients came to the hospital as neglected cases in which the pains had started 12 hours or more. . . . Such cases demanded very urgent intervention which was usually a lower segment cesarean section."[44]

From the perspective of my goal of reconstructing a social history of medicine, a valuable aspect of these mid-twentieth-century medical articles is that they provide us with some clues as to when the custom of packing the vagina with salt came to an end. It seems that the project of large-scale state medicine and the efforts of this cohort of foreign doctors ultimately succeeded in terminating the practice. Underhill wrote that fifty-seven of the sixty-five cases they treated in Bahrain between 1957 and 1963 "were seen between 1957 and 1960, after which numbers rapidly declined and the condition is seldom seen in the younger women." She explained the change: "The practice is being strongly discouraged, and now that facilities for hospital delivery have been greatly increased it is hoped that the barbarous custom will die out. Only 13 patients admitted to having used salt in the past five years."[45] Kamal Fahmy similarly observed in Kuwait in 1965 that "packing of the vagina with rock salt after labour is much less encountered now than some years ago, due to better obstetric service and better understanding of its remote ill-effects. It is now mainly seen in Bedouins, especially in areas where medical care is still lacking."⁴⁶ But despite the measurable achievement in reducing women's pain and reproductive hardships, it seems that many aspects of local health-seeking practices remained beyond the reach of foreign doctors. As Frith observed, "With the new-found oil wealth modern maternity hospitals have been built and all patients encouraged to come in for delivery, but even then rock salt is sometimes found under a patient's pillow, supplied by a thoughtful visitor."⁴⁷

Childbirth in Folk Medicine

Modern biomedicine and professional doctors certainly transformed health care in the Gulf, but it is too simplistic to presume a sudden rupture in local people's health-seeking behaviors between the pre- and post-oil wealth periods. Instead, folk medicine (*al-ṭibb al-shaʿbī*) remained highly pertinent to people's lives. A study of Gulf folk medicine by the Egyptian anthropologist Nabil Subhi Hanna illustrates how, rather than dramatically breaking with existing health cultures, local people creatively interwove multiple medical imaginaries. In the 1980s, Hanna assembled a team of local researchers to investigate Gulf folk medicine. The resulting volume, published in Doha in 1998, was driven by a paradox. Why did people continue to turn to traditional medicine at a time when the welfare state provided modern health services, free of charge? As Hanna posed the puzzle in the introduction: "Folk medicine is a widespread reality among the people. Field studies conducted on the subject have proven the prevalence of folk healers of various types ... and they practice their treatment among the people even in those regions where modern medical services are available."⁴⁸ In bypassing modern medical institutions and turning to traditional healers, Hanna further observed that people drew on a powerful understanding of the material utility of local history. "It also became clear," he wrote, "that people still practice medicine in their homes as treatment for their ailments by following traditional methods they inherited."⁴⁹ Even in the late twentieth century, when large-scale state medical institutions crisscrossed the Gulf and enfolded the welfare state into daily life, local people persistently drew on their medical heritage and sought treatment in their homes.

Flanked by a team of local researchers, Hanna set out to document the enduring world of folk medicine. In 1988, in preparation for fieldwork, Hanna's team listed Qatar's regions, towns, and villages, gathered the names of known traditional healers, and conducted preliminary interviews.[50] Hanna oversaw the compilation of manuals for researchers to use when they interviewed different categories of informants. In describing how they gathered material on women's and children's health, for example, he explained, "a manual has been prepared containing forty-one items related to disease of the mother and the child. Each item deals with a disease or a group of diseases related to a specific system of the body." The manual included further instructions under each item "to help the researcher collect the material efficiently."[51] In addition to the hierarchical workflow, in which local researchers operated under the supervision of Hanna, a professional foreign anthropologist, the labor also was gendered. Qatari women conducted the interviews with female informants and translated terms into the local dialect.[52]

Local conceptualizations of health shaped the book's organization and the selection of informants. Four sections address care of the body and prevention of illness, concepts and traditional methods of folk medicine, the mother and the child, and diving medicine. The team interviewed around fifty informants on women's and children's health, selecting people from different regions of Qatar, both urban dwellers and "those who are still closer to the Bedouin life."[53] The geographical diversity also reflected a range of experiences of the local history of medical development; an Iraqi visitor to Qatar in the 1960s noted that health services in villages lagged behind those in urban areas, such that some villagers complained to him of relatives dying before they could reach a hospital because of the difficulty of communication and transportation.[54] Most of the informants were women. Hanna's team sought out professional midwives (*dayat*) and folk healers who specialized in women's and children's health and childbirth, but they also talked to housewives (*rabbat buyut*), all of whom were "mothers who had given birth and raised children," because they were interested in "everyday folk medicine" in addition to "professional folk medicine." Rather than a clear division between professionals and nonprofessionals, Hanna's team focused on the ages and years of experience of their informants. The women "were chosen from an advanced age group," ranging between forty and seventy-two years of age.[55] Some of them were still working in childbirth and folk medicine at the time of the study, but others had retired due to old age.

As Hanna's emphasis on the informants' advanced ages makes clear, even as folk medicine persisted in practice it depended on the knowledge of the community's elders, those who remembered the old days before modern hospitals and foreign doctors and nurses. Throughout the text, Hanna and the informants signal this temporality through the word *qadīman*, meaning "previously" or "in past times," as a historical milieu and set of cultural experiences that contrast with the informants' understandings of medicalized health in the present. Two examples, one relating to disability and the other to infertility, illustrate this dynamic. One woman informant contrasted the past with the present in terms of the treatment of a person living with disabilities:[56]

> In the past, society used to sympathize with them [*qadīman kāna al-mujtamaʿ yaʿṭif ʿalayhim*], they were treated in a special way, society didn't embarrass them and didn't embarrass their families. And the houses were open to them not closed before them. . . . Now they are expelled from society in isolation in the hospital. In the past [*qadīman*] one of these afflicted people would sit in the majlis normally, observing the behavior of men. . . . He feels as though he is one of the members of society as a result of this kind treatment. But now he feels that he is sick or different from the society as a result of his isolation and the family's and the society's aversion to him.[57]

This woman's comparison between past and present is critical of what she perceives as the current practice of removing people living with disabilities from society and confining them to the modern hospital. But another informant, while also drawing a clear distinction between the two temporalities, recalled the past negatively in relation to the present. In the past, she claimed, the blame of infertility always fell on the woman. She stated that women "were unjustly accused [of infertility] in the past [*qadīman*], because sometimes the fault is from the man. But we believed that he did not get sick when it came to bearing children, and the woman could not say anything to him."[58] This informant suggested that the medicalization of infertility in the present offered more opportunity to place the blame on the man, as opposed to in the past, when women were assumed to be at fault.

As these examples illustrate, the tension between perceptions of health in the past and present structured how informants discussed folk medicine. Woven through Hanna's study is an anxiety that the elders who served as repositories of folk knowledge would soon vanish, leaving the region bereft of a critical source of its heritage. The authenticity of the informants' knowledge largely derived from an (imagined or real) genealogical connection to folk healers of the past. In reference to elderly folk healers who acquired their skills from mothers or fathers, Hanna explained that "the experience of those who have reached the age of eighty contains the experience of their parents and grandparents, which extends back to more than a hundred years."[59] Hanna also believed that his carefully designed research method would lead to factual accuracy: "We deliberately repeated some questions in different parts of the manual in various formats in order to test the validity of the information."[60]

The section of the book on the mother and the child spans more than two hundred pages and is based on the fieldwork conducted by Hanna's women research assistants. Looking back from the present—that is, the late 1980s—the text offers ample space for women to reflect on their experiences with folk medicine. The interviews and quotes are anonymous and organized thematically, so we are left with an impressionistic collective biography of women's perceptions and recollections. Although the interplay between memory and beliefs about the present makes it difficult to pinpoint macro-level change over time in medical practice in this text, four chapters on pregnancy and childbirth allow us to follow the temporal arc of individual women's experiences over the course of critical life events of pregnancy, childbirth, and postpartum challenges.

The discussion of pregnancy begins not with conception, but with a description of the dreaded stigma of infertility. As Marcia Inhorn notes in her study on infertility in Egypt, "Women face the tyranny of social judgement regarding infertility, for they are cast as being less than other women, as depriving their husbands and husbands' families of offspring, and as endangering other people's children through their uncontrollable envy."[61] In 1949, the missionary Ida Paterson Storm suggested that venereal disease was a common cause of infertility in Arabia. She described the benefits of medical work to local people: "Another type of case began to be benefited by us—those women who because of a mild venereal disease that prevails all over Arabia, remain sterile . . . these women consider their barrenness an affliction which causes shame and leads to inevitable divorce."[62] According to 'Ali al-Sayyid Baqir al-'Awwami, syphilis was common in eastern Arabia, but local people did not become aware of the danger of the disease or understand its means of transmission until the oil company started conducting blood examinations for potential employees.[63] Hanna describes infertility as a source of shame, writing, "The word 'sterile' [*aqīm*] is fired at the woman who is deprived of children." This woman might also be stigmatized because "she resembles men who don't give birth." Other women reportedly compared her to "the cow that doesn't produce milk and isn't worth the price when she is sold in the market."[64] As mentioned earlier, before the medicalization of infertility, women shouldered the blame for an absence of children. For a wife to suggest that her husband might be infertile "is considered an insult to him and to his masculinity." According to the women informants, there was only one way for a childless woman to shift the blame to her husband. If the man divorced his wife and then married again and remained childless while his first wife married another man and gave birth, "then they realize that sterility was from the man."[65]

Women's social worlds revolved around the rhythms of childbirth and child rearing, so they experienced infertility as a calamity. People sought to address this problem in a variety of ways. In addition to massages and herbal concoctions, some believed, Hanna tells us, that "a woman giving birth on the feet of a sterile woman, or a woman who has just given birth sitting on the head of a sterile woman, or the cutting of the child's umbilical cord on her leg, all lead to a cure for infertility."[66] In another example, "people prescribe for a barren woman to sit on a hot placenta (that is, a placenta that has just been delivered with the child), and she is without clothes [her skin is against the placenta], and thus her sterility problem will be solved."[67] Such strategies suggest that some people viewed fertility as potentially transmissible through physical contact with a recently fertile woman or the organic evacuation of childbirth.

Women also mentioned strategies for limiting childbirth. Informants associated the first method with "the nature of the woman, as many women do not become pregnant immediately after childbirth," which would allow for some spacing between children. The second method of birth control "related to the nature of economic activity, as the men used to go on pearl diving trips that could extend to four months." Here we gain some insight as to how the rhythm of the region's pearl-diving economy affected women. With men away for months at a time, women were offered a reprieve from their sexual and reproductive labor. Women also reported that they would ask husbands to withdraw before ejaculation.[68] Ending a pregnancy through "violent body movements aimed at removing the fetus," that is, induced abortion (*al-ijhāḍ al-ʿamdī*), was an "abhorrent" act, "and people feel that it is against God's will."[69] Through a story that she apparently hoped would convey a moralizing message, one informant recalled:

> A woman . . . had six children, and when she became pregnant with the seventh she did the impossible in order to end the pregnancy. She was lying on her stomach and told her children to sit or stand on top of her back. She was climbing the ladder and leaping, and carrying heavy things. Praise God, her pregnancy held and she gave birth. But the child was pulled out of her with a machine [*makina*; probably forceps] during childbirth. His head was scratched and he died. Because the ends of the machine squeezed the head. So God left her until she completed her pregnancy then she lost her child. For this is a rebellion against God's grace.[70]

In addition to criticizing attempts to end a pregnancy, this account exemplifies a common pattern in which informants censure certain behaviors by describing the actions of an unnamed third party.

As Hanna's narrative conveys, pregnancy and childbirth involved careful preparations. Women needed to install a pole in the room where they would give birth so that they could hold onto it during labor; "in the case of Bedouins, the tent pole is used for the same purpose."[71] Other required materials included a bundle of sand for the mother to sit on during contractions, a knife to cut the umbilical cord, special herbs, hot water, kohl for the newborn's eyes, clothes for the newborn and rags to clean the blood and secretions from childbirth, and salt.[72] Women also needed to secure access to water and private space. Here the temporality of Hanna's discussion becomes unclear in terms of whether his informants related practices that were in the past or ongoing. For example, in describing the sterilization of tools, he writes: "The water was placed in a small underground tank or in a well in the house. People would extract water from it to meet their needs. Then they wash the tools—like the knife for cutting the umbilical cord and other [tools]—with water and sand. After that the knife and the small tools are boiled in a container over the firewood. Until now, these tools are still sterilized by boiling in water."[73] In the late 1980s women in Qatar would have had easier access to water, but the phrase "until now" suggests that the practice of boiling birthing tools for sanitation persisted. The room for the birth "must be hidden, an interior place where no one can hear her voice."[74] Hanna also mentions the spreading of plastic bags (not widely used until the 1980s[75]) to protect the floor, thus offering another clue that some of these practices endured well after the establishment of state hospitals.

Childbirth represented a climax of women's social life and involved an assortment of women according to their status as respected midwives or their relationship to the mother. In contrast to instances of missionary intervention, when they drew on male authority to access childbirth, men are largely absent in Hanna's discussion.[76] Usually there were at least three other women present for the childbirth, most typically the pregnant woman's mother, her husband's mother, and the midwife, although individual informants provide a sense of variation in the attendees. One mother recalled being aided by her grandmother, a renowned midwife: "The *daya* is my grandmother and she was famous in the 1950s. My grandmother doesn't accept that any other women help her in the [birthing] room. That's why my mother stays outside the room. My grandmother would have me walk about the room until the contractions intensified. Then . . . I sit on a pile of ashes, and I hold her shoulder while I'm sitting."[77] Another mother remembered a childbirth scene with more women in attendance: "The midwife massages me first and puts oil on me. My aunt (my husband's mother) and the midwife prepare me. My husband's mother at my head and the midwife at my legs. The midwife does not let me lie down so I am half lying down to ease the birth."[78]

For some women, the impersonal and alienating state hospital looms in these accounts and serves as a foil to home births, whereas other women integrate hospital births into existing social practices. Hanna reports that one woman went to the hospital to give birth, but she "became frightened and left the hospital and returned to her house," where she successfully delivered her baby without assistance.[79] Another woman recalled the old days wistfully. Even though "our house was simple," she said, and she gave birth in one of her home's two rooms, "our psychological comfort was much greater than it is now, despite everything that is available to the human being."[80] Other historical and anthropological scholarship demonstrates how women carried habits from home births into the hospital. In her 1984 study on women in Qatar, Abeer Abu Saud noted that "in the old days, the expectant mother would go to her parents' house to have the baby . . . nowadays, the hospital provides for such close care and attention, but many mothers still wish to be with their daughters at the moment of childbirth."[81] Describing childbirth in Jeddah in a 1986 article, Mai Ahmad Zaki Yamani observed, "The gathering of visitors at the hospital has become much the same as a formal gathering in the home: the hospital room is transformed into the scene of a formal gathering (*majlis*), where the rules of conduct for a birth are the same as those applicable to other formal occasions."[82] Women thus blended cultures of childbirth to transform medical institutions into more familiar spaces.

In the aftermath of childbirth, families were concerned with the proper disposal of the placenta and the umbilical cord. Some people reportedly believed that if the placenta were thrown out and left for the animals to eat, it might cause harm to the mother. That is why it was "buried underground or thrown into the sea." Hanna also reports that the location where the placenta was buried was thought to carry meaning for the baby's future. The boy's placenta was buried in the mosque or at the threshold of a mosque "so that he becomes attached to the mosque and to prayer and grows up as a religious man," and the girl's placenta was buried in the house or at the threshold of the house so she "becomes a housewife and strengthens her bond with her family." Because the placenta was physically part of the mother, as well as the child, some people also believed that proper disposal was important to prevent its use in "magical practices against the woman."[83]

While the placenta was buried or thrown into the sea, the postpartum mother undertook the business of caring for her baby and physically recovering from the ordeal of childbirth. Hanna's informants commented on the use of salt, but it does not dominate the narrative, possibly because the practice had already been out of vogue for several decades by the time his team conducted interviews in the 1980s. Yet some women remembered salt's pain as well as its sanitizing utility. Hanna recorded: "Salt is considered one of the most important materials that must be used for cleansing after childbirth. Although many women suffer and scream from the effect of salt, it is unavoidable because it is regarded as the strongest of the disinfectants."[84] The use of salt in women's vaginas, Hanna observed, even appeared in "folk humor" (*al-fukāha al-shaʿbiyya*): "It was reported that a large piece of salt was found running towards the sea, returning to it. When they asked the salt, why do you want to return to the sea? He said, 'I can be used to clean and sanitize anything—just not women!'"[85]

Women Navigate Medicalization

Examining childbirth across a range of sources and through the lens of local women's experiences overturns the idea that people in the Gulf and Arabia passively received biomedicine as outside experts shepherded them along a linear path toward development. Instead, the story of the encounter of top-down biomedicine and existing health traditions is one of negotiation between doctors and patients. From the early twentieth century, women proved reluctant to medicalize childbirth, a life event that was saturated with meaning as a focal point of women's social worlds. The boundary between home and hospital remained permeable. Women pursued an assortment of health-seeking strategies even as various medical professionals clamored for control over childbirth. Christian missionaries attempted to supplant local midwives by resorting to male authority. Foreign doctors embedded in state medical projects combined scientific methods and cultural bias to make sense of postpartum vaginal salt packing. Yet even in the 1980s, folk medicine remained relevant to women's lives and provided a way both to critique and to appreciate modern changes.

Focusing on childbirth as a creative process that changed over time allows us to position women at the center of the social historical frame as makers of their own histories, even (or especially) when their menfolk were absent. The next chapter picks up this idea that women, and also men, sought out new institutions and technologies to improve the health and safety of their families. Its status as a colonizing corporation positioned the Arabian American Oil Company (Aramco) to capitalize on local people's health-seeking desires to perform medical experiments in eastern Saudi Arabia.

CHAPTER 4

EXPERIMENTS

FROM THE LATE 1940S, sharply separate and starkly unequal medical care, alongside racial discrimination, inadequate housing, and low wages, inspired popular mobilization in Saudi Arabia's Eastern Province. In November 1953, when the Harvard microbiologist John C. Snyder traveled from Boston to Dhahran to address the Persian Gulf Medical Society's annual gathering, the Arabian American Oil Company (Aramco) was still reeling from a large-scale strike.[1] At the end of the conference, Aramco invited attendees to tour its new Dhahran Health Center. Like the rest of its Jim Crow–inspired facilities, Aramco's medical services were racially segregated.[2] Revealingly, the first hospital, a modern structure, had been in the American senior management camp while separate wooden frame buildings served as the medical facility in the Saudi camp.[3] A tunnel beneath the highway that divided the senior management and Saudi camps connected the facilities. The recent labor action and Aramco's failure to suppress the strike had forced the company to concede improved pay and working conditions for Saudi employees, which included better medical care.[4] The unrest prompted a government commission, and Aramco yielded to some of the workers' demands even as the company collaborated with Saudi authorities to forestall the formation of an organized labor movement.[5]

As Aramco improved health care for its employees, the company simultaneously carried out experimental medical studies. During his 1953 visit,

Snyder learned that Aramco had built a modern laboratory, but the company was still in search of a research project. In a private meeting, Aramco's board chairman Fred Davies asked Snyder, "What would be the optimum use of their new laboratory space?" Snyder suggested that "some of the local health problems should have high priority" and steered the conversation toward the eye disease trachoma, which caused "poor vision especially among local inhabitants serving as employees."[6] Following Snyder's visit to the Dhahran laboratory, in 1954 the Harvard School of Public Health (HSPH) and Aramco signed a contract granting Harvard five hundred thousand dollars for trachoma research over five years. The arrangement entailed "a joint research program financed by Aramco with activities in Dhahran and our laboratories at the HSPH."[7] Aramco later renewed the contract through 1976, and invested upward of two million dollars more in the project.[8]

Aramco's funding for trachoma research reflected an increasingly outdated model among practitioners working in the United States. During the 1950s, medical research and philanthropy in the United States was undergoing a transition during which research foundations began to seek grassroots funding. Jonas Salk's discovery of the polio vaccine in the early 1950s, for example, arose out of the efforts of the National Foundation for Infantile Paralysis, founded in 1937, to popularize fundraising and to seek contributions "from everyone, not just the affluent."[9] In Eastern Province, in contrast, Aramco provided top-down support for medical research, circumventing the need to appeal to a concerned public.

Nevertheless, the Aramco-Harvard collaboration paralleled contemporaneous projects in the United States in other ways. Like their colleagues in the United States, such as those who carried out the infamous Tuskegee syphilis experiments, Aramco-Harvard researchers used nonwhite and disadvantaged populations for medical research and withheld information from them.[10] Aramco's corporate colonialism and company philanthropy bypassed discussing medical research with local people. Instead, the company forged independent relationships with scientists with the conjoined promises of a supply of human subjects from eastern Arabia's local population and funding from Aramco's oil profits.

When the trachoma project started in 1954 the scientific community had not yet isolated trachoma's causative microorganism.[11] As a result, during the initial research phase in Eastern Province, the scientists gathered data by surveying for trachoma prevalence and collecting eye scrapings to send to the laboratories at Dhahran and Harvard. In 1957, the trachoma team benefited from a major breakthrough when the Chinese scientist F. F. Tang detailed the first trachoma isolation.[12] Finally armed with a technique to identify trachoma in eye scrapings, the Harvard team "literally walked across the hall of our Boston laboratory, took [the specimens they had previously collected from children in Eastern Province], did just what the Chinese did, and isolated the trachoma organism."[13]

Once they had managed to identify trachoma in the eye scrapings of Saudi children, the researchers directed their energies toward vaccine development. The team started vaccine trials in Eastern Province in 1962. Their fixation on developing a trachoma vaccine that would eliminate disease with a single shot was consistent with wider discourses of technology and progress embraced by foreign experts and the Saudi state during the period. It was also in line with broader epidemiological thinking of the time, such as the polio vaccination campaigns and the beginning of smallpox eradication efforts. Elinor Nichols, the wife of trachoma project head Dr. Roger Nichols, recalled how the researchers understood the tension between treatment, vaccine development, and the local environment in a 1996 interview:

> They didn't want to treat all these people. I mean, it's easy to treat trachoma: you give them sulfa drugs and they get well. But the reinfection rate if the patient remains in the same situation is 100 percent. All of the Arabs in those days were sleeping on a mat on the floor; they were all sleeping together. A mother wears this aba, and she wipes her eyes and she wipes Fatima's eyes and Mohammed's eyes. They have no running water, no towels, and no soap, washing in a ditch going through the village. So even if you got trachoma and were treated for it, if you go back into the same village, you're going to get it again in six weeks. They had to come up with a vaccine. . . . Roger

and Harvard felt that none of the vaccines could go on the market because they just weren't good enough; so they continued for many, many years to work on a vaccine.[14]

In identifying trachoma as a significant public health challenge during his initial visit in 1953, John C. Snyder had correctly recognized that prevention promised to greatly improve the quality of life for people in the region. But as Elinor Nichols explained, over the course of the trachoma project, researchers used the potential promises of a vaccine and other population-level interventions to justify withholding treatment from individual people and neglecting village sanitation.

From the late 1940s until the end of the trachoma project in 1976, Aramco's health efforts merged the clinic, the laboratory, and the "primitive" village into an expansive medical field. Aramco-funded health efforts targeted ailments that company medical personnel perceived as detrimental to local people's ability to work. Aramco's efforts to saturate Eastern Province's oases with insecticides to combat malaria, as well as the Aramco-Harvard team's absence of communication with local people as to the methods and goals of their trachoma research, bypassed informed collaboration in favor of technological "magic bullets," whether in the form of insecticides or vaccines. The trachoma researchers relied on Aramco's political economy of disparate housing and racialized medical care to conduct their experiments in the shadow of a larger corporate narrative of modernization and development.

Crucially, and in contrast to other large-scale development projects, trachoma research and vaccine testing depended on a politics of health that drew local people to clinics in their search for effective health interventions for themselves and their children. Aramco regularly highlighted its successes in transforming attitudes toward clinical care and vaccination, claiming that enthusiasm for biomedicine was the inevitable result when people experienced health improvements firsthand. A 1951 article reported, for example: "Patients . . . were afraid of the inoculations required by the company to prevent cholera, typhoid, smallpox and other diseases. . . . Today, however, they come to the hospital voluntarily to remind the doctors it is time for a 'booster shot.'"[15] Such narratives elided the fact that, while company benevolence and good intentions among Aramco employees offered many health benefits to local people, improvements to Aramco's services for non-white workers were largely the result of bottom-up organizing and corporate financial calculations.

Disease, Corporate Colonialism, and State Building

After World War II, American technocrats and public health professionals considered public health in Saudi Arabia a blank slate in need of intervention. They sought to advance paternalistic humanitarian concerns, promote the industrial agenda, and accelerate what they imagined to be the inevitable march toward national development. Casting Arabia as an untouched, primitive space, one American official even expressed wonder that indigenous people had survived so long without the advantages of modern medicine and sanitation. He declared, "Saudi Arabia has been a centuries-long testing ground for the survival of the fittest without benefit of medical science."[16]

Public health advances went hand in hand with oil production. Saudi Arabia had granted an oil concession in 1933 to Standard Oil of California. Oil extraction reached commercial quantities in 1938, and during the slowdown of World War II, the Saudi government secured American Lend-Lease funds on the basis of the anticipation of postwar oil profits.[17] In his landmark study, Robert Vitalis has thoroughly debunked the myth of Aramco as a generous provisioner of development aid by demonstrating how the company imported Jim Crow racism and segregation while exploiting Arabian oil.[18] Aramco improved housing, infrastructure, and education for nonwhites, Vitalis shows, only under direct pressure from local labor and political movements. Aramco acted as a colonial power in its modernizing claims and sweeping interventions, all the while extracting oil rents for any development projects. Such modernization schemes resulted in an unequal distribution of wealth and resources across the kingdom.[19] By the 1950s, residents of Eastern Province, and local Shi'a in particular, were voicing their frustration in the local press with the underdevelopment of al-Hasa and Qatif in comparison to the well-funded oil settlements of Dammam, Dhahran, and Khobar.[20]

Aramco's expansion of public health occurred during the final period of 'Abd al-'Aziz Ibn Sa'ud's (1876–1953) efforts to consolidate the Saudi state, followed by the fraught years of his son Sa'ud bin 'Abd al-'Aziz Al Sa'ud's leadership (r. 1953–1964).[21] The Ikhwan, Bedouin who had settled in agricultural areas, emerged as a zealous military force after Wahhabi clerics had targeted them for proselytizing around 1912. Ibn Sa'ud had conquered the agriculturally rich eastern oases of al-Hasa and Qatif in 1913 and, after another two decades of fighting, declared in 1932 that the Kingdom of Saudi Arabia was a unified political body.[22] Ibn Sa'ud integrated health interventions into his projects of conquest and consolidation. When many of Ibn Sa'ud's troops were struck with fever as they camped twenty miles west of Kuwait in May 1914, for example, he requested that Shaykh Mubarak of Kuwait send mission doctor Stanley Mylrea, who diagnosed the troops with malaria, which they likely had contracted while on campaign in al-Hasa.[23] After treating the sick men with quinine tablets, Mylrea visited Ibn Sa'ud in his tent, where they debated "the relative merits of modern and ancient medicine."[24] Four years later, in 1918, Ibn Sa'ud again sought missionary medical services when he summoned Dr. Paul Harrison to travel from Bahrain to Riyadh in the midst of the global influenza pandemic that proved devastating to Arabia's populations.[25] In 1925, Ibn Sa'ud established a Saudi Public Health Authority based in Mecca.[26] As for the Eastern Province, the state sent an Indian doctor and pharmacist to Qatif in 1935. There was no hospital or clinic, so they attended to their patients in rooms on the roof of the old seaside Ottoman fort.[27]

Saudis also started to travel abroad for medical training during Ibn Sa'ud's long reign. By his own account, Yusuf Ya'qub al-Hajiri was the first Saudi Arab professional doctor. Demonstrating the extent of the company's surveillance of rising Saudi professionals, an Aramco report described him as "short, stocky, and wears glasses," and also remarked that he was "cordial, quiet, and soft spoken." Born in Thadiq in Najd, Al-Hajiri studied English in Karachi in 1927–1928. He then traveled to Cairo to pursue medicine in 1929, receiving his MD in 1941. He interned in Egypt for two years and then toured tuberculosis sanatoriums in Europe. An early employee of the Saudi Department of Health, he reportedly resigned because of frustration that foreign doctors were "pushing Saudi doctors around." Al-Hajiri eventually returned to national service to direct the maternity hospital in Jeddah and then the Jeddah Quarantine Isolation Section. In 1961, he received a fellowship from the World Health Organization to study tuberculosis center administration. Al-Hajiri became the minister of health in 1962.[28] Such an illustrious medical career, however, remained an exceptional case in Saudi state medicine. A 1983 study of health services in Mecca, for example, found that at King ʿAbd al-ʿAziz hospital, out of 197 doctors, only 9 were Saudi citizens, and only 21 out of 368 nurses were.[29]

As oil production accelerated after World War II, Aramco's medical team determined that diseases endemic to the oases surrounding eastern Saudi Arabia's vast oil resources threatened the supply of a healthy workforce.[30] Aramco sought to develop public health policies that would render local populations healthy enough for current and future employment. A 1956 article by two members of Aramco's health staff, Richard Daggy and R. C. Page, mapped out the company's investment in preventive medicine in Eastern Province, articulating a bluntly capitalist understanding of sickness as "inability to go to work."[31] "There should be no question," they wrote, "of the valuable returns to industry from an expanded program of preventive medicine and public health, especially in the Middle East . . . where a high incidence of *preventable* disease is a most important factor in labor costs."[32] For Daggy and Page, calculations of profit were intertwined with humanitarian impulses. They hoped for Aramco's health program to "make itself felt throughout the employee family group—and through them—to the general population of the Eastern Province of Saudi Arabia. If we can succeed in this effort, we shall feel we will have made a lasting contribution to improved health in Saudi Arabia. This is our ultimate goal."[33]

Aramco's doctors identified malaria and trachoma as two of the most devastating diseases in Eastern Province. Malaria, which manifests as intermittent and debilitating fevers, is caused by parasites that are transmitted to humans through the bites of infected *Anopheles* mosquitoes.[34] Near Arabia's Gulf coast, endemic malaria was a fact of life in oasis villages where underground aquifers provided ample water and runoff from date cultivation created ideal breeding grounds for the *Anopheles stephensi* mosquitoes that transmitted the malaria parasite.[35] These mosquitoes found blood meals in the densely clustered populations in the oases towns. The threat of malaria rapidly diminished beyond the oases and into the desert, where stagnant water and associated mosquito breeding grounds were nonexistent.

After establishing itself in Eastern Province in the 1930s, Aramco sought to control malaria in order to bolster the local workforce. The company constructed housing for American workers outside of the disease area, but the scourge plagued local labor recruits, even more so after 1945, when the Saudi government drove date prices down to make food more affordable, prompting many farmers to seek waged work with Aramco.[36] In 1946 Aramco rejected 31 percent of local job applicants. The fact that 95 percent of the rejections were due to medical reasons underscores the entangled concerns of disease and labor.[37] Between 1941 and 1947, forty-three people died of malaria in Aramco's hospitals, and in 1942 and 1943, malaria was the single highest cause of death.[38] Controlling malaria also was important to facilitate Aramco's plans to increase expatriate labor. Forecasting the national origins of future Aramco workers, Daggy explained that Aramco "attracts large numbers of prospective employees from all parts of the Kingdom, as well as from other malarious areas in India, Pakistan, Trucial Oman, Muscat, Yemen, Syria, Lebanon, Somalia, Sudan, and others."[39] This comment assumes heightened significance in light of the fact that local Saudi Aramco employees decreased from 21,858 in 1954 to 11,682 in 1959.[40] After conducting malaria surveys, Aramco's health team decided to confront the disease by spraying insecticides in oasis villages. The postwar flurry of oil exploitation coincided with a global push to eliminate malaria using insecticides like DDT, which "seemed like a miracle" until mosquitoes started to develop resistance in response to mass spraying.[41] Qatif received its first oasiswide DDT treatment in 1948, and al-Hasa in 1949.[42] Picking up Aramco's efforts, the Saudi Ministry of Health and the World Health Organization took over the malaria control program in 1956.[43]

Symptoms of trachoma, an infectious eye disease caused by the bacterium *Chlamydia trachomatis*, include discomfort around the eyes, discharges of mucus or pus, and swelling of the eyelids. Cornelia Dalenberg, an American missionary nurse in Bahrain, described how "some sufferers would come to us with pus running down their cheeks. After the problem went untreated for many months, the inside membranes of the eyelid would begin to shrink, causing the eyelashes to be pulled inward, against the eye itself. This led to the wearing away of the cornea, great pain, and eventual blindness."[44] Among communities where trachoma is endemic, infection rates are most prevalent among young children. Reacquisition is common, and visual impairment usually occurs between the ages of thirty and forty.

Trachoma is transmitted through close personal contact and by flies that spread discharge from the eyes or nose of an infected person.[45] Dalenberg described the surgical procedure the missionaries used to relieve some of the pain for patients suffering from advanced cases, a skill she first acquired by practicing on the eyes of sheep heads that the missionaries purchased from the local slaughterhouse. She wrote: "It consisted of cutting a wedge-shaped snippet of skin from the outside of the eyelid, then sewing the edges back together with four or five stitches. This pulled the eyelashes up and out to their normal position." The procedure relieved trachoma patients of "the miserable rubbing of lashes against the eye."[46] Today, curative options include surgery to treat blindness and antibiotics to clear infections. It is generally acknowledged that eliminating trachoma depends on access to clean water, as washing hands and faces with soap and water reduces the spread by removing discharge from eyes and noses.[47]

Eye diseases were pervasive across Arabia, and blindness or partial blindness was common.[48] "Many Arabs had only one eye," Charles Belgrave recalled in reference to the prevalence of trachoma in interwar Bahrain. "Four brothers, who were important merchants, had five eyes between them."[49] In Eastern Province, the local word for trachoma's syndrome was *al-ramad*, referring to pain and swelling in the eyes; later, *al-tarākhūmā* appeared as a vernacularized medical term. One local man recalled putting *al-qirmiz*, a red dye, on itchy bumps in the eyes caused by trachoma.[50] During her 1960 fieldwork in a village in Bahrain, where many Eastern Province Shi'a had relatives, the anthropologist Henny Harold Hansen observed how "the mothers smeared [kohl] along the edge of the children's eyelids to protect the eyes, without, however, waving away the dark swarm of dirty flies which constantly crawled around on the babies' faces." The result of not receiving proper treatment, Hansen explained, "would be a dead, pearl-white, blind eye." Among the villagers she met in Bahrain, "Some people were blind in both eyes, others had one good eye whereas the other shone blind and white."[51] 'Ali al-Sayyid Baqir al-'Awwami also recalled the prevalence of eye disease, along with other ailments, in his autobiographical account of popular movements in Saudi Arabia. For al-'Awwami, poor health was a symptom of neglect. "The general health status of the population—before the appearance of oil," he wrote, "was only a natural result of the general underdevelopment of the region."[52] Eye diseases like trachoma were widespread, and malaria was so common that "seldom was anyone safe from it."[53] Al-'Awwami even references a local poem that assumed the persona of Qatif (*Qatif* comes from a root that means "to harvest") to juxtapose the region's rich agricultural resources with the prevalence of disease. Speaking as Qatif in first person, the poem suggests that no one should expect to depart the region without becoming sick:

> I am al-Qatif, they harvested me
> When a stranger comes, they tell me
> And if he leaves in good health, they blame me.[54]

After World War II, the Saudi Ministry of Health and US development projects expanded public health efforts from Aramco's eastern focus to the rest of the country. In the words of one American, "The east coast oil industry's experience illustrates the difficulty of building up a work force if the local people are unhealthy."[55] In this vision of development, oil wealth offered a direct path to population-level salvation through modern public health and medicine. The endemic prevalence of disease justified ground-level medical excursions into local villages. Such large-scale public health initiatives would lay the groundwork for local people's participation in the trachoma experiments. After witnessing the many material benefits of public health and medical interventions, the residents of Eastern Province were primed to believe that Aramco was offering effective vaccines to their children.

Hierarchical Medical Interventions

While public health workers fanned out across villages to take blood, measure spleens, and spray insecticides, structural inequalities prompted Aramco doctors to perform risky medical procedures on local people even when the doctors lacked necessary qualifications and equipment. The idea that Aramco offered doctors a "medical frontier" was of great appeal for some recruits.[56] Inside Aramco's clinics, hospitals, and operating rooms, doctors pushed the limits of their expertise. Aramco materialized medical difference between white and local employees through their policies of sending Americans to the United States for specialized hospital care. Treatment options for local employees were limited to what was available in Saudi Arabia. From the perspective of Aramco's physicians, the policy made it necessary to perform risky procedures on local patients whom they deemed to have no better recourse. This pattern of high-risk medical interventions also appealed to some Aramco doctors' sense of adventure and medical bravado. But as we will see, an Aramco surgeon's encounter with a local court in the wake of an operating room tragedy would test the limits of Aramco's medical impunity and reveal an undercurrent of frustration with the company's discriminatory medical policies.

The medical provisions Aramco offered to different categories of patients institutionalized racialized inequities between white and local Arab bodies. A gap between the level of medical services available to expatriates and locals developed through differential regulations regarding which patients were sent abroad due to medical need and which patients had to make do with Aramco's on-site services. "We had a rule," the former Aramco surgeon and medical director Julius W. Taylor explained, "that any employee—other than the Saudis—could be returned to his country of origin for medical care if it was necessary." As a result of this arrangement, any American whose medical needs were "too complex" for Aramco's doctors would be sent back to the United States. For example, an American employee with multiple sclerosis would arrange to visit the New York Neurological Center "in connection with a vacation"; when he returned to Eastern Province, the

New York specialists "would send back a whole program for this employee, which we could follow."⁵⁷ In caring for Americans, Aramco doctors adhered to a sharp delineation between the limits of their qualifications and what specialists in the United States could offer.

This correlation between citizenship and level of medical care, in which patients were entitled to the highest level of medicine offered by their state's health system, disadvantaged local patients. But by calibrating level of care with nationality, Aramco minimized company medical costs. "Arabs," Taylor stated, "had to make do with what we could provide. Neither Aramco nor the government would send them out of the country, as this was <u>their</u> country." As a result, Aramco doctors "were doing procedures that were a little beyond what we were set up to do." Taylor's recollection of performing Aramco's first open heart surgery illustrates how they calculated risk when it came to local patients. He represented the surgery as a necessary intervention, despite his lack of qualifications. Taylor explained, "I decided that since there were some serious heart cases around and these patients had serious trouble and were going to die if they didn't have something done, we would see how that went." Taylor admitted that they faced significant constraints leading up to the procedure, including shortages of blood, technical support, appropriate anesthesia, and equipment. The surgery "went okay," he claimed, "but it was a major challenge." Eventually, because of the challenges, "we decided against major heart and vascular surgery."⁵⁸ Taylor also performed the first lung removal for a patient with tuberculosis.

For Taylor, the possibilities offered by the lack of regulation in Eastern Province were something of a professional opportunity. Taylor declared, "I had the right personality for Arabia: I'm adventuresome; I like excitement; I like to do things."⁵⁹ One of the "things" that most appealed to Taylor was performing medical procedures on local patients that were often beyond the scope of his expertise; indeed, the lack of accountability was itself a major attraction. Rather than acknowledging that the local population had little recourse to challenge Aramco's medical authority, Taylor asserted, "Another thing about the Arabs, which in a sense is good: they're very fatalistic." To illustrate this fatalism, he recalled Aramco's hospital corridors in the aftermath of deadly automobile accidents:

> One thing that always used to amaze me: when they had these big wrecks . . . their relatives would come in, and the dead bodies would be laid in the back hall. They'd go down the line until they found their relative, wrap them up in a white cloth and take them away. There was never anything like "Well, what happened here?" or "Whose fault was this?" or "What did you guys do for him?" There was never anything like that; it was amazing. We'd lay them [the dead bodies] over there, and out they'd go. They'd put them over their shoulder, one or two of them would carry the body out and put it in a vehicle of some kind. Gone.[60]

Further emphasizing the exceptional privilege of Aramco's doctors, Taylor contrasted the lack of "medical legal problems" with "a doctor's existence back here [in the United States]," where a subpoena guarantees doctors "a long, drawn-out, miserable affair." Taylor explained: "There was none of that there. That was one of the attractions about being there."[61]

The doctors' assumption that they would be exempt from consequences for risky procedures was challenged when an Aramco surgeon had to appear before a local judge after the death of an employee's son on the operating table. The boy had a brain tumor, and as a dependent, he was entitled to Aramco health care. "None of us were neurosurgeons," Taylor said, but they decided to operate anyway because "that was in the days when Saudis couldn't go anywhere; we had to handle it." Despite their lack of qualifications to perform the procedure, the doctors tried to save the boy's life under circumstances in which they saw no other alternative. The doctors performed "a cerebral angiogram, a blood vessel picture of his brain."[62] Following the angiogram, the boy died.

In the aftermath of the boy's death, a local judge summoned the operating doctor, Michael Juraj, "who was a crack surgeon," to his court.[63] Michael Juraj was probably an Arab expatriate surgeon, one of a large body of medical professionals Aramco recruited predominantly from India and the Arab world to care for nonwhite employees. These nonwhite doctors were paid lower salaries, allowing Aramco to curb costs while providing health care to local employees. As Taylor explained, "In the interval before the government really got their system going, they were a great fill-in, to fill in that gap."[64]

But how did an Aramco surgeon—even an Arab—find himself before a local judge, given Aramco's fiercely guarded status as a corporate colonial enclave? Another account of an Aramco employee who entered the local court system after killing a blind and elderly local man by hitting him with his car offers some revealing perspective. In such situations, Taylor explained, Aramco could either immediately deport the culprit "so that the employee did not get into the Arab judicial system" or "take his chances with the local court."[65] As for the employee who killed the elderly man, his reason for entering the local system rather than fleeing the country was financial. To receive full retirement benefits, Aramco employees had to work for twenty-five years. At the time of the car accident, this employee had clocked eighteen years with Aramco. Even though he expected to be exonerated by the local court, he ended up in prison.

Local judges' willingness to hold Aramco employees accountable despite the pattern of corporate colonial impunity is also evident in the case of the boy who died on the operating table. When Michael Juraj was preparing for court, Aramco reassured him: "Not to worry. We're right behind you." Juraj, apparently confident in Aramco's support, "was taking it all sort of matter of factly, until he suddenly realized that if they decided that he did something wrong, it could be a serious problem." The shift from Aramco's protection to the local court's oversight was a potential source of danger for the physicians, as "once you get in their court and are playing by their rules, if you turned up on the short end of a judgement, you might be subject to their very dangerous sentences." In the end, according to Taylor, they were able to convince the judge that "everybody was trying to do their best," so the judge released Juraj. But the judge issued a stern warning: "In the future, if any doctors like you, Dr. Juraj, are doing things that you're not fully trained to do, there's going to be a bad problem."[66]

This tense court encounter and the Arab expatriate doctor's narrow escape from local prison significantly dampened Aramco doctors' willingness to perform medical interventions beyond the scope of their training. "Those things we had been doing," Taylor said, "which were a little on the margin . . . we quit doing them. That's all. Nobody was going to do them and run a risk like that." Even though the boy died at the hands of a surgeon who was underqualified for the procedure, Taylor insisted that "Juraj was trying to do the best thing for this boy. He was trying to help him if he could."[67] When Taylor looked back on Aramco's medical work in Eastern Province, he maintained that "there was not a real double standard, except for the evacuation part, which was something that was policy." Rather than acknowledging Aramco's unequal medical care between local and expatriate employees, Taylor displaced responsibility onto the Saudi state: "The Saudi government should have approved medical evacuation of Saudis."[68] What is missing from Taylor's account is an understanding of how systemic medical inequality between local and American patients also facilitated this ethos of misguided intervention. While American employees were sent away to state-of-the-art facilities at company expense, local workers and their dependents had to settle for subpar treatment at the hands of underqualified doctors.

Aramco physicians relied on the lack of specialized care to rationalize carrying out procedures on local employees and dependents they were not qualified to perform. Many of the medical activities reflected standard practice of the time. The principle of informed consent was not legally binding in the United States until 1957. It was not until 1972 that public outcry against the Tuskegee experiments began and a series of US court decisions solidified the legal doctrine of informed consent, elevating ethical concerns in discussions of medical research.[69] The extent of Aramco's impunity becomes clear in the provision that foreign employees who were responsible for a local person's death had the option quickly to leave the country. The judge's warning to Juraj, however, suggests that local people did seek to hold Aramco's physicians accountable for the quality of their care—and the deadly outcomes of their mistakes.

Clinical Misogyny

In targeting women for health interventions, Aramco's medical staff intertwined childcare training with the process of categorizing women as dependents of male workers, thus pinning women in a misogynistic and racist frame as nameless and faceless wives and mothers. A *Los Angeles Times* journalist's 1951 description of a visit to Dhahran Hospital captures Aramco's paternalistic exasperation with local women who were reluctant to adhere to their modernizing medical guidelines: "Aramco still has some trouble convincing women to come to the hospital for their babies. Saudi Arab women, who shroud themselves in black veils and stay as far as possible from the American strangers, seldom check in until it is all but too late. Of the three women in the maternity ward, at the time of this correspondent's visit, one had lost her baby after a Caesarean operation, while a second had been delivered of a child who was totally blind. An earlier visit to the hospital might have resulted in healthy children in both cases."[70] Chad R. Parker has noted that Aramco's physicians perceived women's veils as "an unnecessary cultural obstacle to proper medical care."[71] They also struggled to differentiate among women. For example, Bob Oertley, a family physician who joined Aramco in 1963, was concerned with the question of how Aramco's medical records could keep track of employees' dependents. The fact that local employees might have more than one wife fascinated the doctors.[72] The reality that, according to their own calculations, a situation in which a local employee claimed multiple wives as dependents was actually uncommon, does not seem to have dampened their conviction. Oertley explained that employees "could of course have four wives," so the records listed women according to their relation to the employee as "Wife Number One or Two or Three or Four."[73]

A wave of initiatives targeted women and children for care and sought to train women to be better mothers to future workers. In 1958 Aramco opened Al-Khobar Pediatric and Maternity Hospital. The company started a maternal child health program and an immunization program for dependent children in 1960. The program included diphtheria-pertussis-tetanus (DPT) vaccine, oral polio vaccine, smallpox vaccine, BCG vaccine for tuberculosis, typhoid vaccine, live measles vaccine, and cholera and typhus immunization. They performed routine skin tests and chest X-rays to monitor for tuberculosis among dependents, as well as employees. Local people made use of the new services. In 1965, for example, Aramco received more than 460,000 clinic visits.[74]

Oertley conveyed a "funny story" that offers a snapshot of interactions with women in the clinics as "Saudis began to be birth control conscious."[75] During a local woman's visit to an Aramco clinic to be fitted for a diaphragm, the gynecologist was suddenly called away. The patient was left in the exam room. "You know," Oertley mused, setting the scene, "what an ugly instrument the vaginal speculum is . . . this alligator jaw thing, which holds the walls of the vagina open." While the woman was waiting, a nurse came by. Upon learning that the doctor had already seen the patient, the nurse "didn't bother to check," and the woman "was told to dress and that she could go."

The woman left, but the vaginal speculum was still in place. That night, when "her husband brought her back to the clinic," Oertley recalled, "he was irate." Oertley's oral history transcript captures his performance in telling the "funny story": "Literally in a rage, [the husband] said, 'I don't care how effective this instrument of the devil is, but get it out! By all means, get that thing out of there!' And the thing was, with the vaginal speculum, once you screw this little thing open, it stays open. You can't pull it out. He didn't know where to release it. Of course, she's waddling all the way like this when she's coming in! [Laughter]." "I didn't see it," Oertley admitted, "but the story spread through the whole medical group the next day. All four stations knew about it, and everybody was chagrined but laughing."[76] From the perspective of Aramco's physicians, this woman's painful misfortune was humorous collateral damage in Aramco's overarching achievement of measurable improvements in health.

As part of the company's efforts to cut costs and save lives, Aramco's medical leadership sought to shift their resources from clinical to preventive medicine. As Aramco medical officials conceptualized it, preventive medicine depended on first, maximizing the financial efficiency of their medical staff so that patients had more face time with lower-paid, predominantly nonwhite and female, medical professionals, and second, on convincing local people—especially women—as to the benefits of certain behaviors, such as vaccination. Aramco's medical leadership determined that the way to improve the overall health of the population was to educate "the women who are the guardians of the next generation."[77] As Richard Handschin, who worked as chief of preventive medicine (1959–1964) and then medical director (1964–1968), explained, "Literate mothers are really a key to having good health—mothers who establish the family living patterns and mold those—'wash your hands before you come to the table'—all these principles of good health and disease control."[78]

In the oral histories, the former Aramco doctors deploy an arsenal of statistics to argue that, overall, their impact had been indisputably positive. To this end, the clinics' doctors and nurses—that is, the medical professionals who interacted directly with patients actively seeking care—also emphasized preventive health. As proof of their success, Handschin noted that "between 1961 and 1965, the clinic visits per hundred wives or children went up 24 percent. . . . But hospital days per hundred outpatient visits went down by 24 percent."[79] Through the use of comparative figures, Handschin argued that Aramco's activities were responsible for the progressive disappearance of endemic diseases and the universal improvement of health. In 1947, he recounted, there were a total of thirty thousand visits to Aramco's health clinics on account of malaria, but in 1963, there were fewer than a dozen cases among Aramco employees.[80] Between 1960 and 1967, no employees died from tuberculosis, pneumonia, malaria, smallpox, infectious hepatitis, typhoid, "or any viruses." This was in contrast to the fact that, "in the 1940–1950 period, all of these were prominent causes of death."[81] Handschin elaborated: "Comparing 1960–1967 with the 1940–49 period, there was a 98 percent reduction in the communicable disease deaths."[82] In 1952, there were only three non-Aramco physicians in Eastern Province; in 1967, there were ninety-two physicians employed by the Saudi government.[83] In 1957, 40 percent of infants hospitalized in Aramco facilities died within twenty-four hours; in 1967, it was fewer than 10 percent. Between 1962 and 1967, "we saw the deaths among dependent children due to pneumonia, diarrhea, and malnutrition decreased by two thirds. . . . Deaths among children decreased by two thirds."[84] Similarly to the "weapon of statistics" that Mahmood Mamdani analyzes in his examination of a population control study in an Indian village conducted from 1954 to 1960, such figures "built a wall of optimism" and obscured any failures.[85]

For Handschin, Aramco's embrace of population-level preventive medicine that combined cost-efficient clinical treatment, behavioral changes, and environmental interventions explained these statistically measurable transformations. Handschin praised the decision that preventive health experts would work behind the clinical scenes as "staff advisors to line operators." Handschin believed that the preventive health staff "should do the studying, the planning . . . but they should not directly operate most of the preventive programs that were related to clinical care." Implementing preventive plans would be the "curative doctors and nurses" who "were made responsible for the preventive programs in their own clinics." Further decentralizing expertise for the sake of cost efficiency, the system "emphasized using the lowest level of skill which can completely do the job."[86]

This stress on the "lowest level of skill" also reinforced a starkly gendered and racialized labor hierarchy inside the clinic. Doctors worked in a "screening modality" with "several nurses at their elbows." This arrangement allowed the generally white and male (and higher-paid) doctors to cover "maybe a hundred patients in eight hours." Following his rapid examination, the doctor had only to say, "Nurse, do this for the patient."[87] Moreover, nurses involved in health screening were "predominantly Middle Eastern female nurses, Indians doing the more clinical, the more routine aspects of care. But most of these people active in the actual on-the-job training were Palestinian, Jordanian, some Egyptian."[88] Handschin explained how management liked this dependency on nonwhite women nurses because "the nurses that we were hiring cost from one-fifth to one-tenth what physicians cost."[89]

As well as sites of gendered and racialized labor hierarchies, Aramco's dependent clinics emerged as training grounds for local mothers. When women visited Aramco's clinic to seek medical care, they also received hours of additional instruction in child rearing. Over the course of maternal and child health efforts, medical staff lectured mothers on conception, pregnancy, delivery, and childcare; instructed mothers to alter their breastfeeding habits; discussed nutrition and sources of food; and placed infants on a standardized immunization schedule. Handschin's description of the clinic as a space for coaching Saudi mothers offers a window into how women would have experienced Aramco's parenting interventions:

> We developed some day-care units in the clinic, right adjacent to where the curative medicine was being practiced. The mother could be sent by the doctor or nurse to stay in that unit for eight hours to receive education that seemed appropriate for her particular problem. For instance, the mothers would prepare the food for the child there, and they would feed the child under the tutelage of the nurse. And not only once, but repetitively, so that in an eight-hour time period, they would feed the child maybe three or four times. Each time, the activity would be critiqued. A lot of this was group instruction. There'd be ten or twelve or fifteen mothers there in that particular room, and there'd be an interaction in that group—maybe not with neighbors, but with people they could talk quite freely to because they were the same clans.[90]

Aramco health workers also sought to draw women dependents from their villages into Aramco's hospitals to give birth, receive immunizations, and internalize health-seeking behaviors. By 1960, the dependent clinic instituted "a mass immunization program for the children that usually used to come with their parents" that offered BCG, polio, and DPT immunization.[91] Arab and local labor also played a crucial role in this process of communicating to women the purpose of immunization and other preventive health measures. "Predominantly Jordanian and Lebanese" health staff visited public schools with educational movies and pamphlets.[92] In addition to Aramco's expatriate Arab health professionals, "English-speaking Saudi girls," the daughters of Saudi senior staff, "assisted us with visits to homes, talking with parents in particular."[93] According to Handschin, the ultimate purpose of these efforts was "to really develop a willingness among Saudis to both accept and then to maintain health care . . . to understand that health care also involved washing your hands and a variety of lifestyle changes, and try to get them to maintain the things they learned."[94]

As suggested by Oertley's story of negligence during the woman's diaphragm fitting, there is evidence that when it came to accessing birth control, local women actively sought to transcend the limited vision of Aramco doctors who saw them as a faceless mass of wives and mothers. Related to the tantalizing possibility of multiple wives and the adjacent assumption that Saudis took "pride in having a retinue" of children, Oertley claimed that a major change he witnessed was that "Saudis began to be birth control conscious. They sort of recognized that they could never be as wealthy as they'd like to be if they kept on having kids."[95] When local women "found out about" the use of the birth control pill among Americans, "the Arab women who came to these [health education] classes said, 'we want to take the pill.'" But according to Taylor, the "local Qadhi, who were the religious leaders" objected when they found out that women were obtaining the birth control pill from Aramco clinics. Siding with the male religious authorities rather than their women patients, Aramco stopped distributing the pill. In response, "these women raised so much trouble . . . that the religious leaders reversed themselves and allowed the women to have the pill. . . . The only reason they yielded was because the women were so unified in their attitude and demanding the pill."[96]

Aramco approached women's health as an opportunity to transform practices of mothering in ways that would both save the company money through preventive medicine and carry out humanitarian interventions. But when women sought control over their health care by demanding that the company provide them with the same contraceptive options it offered to American women, Aramco's doctors sided with local male religious authorities against the desires of their patients. In insisting on the same access to the birth control pill that they observed among white Americans, local women demanded a role in medical decision-making.

Aramco's practices of village-level epidemiology, medical risk-taking in response to structural inequalities, and clinical misogyny would converge in the trachoma project.

The Trachoma Project

Trachoma research was a transnational enterprise.[97] The movement of bacteria and science in the wake of Tang's 1957 breakthrough paper on trachoma isolation illustrates these dynamics. A British scientist visited "the

Communist Chinese research laboratories" in 1957 to obtain Tang's isolations, and then carried them to London's Lister Institute. Meanwhile, in Saudi Arabia, the Harvard team was struggling to differentiate trachoma from other eye infections. A description of the research process applied to one baby illustrates their methods. In July 1957, in a village near Hofuf, medical researchers examined an eighteen-month-old girl and diagnosed her with trachoma. Then they took a scraping from her eye "for microscopic examination," but in the Dhahran laboratory they were unable to differentiate between the "numerous inclusions."[98] They transferred what was left of the girl's eye scrapings after the initial examination to a small screw-cap vial frozen at sixty degrees below zero Celsius to Boston, where it sat in the freezer for several months alongside other eye scrapings from Saudi patients. Finally, in 1958, as the London laboratory was confirming Tang's virus identification methods, the Harvard-Aramco team removed the girl's sample from the freezers and applied the new isolation technique. Using Tang's method, they identified trachoma from the girl's eye, naming it SA-1, the Hofuf strain. Sadly, Tang did not live long enough to see the global impact of his breakthrough. According to Elinor Nichols, after publishing his paper, he was "picked up by the Communists and put on a work gang and died out there" in 1958.[99]

In Saudi Arabia, the trachoma team designed their research around local women and children who visited Aramco's health facilities. During the village visits, women lined up with their children to attend the trachoma clinics. Their participation suggests that women viewed the clinics as beneficial to their children, having come to associate medical care with improved health. Moreover, it was Aramco's sprawling local presence that granted the trachoma team access to their research subjects. J. Rives Childs, the first US ambassador to Saudi Arabia (1946–1950), conceptualized Aramco as an octopus, with tentacles extending "into almost every domain and phase of the economic life in Saudi Arabia."[100] On the other end of the political spectrum, a 1972 publication by the leftist Arab Support Committee described Aramco as "a state within a state that intervened in nearly every issue having to do with the lives of the people."[101] Trachoma researchers relied on the company's expansive reach to collect data in both clinics and villages. As Dorothy McComb recalled, "We really got a great deal of support from all levels of Aramco." The Government Relations Department, in which the company combined diplomacy and intelligence, was "critical in setting up working relations in the villages."[102] Aramco's medical director allowed them to undertake "visits to the Aramco women's clinic for the Saudi women and children."[103]

Scientific publications provide further evidence of the merging of clinical work and trachoma research, as well as some clues as to what patients might have believed was occurring. A 1960 article that used data from both Saudi Arabia and Egypt described the work in Eastern Province: "The clinical and epidemiological studies were conducted principally among residents of Al Hasa and Qatif, two large oases of eastern Saudi Arabia. In a few instances material was obtained from patients attending eye clinics, either at the Dhahran Health Center, or in the villages."[104] The specimens were from children between four months and seven years old. Twenty of the thirty-nine Saudi children whose conjunctival scrapings they used were "brought to a clinic because of their parents' concern over their eyes."[105] We can infer that concerned parents carried small children to Aramco's clinics, and over the course of their visit they donated eye scrapings to the Harvard team. Moreover, the trachoma researchers appear to have drawn samples from state clinics in addition to Aramco's facilities. A 1963 article referenced taking scrapings from patients attending a government clinic on account of "a variety of complaints, a minority of which were due to eye disease."[106]

Through visits to clinics the trachoma team recruited research subjects already seeking medical care. Village work took the form of population-level surveys and depended on women's cooperation. Researchers posited a gendered explanation of trachoma transmission within the family, an epidemiological framework that persists today.[107] A main driver of cyclical trachoma infection and reinfection, McComb explained, was that "when the mothers would see the children with discharge from their eyes they would just wipe the eyes with their abba or outer garment. So the transfer almost certainly was done a lot by just clothing, from one child to another."[108] McComb further observed, "For those who had experienced [cycles of active disease] over a period of thirty years, many of them had a clouded cornea, and often they would be totally blind in that eye. It was a disease process that was set in motion early in life. When analysis of the data began we found that most of the children were infected by the time they were three months old."[109]

Before Tang's 1957 paper allowed them to isolate trachoma in their collection of Saudi eye scrapings, the trachoma team spent several years surveying local trachoma prevalence and working to find a path to accurate diagnosis. The challenge up until that point was that "under ordinary village conditions," a baby often was infected simultaneously with many agents "during the first few months of life."[110] For researchers in the early to mid-1950s, this inability to distinguish trachoma from other viruses justified a study in which "five blind children were experimentally infected" with trachoma and other viruses to compare the clinical and laboratory results.[111] The "infection was accomplished" by dropping "bacteriologically sterile lines" of fluid "into the conjunctival sac of each eye" and finishing with "gentle rubbing" of the eye using a sterile cotton swab.[112]

But after 1958, once they had a methodology to identify trachoma under the microscope, the team could devote itself to developing a vaccine. Indeed, manufacturing a trachoma vaccine had been the project's agenda from its beginning. A 1954 article on the start of the Harvard-Aramco collaboration declared, "The ultimate goal will be the production of a safe and effective vaccine."[113] The prioritization of a technological innovation in the form of a vaccine that could eliminate endemic disease was consistent with Aramco's strategy of pursuing "various modernization programs" that merged "everyday operations with broader notions of development."[114] A successful vaccine would also offer a wide-reaching humanitarian intervention while providing a globally prestigious discovery for the Harvard researchers.

Throughout the research period they produced a series of academic publications that advanced their careers as well as offered care to patients. Had they successfully developed a vaccine, many children would have avoided pain and loss of vision, and treatment would not have been necessary. But it is also important to note that even at the beginning of the vaccine trials, the research team understood that trachoma was treatable and that environmental improvements had a powerful preventive effect. As three of the researchers wrote in a 1963 article: "It is generally accepted that, in areas of high endemicity, the control of trachoma by mass treatment campaigns is unlikely to eradicate the disease, even if it should prove economically feasible. As living standards are raised, trachoma tends to decrease in incidence and severity of its own accord. Despite the apparent lack of natural immunity associated with this disease, it has seemed to several groups of investigators that an immunologic approach to control has more intrinsic merit than the therapeutic approach."[115] Here they acknowledged and then dismissed the benefits of treatment and improved living standards, instead insisting on the as yet unrealized utility of a vaccine. The potential of immunization was almost magical, in that it might "(1) prevent the disease, (2) diminish the incidence so as to lower the transmission rate, (3) reduce its contagiousness by affecting the amount of virus in the eye of an infected person, and (4) prevent the serious sequelae of trachoma."[116] In the 1950s and 1960s, the successes of polio and smallpox vaccination appeared to promise the most rapid and comprehensive means to control infectious diseases around the world, and this context shaped the researchers' thinking about trachoma. Without knowing their search would prove unsuccessful, over the course of the 1960s the trachoma researchers disregarded large-scale treatment options and environmental improvements for the indigenous population of Saudi Arabia in favor of pursuing the still nonexistent benefits of vaccination.

Even though a 1954 Aramco publication declared that "no vaccine will be used in human beings until appropriate safety tests have been made on apes," by the early 1960s, the scientists had decided that Saudi patients were suitable recipients of experimental vaccinations.[117] The vaccine trials started in the spring of 1962, tested four different vaccines, and involved 3,282 subjects in eastern Saudi Arabia, the majority of whom ranged in age from a few days to two years old.[118] The scientists used approximately the same number of boys and girls. Using a system of randomization, half the subjects received trachoma vaccines at three dosage levels while half served as controls and received a placebo.[119] Following experimental vaccination in 1962, the researchers returned in 1972 for follow-up investigations. By then it was clear, as McComb admitted in 1996, that "the vaccine didn't work."[120]

What did research participation involve for the subjects? In a photograph from the early 1960s, Roger Nichols squats and tilts a boy's head back, holding open his eye (fig. 4.1). We see the arm of another white adult man reaching down from beyond the captured frame, firmly holding the boy's head in place. They are outside on the sand, and a goat in the background seems to be watching the eye exam. In preparation for the visits, the team would send advance word so that villagers could prepare for their arrival. "Everybody knew we were coming," McComb recalled. The benefit of this strategy was that, "by announcing we were coming back for a visit, the children and parents would be lined up waiting for us when we arrived." The interviewer interjected, "They didn't object to this?" McComb reassured her, "Oh no, they were really very good. Very, very good." She elaborated:

> In fact when we went back for a ten-year follow-up, there were women who brought with them the IBM number tag that we had assigned to that child on the first day. It was a linen tag which we tied around the wrist of the child. It had the IBM number stamped on it for easy reading. If the family showed up with the numbered tag we would still ask them all of the information to make certain we had the right child. Most often we were working outside of any building; in the primitive villages, there was no place big enough for us to work inside.[121]

To obtain conjunctival specimens, researchers would hold the upper eyelid everted and then scrape the inner surface with a sterilized steel instrument that was "intermediate in sharpness between an ordinary table knife and a surgical scalpel." Directing the instrument at a sixty-degree angle, "The scraping stroke was very light, and was intended to obtain only the superficial conjunctival cells on the outside edge of the instrument." There was generally not bleeding "unless the conjunctivae were severely inflamed" and "no anesthetic was used." Then, screw-cap vials carried the conjunctival scrapings "by air from Saudi Arabia to the laboratory at the Harvard School of Public Health for study."[122] In the follow-up village visits in 1972, the researchers required participants to enter "a darkened van that had a slit lamp in it for examination of the eyes." McComb explained,

"The routine was that you checked the people in, you did the preliminary exams of the eye, and then the child went into the van and had a slit lamp exam which provides a very precise measurement of the clinical status."[123]

To illustrate the dynamics in the interactions between the research team and local participants during the vaccine studies, McComb shared a story from Abqaiq, an Aramco townsite some fifty miles south of Dhahran. A woman came through the line with a child, but "she didn't have the child's record in hand." The team "went through the stack of patient records," but still couldn't find the missing document. McComb recalled, "We'd never lost a record before, and there was some consternation in the group!" Because without the record they were unsure of the child's vaccination history, they decided "to inoculate the child with a placebo—we always carried sterile saline with us." But then, when "the child's garment was raised," they were surprised to discover "the patch of iodine indicating the child had been vaccinated!" The mother and child had "already been through

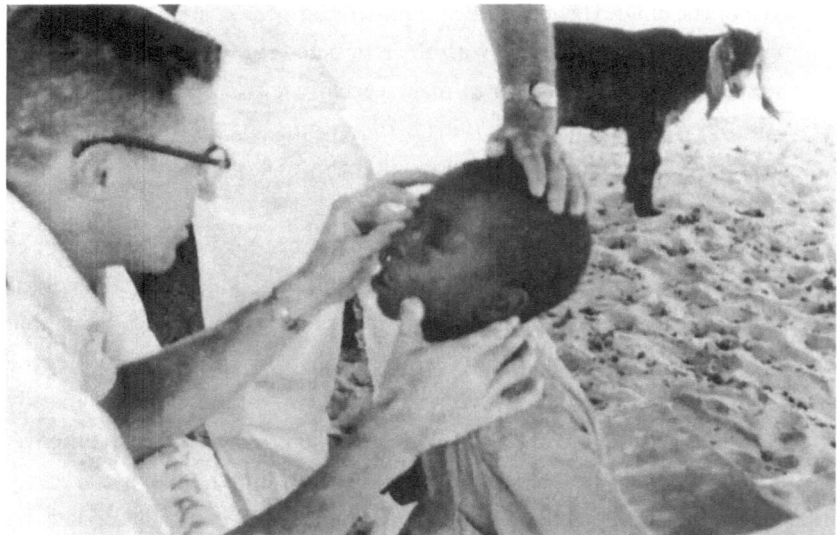

FIGURE 4.1. Roger Nichols examining a child's eyes in Saudi Arabia in the 1960s.

SOURCE: "Health and Disease in Saudi Arabia: Oral History Transcript: The Aramco Experience, 1940s–1990s/1998,"BANC MSS 2000/41, Bancroft Library, University of California, Berkeley, CA.

the line. Somehow the mother had gotten confused and thought there was more to it and got back in line" and so the child's record "was already in the 'out pile'!"[124]

The trachoma team included assistants from the local community as well as scientists and physicians from other Arab regions. Nadim Haddad was a coauthor on some of the scientific publications. An ophthalmologist, Haddad was a Palestinian Christian and, McComb divulged, "among the group that lost their land in the 1948 war with Israel."[125] Ali Abdul Rahman worked as a laboratory technician, and a photograph of him distilling water was even featured in a 1960 *Aramco World* article on the trachoma project.[126] A Saudi woman, Tahiya bint Hemd, joined the village visits in 1972 after completing her medical degree in Scotland.[127] The group that went to villages to administer vaccines also included three male Saudi nurses and several bilingual clerks.[128] The presence of local people and Arabic speakers on the research team would have reassured the villagers and facilitated communication and recordkeeping. Middle Eastern scientific actors, as Elise Burton writes, "imagin[ed] themselves as collaborators in a global scientific enterprise" and viewed such projects as professional opportunities.[129] The participation of this diverse group of Middle Eastern researchers and assistants illustrates the extent of the trachoma project's integration into Aramco's medical work.

Did Saudi state officials know that Aramco and Harvard were carrying out vaccine trials using Saudi citizens? There is some indication that Roger Nichols's competitive spirit prompted him to report on his vaccine work to Riyadh. Elinor Nichols recalled a party she attended "somewhere in the sixties" at which a "tall doctor, an Arab," told her that "the Italians have come up with a vaccine. The king is going to buy all the vaccine they have, and we are going to vaccinate every single person in Saudi Arabia." Back at home later in the evening, she repeated to her husband what the Arab doctor had said. Roger was "horrified" and rushed to Riyadh to "talk to all the medical people over there, including the King." According to Elinor, Roger framed his visit as an update on Harvard's activities: "He said: 'You know, I feel bad. I haven't kept you all current with what Harvard is doing. I'd like to come over . . . I'll bring all of our material with me, and spend a day with all of your medical people.'"[130] Elinor said, "he did it brilliantly . . . He went over there with all of his documents, all of the information about their vaccines . . . where they were, what the problems were with each of the vaccines." To make his case against the Italian vaccine, Elinor mused that Roger Nichols "may have mentioned: 'Other labs are working on this, and we are nowhere close to holding a vaccine that I feel is safe enough to announce to the world.'"[131] Elinor's story, recounted decades later, perhaps overestimates the competence of her husband. She repeated the narrative she received from him that the Italians had "made a terrible vaccine! It was absolutely worthless."[132] It is also revealing that the potential loss of a lucrative vaccine contract to rival researchers is what prompted Nichols to report on Harvard's activities to Saudi authorities. It seems likely that Saudi officials were ill informed about, if not totally ignorant of, the scope of the Aramco-Harvard trachoma research.

Over the course of the study, it became increasingly clear to the researchers that the living conditions Aramco had produced in Eastern Province created clear distinctions between trachoma levels among the children of Aramco employees and other local children. Even as they continued to rely on racial categories for population groups, they embraced environmental differences as the principal explanation of trachoma prevalence. For example, a 1969 study of trachoma antibodies in eye secretions examined samples from eighty-one "Saudi Arab" children and used thirty "Caucasian children with normal eyes living in Saudi Arabia" as controls.[133] It is important to note that they do not seem to have used white children on account of presumed biological difference but rather because they understood that white children lived in healthier conditions and would not have been exposed to trachoma. By this point, the Harvard-Aramco team's previous publications had already argued against race as a determining factor in trachoma, pointing to their findings that, in Eastern Province, "wide differences in trachoma occurred within a very limited geographic area, in populations with similar physical environments of climate and geography, and with ethnic and cultural backgrounds which were quite homogenous."[134]

Rather than racial difference, the primary variables the researchers settled on were running water and access to medical care. They characterized the population under study, first, by type of housing, and second, according to whether they were Aramco dependents or nondependents. The study took place in ten villages. The researchers categorized each village as a townsite, an oasis village, or an intermediate village. Two townsites were "constructed with the planning and financial assistance" of Aramco and "offered the most favorable living conditions," including electricity, running water, window screens, and sewage and garbage disposal (fig. 4.2).[135] Six oasis villages were "traditional in construction, consisting of baked mud and stone houses or of palm thatched huts," suffered from high fly counts, and rarely had electricity or running water (fig. 4.3).[136] Two intermediate villages featured a combination of these conditions. Townsite residents were mostly Sunni, and oasis residents were mostly Shiʻi.[137] Yet consistent with other contemporary development narratives, the trachoma researchers "systematically ignored the complicated sociosectarian relations" of Eastern Province in favor of the notion that "traditional culture . . . was a source of the region's threats."[138] Contrasting the conditions of village life with the material improvements Aramco provided

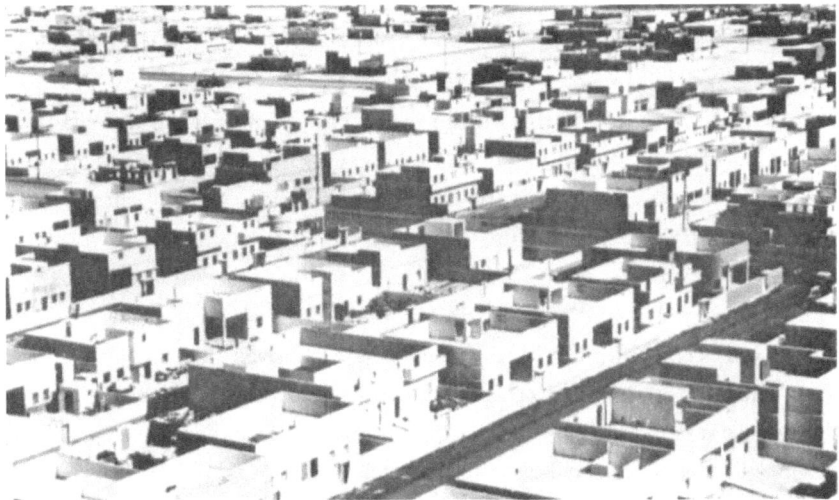

FIGURE 4.2. A townsite village in Saudi Arabia.
SOURCE: Roger L. Nichols, Arthur A. Bobb, Nadim A. Haddad, and Dorothy E. McComb, "Immunofluorescent Studies of the Microbiologic Epidemiology of Trachoma in Saudi Arabia," *American Journal of Ophthalmology* 63 (1967): 1374.

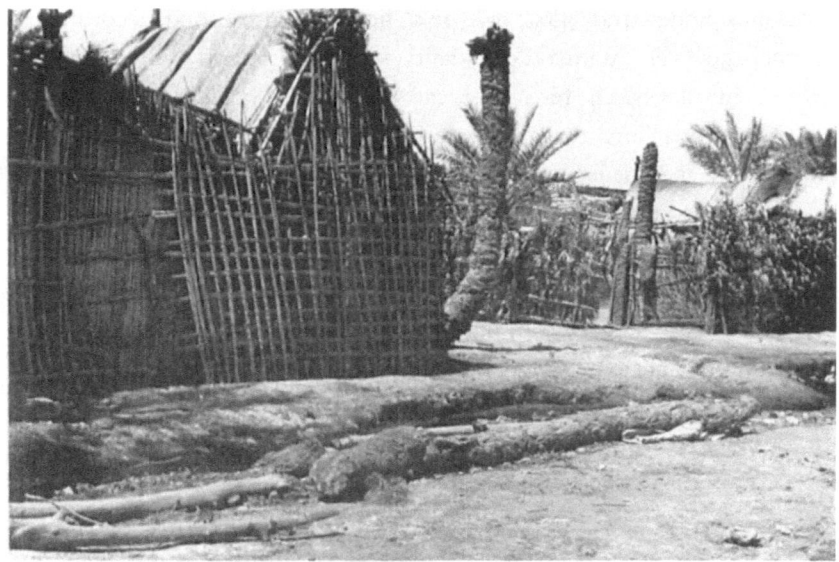

FIGURE 4.3. An oasis village in Saudi Arabia.
SOURCE: Roger L. Nichols, Arthur A. Bobb, Nadim A. Haddad, and Dorothy E. McComb, "Immunofluorescent Studies of the Microbiologic Epidemiology of Trachoma in Saudi Arabia," *American Journal of Ophthalmology* 63 (1967): 1375.

to its workers, they found that village versus townsite residence and whether a child's father was an Aramco employee were the principle factors that predicted trachoma rates. "Industrial employment of the father," they wrote, "permitted attainment of a higher standard of living, whether in townsite or oasis, and gave access to modern medical care to families of employees."[139] Later, McComb would recall the dramatic differences between townsite and village children: "You could tell easily which children had grown up in a town-site home. The children appeared to be taller, their health was better, the disease was milder."[140] The scientists framed disease differences between towns and villages as separate rungs on a developmental ladder rather than as environmental conditions that Aramco produced, sustained, and made available for comparative medical research in Eastern Province.

It is evident that village parents actively struggled against this pattern and made an effort to treat their families' eye ailments with whatever medical services they could access. One study noted that even though it was the families of employees, the predominant group in the townsites, who enjoyed the privilege of free company medical care, "it was interesting to find antibiotic ointment for the eyes in twice as many homes in the oases as in the townsites." But sadly for those children, the researchers felt that they were not using the ointment "in a manner adequate to constitute effective treatment" and that the differences in trachoma between townsites and villages "cannot be ascribed . . . to medical treatment, whether at home or in clinics."[141] In contrast to the inadequate medications the researchers found in village homes, when Roger Nichols accidentally infected himself with trachoma, he immediately treated himself with sulfa so that he did not have to miss a vacation to the Himalayas.[142]

To trace the life cycle of the disease and the effects of the vaccines, the scientists relied on environmental differences between Aramco and non-Aramco housing and medical care. In 1969, one article even presented Aramco's differential living conditions as a particular strength of the research: "In comparing townsite versus oasis villages, we were fortunate to find a situation in which many of the epidemiologic variables alleged to influence trachoma—race, cultural patterns, climate, geographical separation, nutrition, extrinsic contacts—were minimized or eliminated."[143] A comment Taylor made during his 1996 oral history suggests that Aramco and its Harvard collaborators chose to overlook the knowledge that better housing would do away with trachoma in favor of continuing vaccine tests. "One time," he stated, "I seriously proposed that instead of spending all this money on the trachoma research, we should put water systems into these areas and we'd knock out trachoma. That happened, but by accident, not planning."[144] When McComb returned in 1972, it was clear that "the vaccine really had not been effective."[145] The project ended quietly, as trachoma receded as the result of modern housing, sewage, and sanitation. McComb explained the acceptance of the project's end: "What you really do [after the vaccine fails] is what Aramco had already started to do, i.e. change the environment and personal habits. When I went back to the Saudi study village of Al-Mallahah in 1976, and closed the laboratory, the narrow streets had already been paved."[146]

Medical Experiments and Popular Participation

In the context of accelerating popular pressure on Aramco to improve its services for nonwhite workers and demands that the Saudi state provide a more equitable distribution of health services, local people approached health care as a hard-won privilege. Both locally and globally, health projects generated optimism about the potential to eliminate disease. The researchers in Eastern Province made use of local people's increasingly enthusiastic attendance in medical facilities to recruit research subjects for the trachoma vaccine trials. In particular, researchers took advantage of concerned parents, who were not informed about the experimental nature of the trachoma clinics before deciding to enroll their children and permitting them to receive vaccines.

The trachoma project ended in 1976. After more than twenty years of research in Eastern Province, the scientists had failed to create an effective vaccine. In fact, when they returned to one of the villages for a ten-year follow-up survey in 1972, they found that 20 percent of surveyed participants were blind in one or both eyes.[147]

Aramco's racial segregation resulted in comparative population samples, and the trachoma team determined that the divergent environmental conditions created by inequalities—rather than racial differences—best explained dissimilar trachoma prevalence. The researchers instrumentalized the differential environments that Aramco had produced in Eastern Province to study trachoma's life cycle and to search for a vaccine. Yet even as they moved away from racial determinism in their arguments, they embraced, rather than criticized, racial and religious discrimination because it was precisely the discriminatory practices that provided them with a clearly delineated variety of testing sites and populations. Researchers capitalized on Eastern Province's uneven development and structural discrimination to examine interactions between environmental conditions and disease. Embracing unequal access to resources as a scientific advantage resulted in the further elision of discrimination into stages on a developmental ladder, as illustrated in their distinction between villages and townsites.

Although it failed in the stated goal of discovering an effective vaccine, the trachoma project succeeded in producing several academic publications and advancing scientific careers. In the published proceedings of a 1970 Boston symposium on trachoma edited by Roger Nichols, several papers by Harvard-affiliated researchers listed Aramco as an affiliate or sponsor, or both.[148] Nichols evidently shared the eye scrapings of Saudi children with his Harvard colleagues; as J. Dennis Mull and John H. Peters wrote in their acknowledgments in their paper comparing eye secretions of infants and children in regions with and without endemic trachoma, "Prof. Nichols provided all of the Saudi Arab eye secretions tested in this study."[149] In 1970 Nichols became head of the Department of Microbiology at Harvard School of Public Health, and in 1977 he was named director of Boston's Museum of Science, a position he held until his death in 1987.[150]

When she was interviewed in 1996, Elinor Nichols struggled to reconcile her pride in her deceased husband's career and his humanitarian efforts with her realization, through the act of remembering, of what the trachoma research had entailed for the people of eastern Saudi Arabia:

> I went with him on a lot of trips to the villages, where he was scraping eyes. But I started to tell you earlier on: the one thing that was sort of difficult was that if they treated all these people with trachoma, then they were no longer useful to develop the vaccine. So we had a problem. You sort of had a moral problem here: are you going to treat all of these people who have trachoma, or are you going to use them to get a vaccine? And I'm sure that he must have treated—he must have—I cannot believe that through all those years, that they weren't also treating people. But the only way to do a study and to follow children is to go back out regularly and scrape the eyes and see what's going on. So I think there was sort of a moral dilemma there.... I honestly don't know how they resolved that. Because we had to have real trachoma going on. Obviously, they'd never let people go blind from it; they would treat it before it got too far advanced.[151]

Grappling with the tension between long-term advancements in public health and the immediate benefits of individual treatment, Elinor Nichols captured the changing dynamics of late twentieth-century research ethics.

In the field of medicine in the 1950s and 1960s, it was all too normal to target vulnerable, nonwhite communities for experimental research. In the United States, news of the Tuskegee syphilis experiments, in which scientists withheld treatment from Black participants in Macon County, Alabama, broke in 1972, the same year the trachoma team was carrying out its ten-year follow-up visits to the villages where they had tested vaccines. But in the 1990s, it was unimaginable to Elinor Nichols that her husband would not have treated Saudi children for trachoma.

Finally, it is worth reemphasizing that the trachoma vaccine experiments depended on popular participation. Aramco's efforts to promote vaccinations among employees and their families facilitated the trachoma team's medical research. In the years of accelerated oil exploitation following World War II, local people were coming to associate vaccinations and other curative and preventive procedures with positive health benefits. By the time the trachoma researchers started testing vaccines in the early 1960s, the people of Eastern Province were accustomed to receiving vaccines from Aramco's medical staff, and even viewed such medical care as a privilege of employment. To study trachoma and test their vaccines, the scientists relied on the willingness of local parents, particularly mothers, to bring their young children to the trachoma researchers. As the trachoma researcher Dorothy McComb recalled villagers waiting in anticipation of the researchers' visits, "there would be a lot of people who would stand in line for a long time, and we'd just take them in the order in which they came."[152]

The next chapter picks up the thread of gendered medical labor but switches from Aramco's corporate paternalism to state welfare in Kuwait. As health services emerged as integral to the postwar development state, noncitizen nurses arrived from across the Arab world to staff the expanding medical infrastructure. Although these women were state builders, patriarchal norms and hierarchies of citizenship constrained their professional and personal lives.

CHAPTER 5

NURSES

IN 1965, the menace of cholera gave Kuwait an opportunity to deploy its expanding medical infrastructure. Cholera had appeared on Iran's Afghan frontier in July, and Iran responded by shutting down communications with its eastern regions, dispatching 1,428 medical workers, closing schools, banning public gatherings, and imposing quarantines on its borders.[1] In stark contrast to the Sultan of Oman's lackluster response in 1899 to warnings that cholera would likely make landfall in Muscat if he did not take precautionary measures, by 1965, the Kuwaiti reaction to news of cholera in Iran exemplified how drastically government attitudes toward preventing disease had transformed. When Kuwaiti authorities learned of the outbreak, they halted travel between Kuwait and Iran and prohibited the import of food. The government requested additional vaccine from abroad and ordered vaccination for "the entire population of Kuwait."[2] Moreover, Kuwait's residents were willing participants in these public health measures, perhaps thanks in part to the long history of vaccinations in Kuwait.[3] According to the director of the Ministry of Health's preventive services, "Vaccination is currently being done without resorting to force and compulsion because health awareness in Kuwait has reached an impressive level . . . the people are coming for vaccination in a manner that is reassuring."[4]

Nurses, the largest population of medical professionals, were on the front lines of these sweeping vaccination efforts. Jamila Fadil Khoury, the Syrian woman who directed Kuwait's nurses throughout the 1960s, seized on the cholera epidemic to argue forcefully that Arab women nurses were state builders, comparable to—and in no way less than—skilled male professionals and even patriotic soldiers. Using military metaphors to explain disease, Khoury declared, "In my opinion, as far as Kuwait feels the need to build a strong modern army to protect its borders and defend them from the enemy, there is also a need for another army of Kuwaiti Angels of Mercy to keep the country safe from the invisible enemy of disease."[5] Emphasizing the central role of the nurses in Kuwait's response to cholera, she continued, "This [need] became clear in recent days when this army—I mean the female nurses and the male first aid responders—played their honorable role in immunizing citizens to stave off the danger of cholera."[6] The role of the nursing staff, she elaborated, "was exactly as the role of the army in a state of antagonism and war . . . side by side, day and night, with full attention and desire to vaccinate the citizens."[7]

Khoury's comparison of nurses and soldiers suggests that she understood how a sizable population of working women, many of whom were unmarried, sat uneasily with patriarchal norms and anxieties surrounding citizenship, family, and sexuality in Kuwait's rapidly changing social world. Throughout her interviews in Kuwait's vibrant press, Khoury combated such tensions over the professional status of women nurses by presenting her own migration to Kuwait—and the migration of other women Arab nurses—as a political act. Nurses, in her view, helped to stitch the newly minted sovereign state (Kuwait gained independence in 1961) into the Arab world and to integrate it into a particular transregional vision of decolonizing modernity.[8] More than a medical administrator, in her interviews she used her personal narrative to advocate for the professional virtue of women workers. Khoury was born and completed primary school in the town of Mashta Al Hilu in northwestern Syria. She moved with her family to Tripoli, where she finished secondary school, and then enrolled in the nursing program at the American University of Beirut.[9] After graduating at age nineteen with a nursing certificate, she worked in Tripoli and Homs. With the outbreak of the 1948 war, Khoury rushed to Lebanon's border with Palestine so that she could "provide first aid to the *mujāhidīn* and fighters."[10] The war proved a formative experience, solidifying her sense that nursing was a patriotic duty.[11] The fact that Khoury had worked as a nurse in the 1948 Palestine war also would have endeared her to Kuwait's expanding professional class who were deeply involved in Pan-Arabism and the Palestinian issue.[12] In a 1963 interview, she explicitly linked her work as a nurse to her political awakening in 1948, stating, "In this war, painful calamities occurred that affected my soul and pushed me to devote myself more and more to the profession."[13]

After the war, Khoury was head nurse at a hospital in Jeddah. Her next stop was Syria, where she also taught nursing. Khoury then traveled on a Rockefeller Foundation fellowship to the United States, where she earned a bachelor of science in educational and administrative nursing before returning to Syria. Kuwait's Department of Public Health, at that time headed by Shaykh Fahad al-Salem Al-Sabah, offered her a position in 1959. She worked as the director of nurses in Al-Amiri and Al-Sabah hospitals before being promoted to lead the country's nursing staff, a position she held until the 1970s.[14] Although in her public narrative she emphasized her credentials as an Arab woman dedicated to serving the pan-Arab community, her American education—both at the American University of Beirut and in the United States—facilitated Khoury's professional mobility in the Arab world and authorized her to promote an Arab version of this universally feminized profession.

Gulf migration is regularly presented as an explanatory mechanism for twentieth-century transformations in the Arab world. But histories of state building and multidirectional migration within, to, and from the Gulf have yet to fully explore the ground-level interactions that populated large-scale economic, social, and political changes, let alone how people understood the meaning of their own migrations. Largely because of the focus on the oil industry, there also has been scant attention to how Arab women's labor shaped these demographic and social processes or to the gendered experiences of Arab women migrants. As state agents, nurses were tasked with translating, standardizing, and implementing biomedicine into local health practices. As migrant and professional women whose jobs entailed intimate interactions of physical touch and personal care with Kuwaiti residents from all walks of life, nurses also contributed to shifting dynamics between women and men. Their specialized training made them essential to the state's modernizing project, but their status as women resulted in systemic economic devaluation of their labor, frequent workplace harassment, and paternalist laws that regulated their movements and leisure.

The focus on elite and male foreign experts and on economic causality rather than social processes has elided an important reality: migrant women mediated the majority of residents' interactions with the state's medical infrastructure. These women's labor was crucial to building the modern welfare state. Moreover, Khoury's argument for the moral and professional role of Arab women reminds us that, as Andrea Wright states, "migration is not a simple economic calculus," and "much is lost in using supply and demand, surplus and scarcity" to explain the migration of workers to the Gulf.[15] Khoury did not conceptualize the presence of noncitizen Arab women nurses as the result of a surplus of people in Egypt, Lebanon, and Syria and a shortage of medical workers in Kuwait. In 1963, when a reporter asked Khoury, "What is your view of the Arab girl and what is your advice to her?" Khoury replied: "The Arab girl is distinguished by her strong morals and her ambitions. She is now working in all fields. She has proven her great merit and her ability to master every job that is entrusted to her. My advice is to avoid vanity and to learn a lot from science."[16] Khoury adeptly used her position of medical leadership to promote the idea that women had a duty to participate in the Arab national project as nurses, that their efforts demanded specialized training and expertise, and that they deserved society's respect. She offered up Arab nurses as agents of social change in a newly independent Kuwait.

Health Care and State Building in Kuwait

In the period between the end of World War II and the 1973 oil boom, health care, along with education, housing, and infrastructure, emerged as a hallmark of the Gulf welfare state. As escalating oil revenue flowed directly to the region's rulers, the "public sector was the natural driver" of development.[17] Central to modern Gulf history is the question of how a particular form of state largesse emerged as a universal expectation. Did the region's British-backed autocrats distribute services to a passive population as a calculated strategy for placating political dissidents and squashing demands for popular representation? Or, in a similar mode of economically driven political causality, did local people naturally and inevitably lose interest in political rights as a result of state jobs, modern infrastructure, and generous welfare programs? Although such framings persist in some quarters, recent scholarship decisively has dismantled two interconnected ideas that long have haunted Gulf studies: first, that the region's elites voluntarily redistributed oil wealth in a series of top-down decisions that ricocheted around the region, and second, that Gulf residents, citizens and noncitizens, have been politically submissive in the oil era. As Alex Boodrookas writes in his study of the labor movement in the Gulf: "The benefits of the Kuwaiti welfare state, including universal healthcare, education, social security, and housing, were not the free gifts of a benevolent autocrat. Nor were they merely the result of a cynical ploy to 'buy off' the opposition. Rather, these benefits had to be won."[18] Far from a sudden inundation of overnight riches hoisted onto a docile, expectant population, the process of directing state resources toward national development and welfare was incremental and contentious.

Most scholarship addresses the welfare state as an assemblage of interconnected benefits and institutions. Instead, I set the stage for my argument that nurses were central to the welfare project by unraveling health from the tightly coiled bundle of state services that have come to characterize mid-twentieth-century development. I demonstrate that the Kuwait Municipality's intervention into health in the early 1930s—that is, before the large-scale exploitation of oil—altered local people's expectations and thus laid the groundwork for later state projects. Global trends of postwar welfare intersected with local politics of oil production to embed health care at the heart of Kuwait's development state.

A survey of Kuwait's vibrant political scene in the 1930s and the pre-oil history of state health care illuminates how local politics established the foundations for a dynamic relationship between governance and health prior to the influx of oil wealth. The merchant-dominated Kuwait Municipality, founded in 1930 and considered a foundational institution for Kuwaiti democracy, constructed early polices around sanitary reforms. In its first year, the municipality sought to train Kuwaitis to keep their streets clean, defecate privately, and dispose of their waste in designated locations or outside of the township. The sanitary situation at this point was foreboding. "Many large heaps of accumulated rubbish" and "some fifteen deep and unsanitary pits resembling enormous 'shell' craters" that had "become the recognised latrine areas for the poor" checkered the city.[19] The 1930 order forbade residents from throwing dirt and waste from their homes onto common garbage heaps. Instead, they were to use the municipality's garbage bins or to throw their waste (including the remains of dead animals) into the sea or outside the township. People were forbidden from blocking the streets with rocks or mud for an extended period of time. There was to be no defecating on the roads. The announcement was not a mere suggestion; anyone caught violating the order "must be punished."[20] The efforts were remarkably effective: "Within weeks of the Municipality's inception, nearly five thousand tons of accumulated street refuse had been removed from the inner neighborhoods."[21]

On the heels of these attempts to manage waste, the municipality's formative years intersected with a devastating smallpox epidemic in 1932 which claimed the lives of around three thousand Kuwaitis. According to one observer, "The child population between the ages of three and ten was almost wiped out."[22] The year 1932 was also the first one in which the Municipal Council held elections.[23] As smallpox cases soared in the spring, the municipality, chaired by Shaykh ʿAbd Allah al-Jabir Al-Sabah, sprang to action. It offered smallpox vaccinations (sometimes by force), cooperated with the ruler to transport vaccinations from Basra by car, papered the markets with public health announcements, and recorded daily deaths. The municipality also decided to deport recently arrived Iranian migrants as an anti-smallpox measure.[24] Kuwait's elites viewed this group as a destitute population in search of relief from the economic depression, and this epidemiological measure was politically consistent with the ruler's decision to deport hundreds of poor Iranians to the Shatt al-Arab.[25] The municipality thus simultaneously responded to perceived epidemiological and economic risk by partitioning the population according to a calculation that privileged nativist political interests. In the wake of the 1932 smallpox epidemic, public health emerged forcefully as a field of intervention for Kuwait's local representative government.

The arrival of the Kuwait Oil Company (KOC) in the 1930s introduced a new player to Kuwait's medical field. The ruling shaykh's wealth and legitimacy quickly were welded to his relationship with the oil company, granting him unprecedented control over how rising prosperity would be redistributed to the population. The political agent H. R. P. Dickson captured how the oil concession resulted in Shaykh Ahmad al-Jabir's (r. 1921–1950) rapid political promotion and increased intimacy with London: "On 23rd December 1934 Shaikh Ahmad, with the approval of His Majesty's Government, had given an oil concession to the Kuwait Oil Company, a joint Anglo-American concern. In the summer of 1935 the shaikh had paid a private visit to London, where he had been very well received. On 1st April 1937 he was granted the title of His Highness by His Majesty's Government, and was shortly after given the K.C.S.I. [Knight Commander of the Order of the Star of India]."[26]

As in eastern Saudi Arabia (see chapter 4), an acceleration of medical work accompanied the exploitation of oil. Both oil companies' desire to ensure the availability of able-bodied workers and local people's swelling demand for medical services drove centralized health efforts. In 1935 in Kuwait, KOC employed its own doctor, provided "a good stock of drugs and dressings" for company use, and recruited Doctor Mylrea of the American mission to their medical staff.[27] Separate from the township, the mission hospital, and the British dispensary, the oil company provided its own health services for employees and their families.[28] But there was an additional population that benefited from the company's medical care, an arrangement that would prove contentious in the coming years. The 1934 KOC concession included the provision that "the Company shall provide free of charge medical service for its employees, and the Sheikh and his family (at present around 400 members) shall have the right to such medical service and necessary medical supplies free of charge."[29] While the shaykh and his household had received free treatment at the American mission hospital since its establishment, the same services were still available to the rest of the community, albeit for a small fee. In effect, the oil concession separated the ruling family's medical care from that of the rest of the population.[30]

Moreover, the role of the merchant-controlled Kuwait Municipality as a check on the shaykh's power would come under attack with the onset of oil revenues. KOC, established as a 50-50 holding between the British Anglo-Persian Oil Company and the American company Gulf Oil, discovered commercial quantities of oil in Kuwait in 1938.[31] Oil revenues reshuffled the political balance of power because "unlike taxes, oil revenues did not go through the pearl merchants on their way to the Shaikh but went directly from the oil companies to the ruler."[32] The merchants' desire to maintain political influence and to disrupt the direct relationship between KOC and the ruling family laid the groundwork for the Majlis movement. In early 1938, "a group of merchants met secretly to draw up a list of reforms which they then circulated in leaflets and anti-government wall writing."[33] In June they elected a legislative assembly of fourteen. Abdalla Salim, Shaykh Ahmad's cousin and rival within the royal family, headed the assembly. In July, the assembly presented the ruler with concrete demands and prepared a basic law that granted the assembly control over state institutions and legislative rights. Ahmad initially agreed to the demands, but after they stipulated that he submit his revenues from the oil company, he dissolved the assembly on December 17.[34] As Jill Crystal describes the events, "The members did not accept the dissolution without a fight. As Ahmad collected his supporters, the Assembly members locked themselves into a fortified building, accompanied by their guards and supporters. This was a strategic error. Although Abdalla Salim tried to negotiate a settlement, in the end the matter was settled by force. The ruler called in his beduin supporters. . . . Outmanned, the Assembly conceded defeat."[35] At the heart of this dispute was who would control the projected oil wealth. The shaykh violently disbanded the representative body rather than negotiate this point.

Yet the Majlis movement lived on in local memory and political formations as an aspiration for representation. It also indicated the growing influence of transnational imaginaries in Kuwait. In addition to protecting their long-standing domestic political influence, Arab nationalism was the "guiding ideology" of the merchants' political movement.[36] The Educational

Council, founded in 1936, exemplified the growing Arab influence on Kuwaiti institutions and ideologies. For the following several years, as Talal Al-Rashoud has demonstrated, Palestinian teachers "increased awareness of Arab nationalism and the Palestinian cause" and relied on an imported Iraqi curriculum, the combined effect of which heightened Arab nationalism's local cultural currency.[37] Ahmad al-Khatib, future opposition leader, Kuwait's first university-trained doctor, and founder of the first official branch of the Arab Nationalist Movement in Kuwait, "credits his first stirrings of Arab national sentiment in the late 1930s to the influence of his Palestinian teachers."[38]

In this political setting, emerging understandings of an Arab state's responsibility to ensure the health of the Arab people was also a driving ideological motivation for the Majlis movement and its sympathizers. During the events of 1938 and 1939, the Iraqi press maintained a heated attack on the Kuwaiti government. In a 1938 speech in parliament, the Iraqi foreign minister referred to Kuwait as "an inseparable part of Iraq, Iraq's natural outlet to the sea."[39] In April 1938, the Iraqi newspaper *Al Istiqlal* opined, "It pains Iraq to behold on her borders an Arab territory with an excellent geographical position and yet in a backward state, deprived of means of education and of health and economic organisation."[40] Such sentiments also found voice on the local level. A British report on the motivations of the opposition explained, "It is a grievance of the people of Kuwait that while the Shaikh has taken care to secure free medical attention and supplies for himself, the poor and others have to pay for hospital attention."[41] The Majlis's July 1938 basic law had included "The Law of Public Health, the purpose of which is to establish Laws of Health which will protect the State and its inhabitants from the dangers of ill health and diseases of all kinds."[42] Finally, in the opposition's formal demands, they listed "A Free Hospital" in second place, behind only "Fiscal power, an annual Budget, and various Administrative reforms."[43]

In short, the Majlis movement sought to enshrine the government's responsibility to provide health care. Reflecting the fluid categories of Kuwaitis and foreigners of the 1930s, the movement did not limit this state responsibility to Kuwaitis but extended it more broadly to include "inhabitants."

Through such measures, the Majlis movement directly challenged the royal family's privileged access to free health care and made plans to modernize state medicine and public health. The Kuwait Municipality and the Majlis movement established the ideological and institutional foundations from which Kuwaitis would demand health care from their state, whether it was run by an elected body or an authoritarian monarchy. By the end of the 1930s, representative government had transformed the fabric of daily life in Kuwait, and it had done so in the name of public health. It was no longer acceptable for the people to languish from preventable or curable diseases while the ruling Al-Sabah family received free medical care.

International trends validated and enforced the belief of people in Kuwait that the state should provide health care. World War II precipitated a global shift in which health care came to signify the promise of development and the state's ability to govern; as Sunil Amrith writes, "In a very short space of time, to possess a health service had become a universal element of the functions of a state; any state."[44] In Britain, Kuwait's imperial patron, the transformed expectations of the postwar period and the Labour Party's outright victory in 1945 resulted in "a genuine 'Welfare State'" characterized by state monopolies over public provisions.[45] Seeking to reconcile with the members of the Majlis movement, Shaykh Ahmad appointed leading merchants to new government institutions in the early 1940s, including a Health Council which he formed in 1943.[46] With the resumption of oil production following World War II, the consolidation of power in the hands of Kuwait's ruling elites ran parallel to the expanding influence and profits of the oil industry as payments were delivered to the ruler. During his first year in power, Shaykh Abdullah al-Salem (r. 1950–1965) directed nearly a fifth of state revenue toward health and education.[47] In the wake of the Saudi 50–50 profit-sharing agreement and Iran's nationalization of oil, Abdullah negotiated a 50–50 profit-sharing agreement with KOC in 1951. British Petroleum increased oil production in Kuwait in response to the loss of facilities caused by Iranian oil nationalization. The result of the skyrocketing revenue was that Kuwait "rapidly took on the characteristics of a boomtown, with an explosion of construction, migration and consumption that, to many inhabitants, seemed to have taken place almost overnight."[48]

Over the same period, the popularity of Arab nationalism swelled in the wake of the 1952 Egyptian Revolution. Al-Rashoud explains the "widespread veneration" of Gamal Abdel Nasser's image as "a symbol upon which people in the Gulf of various backgrounds projected their hopes and dreams."[49] When Nasser nationalized the Suez Canal in 1956, Kuwaitis enthusiastically participated in the region's pan-Arab and anti-imperialist movements. Kuwait's residents carried out a general strike, boycotted French and British goods, and planted a series of bombs in oil-producing areas.[50] In 1959, following a protest at which opposition leader Jassem al-Qatami challenged Al-Sabah leadership and called for democratic rule, Shaykh Abdullah stifled opposition activity by closing social clubs and civil society organizations, suspending the press, and banning public demonstrations.[51] In the same year, a new nationality law extended the definition of those who were "originally" Kuwaiti to include descendants of residents of Kuwait since 1920 (rather than 1898) but restricted naturalization.[52] Such measures both weakened internal opposition and exacerbated distinctions between the increasingly rigid category of Kuwaiti citizens and the growing Arab migrant population. As Kuwait moved toward its 1961 independence, "the ruler apparently felt that the opposition's educated cadres and pan-Arab credentials would help attain regional recognition for his fledgling state," and the clubs and press regained some of their freedoms.[53] This strategy paid off when, as Iraq threatened to invade Kuwait in the days immediately following its official independence, Abdullah enjoyed unprecedented popularity. In the face of the Iraqi threat, Kuwaitis even expressed their patriotism in their medical facilities, as volunteers poured into Kuwait's central laboratory to donate blood during the crisis.[54] The 1962 constitution declared the state's responsibility for public health, preventive medicine, and treatment of diseases and epidemics.[55] The elected National Assembly, rooted in the 1938 Majlis movement, further institutionalized divisions between the ruling family, Kuwaiti citizens, and the noncitizen population. Ruling family members could not serve in the assembly, and noncitizens were not eligible to vote.[56]

As these political events unfolded, Kuwait's population increased from 70,000 in 1944 to 467,000 in 1965.[57] Labor recruitment pivoted toward the Arab world, and health services developed in dialogue with emerging categorizations of Kuwait's growing population. KOC and the state hospital alike sought to recruit Arab medical staff; pharmacists and doctors began to arrive from Lebanon, Iraq, Syria, and Egypt. In 1939, the first state-employed doctor and pharmacist were Lebanese brothers. The first state clinic imported most of its medicine from Iraq and Syria. Although the Lebanese brothers lasted only a month in Kuwait, they were replaced by a Syrian doctor, Yahiya al-Hadidi. In 1942, the Department of Health employed an Egyptian as its first Arab woman doctor. The first state hospital, Al-Amiri, opened in 1949.[58] A decade later, Kuwait had four hospitals and seventeen clinics, five of them specializing in mother and child care.[59] Tuberculosis was one of the leading causes of death. A men's tuberculosis clinic was opened in 1951 and a women's clinic in 1953, and they were followed by other clinics and centers to combat tuberculosis through the 1950s and 1960s; by 1962, approximately one thousand beds were reserved for tuberculosis treatment across Kuwait.[60] The modern Al-Sabah general hospital, with a capacity for six hundred beds, was completed in 1962.[61]

Like earlier mission hospitals that drew in visitors from far-flung regions (see chapter 2), state health services, available to Kuwaitis and non-Kuwaiti residents alike, attracted patients from across the region. According to one observer, in 1954, patients in the tuberculosis sanatorium were predominantly from Saudi Arabia, Iraq, and Iran, while only 5 percent to 10 percent of total hospital patients were Kuwaiti.[62] The Ministry of Public Health's reporting on the years 1958–1962 recorded Kuwaiti birth and death rates, but their calculation of the population also accounted for the numbers of incoming and outgoing migrants.[63] In 1962, the government introduced a health registration system that divided the state's territory and residents into eleven districts, assigning each family to a clinic in its residential area. Individuals were issued health identity cards, and the clinic kept records on each family. If the clinic staff found that a patient required specialized treatment or tests, they referred the patient to a hospital. Newcomers to Kuwait received information about their health care upon arrival and were issued temporary registration to a clinic.[64]

The expansive reach of disease across binaries of citizens and noncitizens informed early state health projects. Consistent with post–World War II trends around the world, Kuwait's ruling elites, responding to popular expectations, integrated health care into their state-building apparatus as a mechanism of control and a redistributive service. Although there was growing differentiation between the health care offered to citizens and noncitizens, the distinction was fluid and took into account modern ideologies of contagion, medicine, and population-level vulnerabilities. Incoming noncitizens, as well as Kuwaitis, factored into state calculations of the population and an expanding medical infrastructure.

Nurses as Workers

Who worked in this growing health system, and what was it like for them to interact with Kuwait's diverse population of patients? The politics of state health derive from the fact that health care is a lived experience that changes over time across shifting fault lines of men and women, citizens and noncitizens, workers and patients. As one of the first points of contact between the population and the newly independent nation's nascent welfare system, nurses were at the forefront of Kuwaiti state building.[65] The number of nurses at work in the country expanded alongside Kuwait's population (table 5.1). In the early twentieth-century American South, the development of the welfare state through health reform targeting Black communities depended on "the work of women at the bottom of the

TABLE 5.1. Population, medical staff, and beds in Kuwait, 1965–1970

Year	Population	No. of government-sector physicians and dentists	No. of government-sector nurses	Population per bed (government)
1965	467,339	490	2,026	165
1966	511,557	507	2,034	171
1967	561,047	533	2,185	173
1968	613,988	558	2,253	182
1969	673,244	571	2,367	195
1970	738,662	585	2,442	208

SOURCE: *Statistics Abstract in 25 Years* (Kuwait: Ministry of Planning Statistics & IT Sector, 1990), 305, 307.

medical hierarchy"; similarly, Arab migrant nurses, as the majority of the government's medical labor force, were the backbone of health care in Kuwait's welfare state in the 1960s.[66]

Unlike women teachers, the other large female professional staff in Kuwait during this period, the very nature of nurses' work brought them into close contact with all categories of the Kuwaiti population, regardless of gender, social class, or age. Because the overwhelming majority of nurses in Kuwait were migrants, as well as women, they faced multiple barriers when they tried to express their frustrations. In this sense they resembled Indian migrant nurses in the twentieth-century United States, who enjoyed "the possibility of professionalization" but were an "inherently unstable (due to immigration/citizenship status), part of the workforce."[67] As residents whom the state categorized as transient and temporary, long-term occupational health issues caused by the nurses' work would not have been as visible or concerning to the state as were the complaints of citizen patients.

Recruiting nurses demanded diplomatic efforts. Throughout the 1960s, as health facilities struggled to provide enough nurses to keep pace with the growing population and its medical needs, the Ministry of Health regularly sent representatives to Amman, Cairo, Beirut, and Damascus in search of nurses.[68] Yet the Kuwaiti Ministry of Health pursued transregional nursing recruitment despite a nursing shortage throughout the Arab world. In 1963, for example, when the Ministry of Health of the United Arab Republic stipulated that "members of the nursing staff should not travel due to the urgent need for them there," authorities in Cairo made an exception for Kuwait.[69] Sixty new nurses arrived from Egypt that spring, selected from a pool of eight hundred applicants. As Jamila Fadil Khoury explained in 1965, "We often encounter difficulties obtaining nurses from Arab countries . . . we find, for example, that there is a surplus of lawyers and graduates of other institutes, but in the Arab countries strict procedures are imposed on nurses before they leave."[70] This dynamic was part of a global process in which worldwide shortages resulted in the movement of nurses from poorer countries to richer countries. As Catherine Ceniza Choy argues, transnational nurse migrations are "inextricably linked to the larger processes of global restructuring in which the increased demands for services in highly developed countries . . . have contributed to increasing worldwide mobility" and exacerbated global inequalities of health services.[71]

But what health officials viewed as a nursing shortage was largely the product of nurses' low wages and poor working conditions. This pattern of labor policies mirrored the corporate strategy of the oil industry.[72] As Boodrookas writes, "Unwilling to train their employees, pay a living wage, or treat women as paid workers, oil companies turned to recruitment abroad, where they could find already trained, low cost, and easily deportable men."[73] Nurses additionally were burdened by the fact that the gendering of nurses as women further justified low salaries. Nevertheless, nurses in Kuwait actively sought to renegotiate the value of their labor and to improve their working conditions. The discrepancy between the need for nursing staff in the growing number of hospitals, clinics, and sanatoriums in Kuwait and the condition of a perennial "shortage" of nurses could result in labor disputes between the nurses and the ministry. In 1963, as part of a wave of labor activism around Kuwait, nurses carried out a brief strike at Al-'Azam hospital.[74] They were reacting to the Ministry of Health's recent move to apply a two-shift system in all hospitals.[75] The nurses' demands included working a single shift, receiving compensation for additional work, and being allowed to eat a meal at the hospital during their working hours. The strike ended when a government representative agreed to consider their demands, but he warned that nurses working a single shift "delays work for citizens."[76] *Al-Tali'a*, the pro-labor mouthpiece for the Movement of Arab Nationalists, picked up the nurses' demands. To strengthen its case, *al-Tali'a* connected the nurses' working conditions to the well-being of the patients. *Al-Tali'a* argued: "As much as we are concerned with work, we should care for those who perform that work. Otherwise, our interests will be imperfect, unhealthy, and subject to permanent setback and failure."[77]

The labor dispute captured the unique role of health professionals and the persistent discourse of their "shortage." According to *al-Tali'a*, the nature of state medicine in Kuwait, "where medicine and examination are free," meant that the relationship between the Ministry of Health and the general population "is much stronger, it is direct and daily, and includes all categories of citizens, and everyone who lives in this country."[78] The article pointed out that "[the nurses'] numbers are increasing, and their responsibilities are increasing, and their problems grow more complicated by the day," characterizing nurses' work as "dangerous and delicate."[79] The two-shift system the Ministry of Health sought to impose "does not provide [nurses] with adequate and necessary rest to carry out their skilled and challenging work."[80] As for the striking nurses themselves, the ministry's reply to *al-Tali'a* was to point out "the great shortage in numbers of nurses" and to claim that "it has been trying for several years to fill this deficiency but it didn't find enough [nurses]." As a result, "the ministry is unable to commit to a specific time when it will overcome this deficiency."[81]

The debate between *al-Tali'a* and the representative from the Ministry of Health as it played out in Kuwait's press highlights the nurses' challenges in representing their working conditions and their personal safety within the framework of labor rights. The difficulties of capturing the gendered hardships of work usually performed by women were not particular to Kuwait. In the United States, "For most people, the phrase *occupational hazard* brings to mind blue-collar men, not women; heavy industry and not service work . . . the primary association of dangerous work with white men in mining, manufacturing, and construction obscured the work experience of women and minorities."[82] In Kuwait, labor organizing was concentrated around the oil and government sectors. Oil companies recruited male workers. Grounded as it was in male-dominated industries, much of the labor movement conceptualized labor concerns as male.[83]

It is not surprising, then, that even as *al-Tali'a* demanded better working conditions for nurses, it also effaced the fact that nearly all the nurses were women. Its coverage stands out in discussions of nurses in the media in this regard. Usually, coverage of nurses emphasized their feminine qualities as self-sacrificing caregivers and compared their working conditions to those of other women. When a reporter asked the head doctor of Al-Sabah hospital about nurses' status, for example, he replied, "Yes, she is treated unjustly in relation to her female colleagues in other professions."[84] Another (male) official echoed this sentiment, "The nurse has human lives in her hands whereas the secretary has papers in her hands. . . . In terms of the work [the nurse] does and the salaries of her female colleagues in other fields, [her salary] is not rewarding."[85] In contrast to representations of the nurse that framed the value of her work in relation to other women-dominated professions, *al-Tali'a* used both the male and female constructions of "nurses" (*mumarriḍīn/mumarriḍāt*) throughout its article, even as it included photographs that depicted nurses exclusively as women in crisp white dresses. *Al-Tali'a* proved unwilling to reconcile the reality that nurses were predominantly women with the idea of nurses as workers.

Although *al-Tali'a* failed to capture the breadth of their concerns, nurses themselves managed to convey the strenuousness of their labor in language that took into account their gendered realities. They emphasized the challenges of their lack of authority over hospital visitors, the constraints of feminized caregiving, and the hardships of the double responsibilities of marriage and employment. They recognized that rising patient-to-nurse ratios and longer working hours that resulted from the nursing shortage "placed greater strain on nurses . . . which often led to higher incidence of workplace stress and injury" and inevitably worsened patient care.[86]

In a 1968 conversation with a woman journalist, the Sudanese nurse Fawziyya Dawud, who had been working in Kuwait for four years, explained that "the salary is low in terms of the hard physical and psychological efforts."[87] She described how the nurses struggled with "the visitor who doesn't respect appointments and brings food from outside and carpets and televisions and disturbs the rest of the patients."[88] A Jordanian nurse, Sara al-Afghani, recalled her decision to enter the profession: "My mother got sick and I stayed beside her. I promised myself to serve the patient if God healed my mother, and I fulfilled the vow." Her vocational narrative was consistent with the gendered view of the woman nurse as caregiver. This expectation that nurses were realizing a naturalized gendered role both made it more difficult for women to seek financial remuneration for their work and overlooked the possibility that better working conditions and higher salaries would alleviate the nursing shortage. If it was their femininity that made nurses ideal caregivers, this assumption also constrained them from demanding increased pay for work that was supposedly in their nature. But even Sara al-Afghani, who had made a vow to God to devote herself to patient care, had not anticipated the combined burden of work and marriage.

Al-Afghani described the night shift, during which the nurse had to remain alert in the hospital from seven in the evening to seven in the morning in total silence (activities like listening to the radio and knitting were forbidden) as the patients were sleeping, as a "slow death for the nurse." But she acknowledged that she could not stop working as her family depended on her salary. She declared: "I was married so I was exhausted from work and home. If I had known of these troubles, I would have chosen one of the two paths—marriage."[89]

How did the state regulate this expanding population of noncitizen nurses? According to a 1964 law, nurses practicing in Kuwait were required to hold a nursing license from the Ministry of Public Health. To obtain this license, the applicant had to have a recognized certificate or diploma. The application for the license required nurses to submit a birth certificate or a certificate of age issued by two doctors who were licensed to practice in Kuwait, proof of academic qualifications, testimony of good conduct and verification that the applicant's record was free from past crimes, a medical certificate verifying sound health, and a nationality certificate or passport with three photographs attached. The licensing process included a fee of five dinars. If the Ministry of Health's committee accepted the applicant, the nurse would be added to an official register. The ministry required nurses to keep them apprised of their place of residence. Nurses were subjected to a tiered punishment structure for breaking any of the regulations, which at its final stage could result in "revoking the license and striking the name off the register."[90]

Hospital administrators aimed to regulate the nurses' education level so that they were qualified to care for patients effectively, but not to the extent that they would challenge the authority of (predominantly male) doctors. The 1964 law stipulated nurses' subordination to doctors, stating that "anyone who is authorized to practice the nursing profession may not examine any person with a view to diagnose the disease nor may he provide any medical advice except by order of a physician authorized to practice the profession of human medicine or dentistry in Kuwait."[91] In 1965, Barjas Hammud al-Barjas, assistant undersecretary of the Ministry of Health and the official in charge of supervising Kuwait's nurses, declared that "nursing is in high crisis."[92] He noted that on his visits to Europe, he had observed how "the nurse has her dignity and respect in the street, in the society, and in the hospital among the patients and the doctors and the nursing staff." In Kuwait, in contrast, he declared that the nursing shortage and the poor quality of those nurses currently employed was due to "society's perception of this profession" (omitting the possibility that low salaries and poor working conditions hindered the recruitment of nurses). He acknowledged Egypt's leading role in producing nurses, but he also pointed to a "major problem" in Egyptian nurse training. "All the female graduates from the Higher Institute of Nursing," he explained, "demand equal treatment with doctors, and the women demanded leadership positions in the hospitals." By seeking higher education, he argued, nurses were forgetting their mandate to care for the basic needs of the patient—and to remain subordinate to the doctor. When the journalist asked al-Barjas what he thought about women who received advanced degrees in nursing in the United States, he laughed and replied, "This poor guy is sick, he can't leave his own bed, what is he doing with someone who has a doctorate?"[93]

Such attitudes mirrored post–World War II hostility toward advanced education for nurses in the United States, where health officials sought to discourage nurses from "legislating and educating themselves out of jobs."[94] While nurses, in al-Barjas's view, were missing the point of their profession if they obtained too much education, he also complained, "Our nurses are ignorant, and not interested in culture."[95] As evidence, he noted that Kuwait's nurses did not show interest in the magazines "specializing in the nursing profession" that the ministry provided in the nurses' housing. Instead, as we learn later in the same article, the nurses "tear the magazine and wrap their sandwiches in it."[96] Constrained by low salaries, limited rights as temporary residents, gendered expectations of patient care, and institutionalized ceilings limiting their education, it is little surprise that Kuwait's nurses fell short of al-Barjas's ideal.

The Exemplary Virgin Nurse

Consistent with standards for nurses around the world, Kuwait's unmarried nurses were subjected to a highly gendered set of expectations regarding their private, as well as professional, deportment. Charlotte Dale's summary of these attitudes in the Anglo-Boer War in Southern Africa also reflects the situation in Kuwait. She writes that "there were only two types of nurse: the 'good nurse,' presented as a self-sacrificing angel, a woman ready to deny all in her dedication to those within her care; or her polar opposition, the 'bad nurse.' This was a woman willing to abuse her position of 'power and authority' for her own means." In this rhetorical dichotomy, "nurses were often depicted as 'sexless white angels' or as 'predatory' and 'highly sexualized' women."[97]

Sexually compromising situations—or the appearance of such situations—was an unavoidable and constant concern for Kuwait's nursing staff. As one older nurse, expressing a sense of maternal responsibility for her younger colleagues, stated: "Every young woman was exposed to indiscretion and in need of advice. And everyone who opens her heart to me and considers me as her mother, I give her advice to avoid incidents that damage her reputation."[98] One young nurse who seems to have followed such advice to "avoid incidents that damage her reputation" was Nawal al-Mir'ibi. In a 1966 article titled "Angels of Mercy: Nawal al-Mir'ibi is an Exquisite Example," a sly male journalist posed as a patient to capture a candid interview with the reticent nurse. "In Kuwait," he tells us, "a very large number of angels of mercy are distributed among all the hospitals, sanatoriums, and clinics . . . in humanitarian service, silently, conscientiously, and willingly." The newspaper, apparently, had attempted several times to obtain an interview with this particular "exquisite example of the human female nurse," but she "always apologized, avoiding the questions with tact, courtesy, and kindness." Despite her persistent refusal, one journalist finally managed to have a "brief meeting with her" by claiming to be a patient in her ward.

The ensuing interview, as it was reported, captured both the idealistic professionalism and sexual allure and innocence of the young nurse. Nawal al-Mir'ibi responded to questions "with a lively smile" and "in her lovely Lebanese accent." Nawal al-Mir'ibi had studied nursing in Syria. Echoing Jamila Fadil Khoury, she tells the journalist-patient that nurses are "akin to anonymous soldiers, doing their humanitarian duty silently." The ideal nurse should "shy away from the limelight, avoiding attention," just as

Nawal al-Mirʿibi did by refusing a formal interview. Even if she saw herself as a soldier, the journalist, speaking with the authority of one of her patients, described Nawal al-Mirʿibi as "extremely sensitive, her feelings are delicate. If a patient cries, she cries with him. And if he is hurt, she shares his pain." Moreover, even when the patient "complains and grumbles," her response was to "be more patient, and calm, and faithful, to serve him and to mitigate his suffering." Her greatest wish, she told him, is for "humanity to triumph over every disease, and for the world to live in health and wellness and understanding and peace!"

After capturing her views on these lofty ideals, the journalist pushed the conversation toward more personal matters. He asked her about love, and she replied, "I don't know anything about it, because I didn't experience it." Then he asked about marriage: "Not yet, she said in her Lebanese mountain dialect, her cheeks turning red!" But by the time he got around to quizzing Nawal on her ideal man, she finally realized what was going on. "Suddenly, before she could answer the ring of the bell from one of the patients' rooms, she asked with surprise, 'Why all these questions and answers? Is it for publication?'" The article ends ironically with the journalist-patient's quick reply, "It is not for publication. Never!" The tabloidesque entertainment of the "patient" interview is in the pursuit of an ideal but inaccessible, young, and sexually inexperienced woman nurse. If she had openly agreed to an interview, she would have lost the allure of retiring modesty and exposed herself to reprimand from her superiors. Instead, he must trick her into speaking in the hospital corridors by lying to her.[99]

While the "patient" depicted his hallway conversation with Nawal al-Mirʿibi as harmless flirtation, other accounts reveal the great lengths that nurses had to go to toward protecting their reputations—as well as their personal safety—from any taint of sexual or romantic encounters in the workplace. In 1968, a woman journalist, Mufida Hilmi, conducted a long investigative report on the state of Kuwaiti nursing, provocatively titled "The Angels of Mercy Are in Hell!" She met with a group of nurses at Al-Sabah hospital, including their director Wadiʿa Harb and nurses from Lebanon, Sudan, Egypt, Jordan, and Kuwait. But Hilmi ventured into uncomfortable territory when she asked the assembled nurses, "How does the nurse respond when she is exposed to the patient's flirtation—or the doctor's pursuit?" Harb, the nurses' supervisor, immediately swooped into the conversation, cutting off the possibility of the younger nurses responding. She declared: "Ignoring is the right way. No rejection and no reaction. As for the doctor, if he allows himself, and his morals are such that he flirts with the nurse, it is upon her to do her work and leave the place to him empty." Harb further revealed that "there is an alert for sisters if the doctor enters their room." When nurses became aware of the presence of an ill-behaved doctor, "they leave the room and busy themselves with the patient." Evening shifts were of particular concern, so one nurse "is not left alone." Harb's instructions covered every possible hospital space: "If the doctor gets on the elevator, the nurse takes the stairs to avoid embarrassment." If a doctor persisted to the point that the supervisor took notice, then "without her knowing and without her making an issue out of it and in order to preserve her reputation, [the nurse would be transferred] to another department on the pretext that she is gaining new experience."[100]

Young and unmarried nurses were expected to maintain a virginal ideal while not drawing attention to any predatory behavior from men they encountered in the hospital, whether doctors or patients. A defining concern of professional life for the nurses entailed arranging their movements, their behavior, and even care for their patients in ways that would reduce the risk of potentially dangerous and reputation-threatening encounters with men. When undesirable overtures did occur, the official response was to remove the nurse without drawing attention to her, all the while making every effort to avoid causing any friction with the perpetrator. Kuwait's nurses were under constant scrutiny as potential sexual deviants, but men who might place them in compromising situations were carefully shielded from blame or embarrassment.

Nurses at Home and on the Town
The combination of gendered tensions over the intimate nature of hospital care, stereotypes of sexually loose nurses, and a patriarchal and family-centered citizenship structure generated anxiety among health officials.

At work, nurses followed an intricate—if unwritten—set of procedures to avoid reputation-damaging mishaps. Outside of work, the state controlled their movements and interactions through a list of regulations on permissible and forbidden activities. The Ministry of Health's assistant undersecretary Barjas Hammud al-Barjas clarified the logic behind these rules: "The motivation for this is so that the nurses feel safe, and also so that the family feels safe that their daughters are under supervision." For al-Barjas, "The Ministry plays the role of mother and father." He explained, for example, that the nurse must return to her housing by nine at night because "I do not think that a girl living with her family would be allowed to remain out of the house later than 9:00 in the evening."[101]

Unmarried nurses lived in housing provided by the Ministry of Health. The health zone of Kuwait's 1959 Hospital Master Plan included hostels for nurses and doctors.[102] An anonymous 1968 letter to a newspaper from a nurse residing in state housing demonstrates that not all the nurses appreciated the ministry's paternalism. She complained, "We are working hard all day and if we go back to our housing there are strict laws that make housing an air-conditioned prison!" She sent the newspaper "a copy of the system applied in the residence" so that the reader might "see for yourself the extent of the 'harassment' that puts pressure on our nerves, in addition to the torment of alienation." The article analyzed some of the enclosed regulations for the paper's readers, which included a total of eighteen rules. For example, nurses were allowed to extend the nine o'clock curfew by half an hour twice a month "with the intention of attending the cinema, and woe to the nurse if the film is a little bit longer than the time allowed in the system." Nurses could leave the residence in the company of a single man only if "this man carries written consent from the Ministry" or if he had a marriage contract approved by the ministry or was engaged with the knowledge and approval of the ministry.[103]

A notable—and much debated—difference between rules for single female nurses and teachers working in Kuwait had to do with means of transportation. Nurses were forbidden from riding in taxis, and a nurse could ride in a private car only if "she is with a family and this family should be familiar to the director of the residence, and write its name and the number of the car in the notebook prepared for this purpose."[104] Teachers, in contrast, were allowed to take taxis but were forbidden from riding in private cars unless they were with a relative, but they also had to return to their housing by six o'clock, a full three hours earlier than nurses. Kuwaitis regularly took taxis in the 1940s, but by the 1950s "citizens found it socially 'demeaning' to use such forms of public transportation, though it was acceptable for foreigners."[105] When a reporter asked Jamila Fadil Khoury about the discrepancy between transportation rules for single female teachers and nurses, she replied diplomatically that the Ministry of Health had "improved many of [the nurses'] social and housing conditions."[106]

The journalist writing in response to the anonymous nurse was more critical: "The designer of this system intended—no doubt—to protect the morality of the nurses and to not give them the opportunity to communicate with others." But the journalist expressed suspicion of the ministry's motives, "It appears that the ministry does not trust the morals of all the nurses it hires. Even those who have been around for a long time.... And we ask the officials, if you do not trust the old nurses who have been among us [for a long time] then why do you keep them? How do you allow those whose morals you do not trust to enter our homes and nurse our women?"[107]

Moreover, the Ministry of Health had recently made its rules more stringent in response to an undesirable (from its own perspective) event. While out with a family—which was permitted—a nurse "was introduced to the family's son" and they became engaged. The man "came to the ministry for approval as the system requires, and they got married." But following this incident, "the ministry issued its announcement forbidding [nurses from] going out with a family in case she gets to know his son and marries him." The journalist found that this was "strange logic." The article concluded, "All that remains is for the employees of the Ministry of Health to carry out night inspection campaigns in the nurses' residence to ensure that everyone is in their rooms—as morality police in Beirut check foreign women working in cabarets and bars."[108]

It is striking that a nurse's marriage to a (presumably) Kuwaiti man caused so much consternation that the Ministry of Health would alter its rules concerning nurses' socializing with families. Chris Rominger points out that for North Africans during World War I, "The kind of intimate contact already dangerous within the confines of the hospital could prove even more so when it moved to the civilian spaces of France," and by compromising the prestige of white women, "such encounters could overturn the entire colonial order."[109] In Kuwait, after the passage of the 1959 nationality law, "the Kuwaiti press was gripped by a panic over a rash of young Kuwaiti men marrying 'foreign' women."[110] Drawing on French, British imperial, and Ottoman precedent, and reflecting a framing that the British first introduced to the Gulf through the Bahrain nationality law, Kuwait's gendered citizenship laws defined "the family, rather than the person . . . as the basic unit of society."[111] By 1965, three years before the newspaper reported this incident of a noncitizen woman nurse marrying a Kuwaiti man, Kuwait's third national census had indicated that Kuwaitis were the demographic minority. In this context, "restrictions on female citizens' entitlements and the imposition of penalties on Kuwaiti women who married non-Kuwaitis also became policies aimed at social control and national boundary demarcation."[112] Unmarried noncitizen nurses appeared as a threat to the Kuwaiti family and, by extension, to Kuwaiti national cohesion.

The Fallen Nurse

The specter of illicit sexual contact and the terror of nurses mistreating helpless patients hovered over representations of the nurses in the press and in the laws and policies regulating their movements and interactions. As Sujani Reddy observes, "The stigmatization of their labor as both workers and (potential) wives" is "one of the primary ways in which nurses have appeared in the historical record."[113] But what happened when, despite the elaborate precautions in place to safeguard their reputations and prevent undesirable encounters, an unmarried nurse chose to participate in or was coerced into a romantic or sexual relationship? According to an article that asked, "What is behind the bold accusing hand that points to the nurses?" it seems that such an incident occurred in a rural clinic in 1964. Unfortunately the article never directly answers the tantalizing question that it poses in its title. But its vagueness is itself an indication not only of the sensitivity of the subject, but also of the fact that the Kuwaiti press was in the process of formulating a vocabulary through which it could articulate the intersecting problems of professional women and workplace sexual harassment.

The article's anonymous author set out for "the distant al-Maqwa village clinic in the desert" to meet with the clinic's director Regina Hadad, who "denied that one of the nurses was the type to warrant accusation." The reporter asked, "Why was a nurse put on trial?" Hadad explained, "The reasons that prompted the Ministry of Post and Telegraph to put the employee who works on the clinic's telephone and the nurse on trial were the employee's harassment and constant pursuit of her." The reporter was not satisfied with the explanation, especially after the director and the head doctor claimed, in contradiction to recent events, that "no problem has occurred in the clinic." The reporter declared that "the solution is to remove single women from the clinic" so as to "preserve [their] reputation and dignity." He further supported this proposal by claiming that single women's labor is not needed in isolated areas, as "the first aid man does the women's work, and even more. In that remote clinic, only some married nurses who are responsible and take their husbands into account should work." The solution, in short, was to "move [the single] women to the women's clinic where there is a need for more nurses" and thus "prevent the nurse from falling into immorality." The reporter was quick to point out that *he* was not trying to degrade nurses, but rather to protect them from negative assumptions. He explained, "This is a backwards view of women . . . the nurse's condition demands a comprehensive and thorough social study, and in light of this study, the Ministry of Health should carry out measures to preserve the dignity of nursing and the reputations of those who work in it!"[114]

Women nurses, gendered as caregivers, also came under attack when they were perceived as falling short of idealized feminine qualities in their treatment of patients and interactions with the public. On a visit to the women's sanatorium, one columnist was outraged when he found "my sick mother . . . sprawled on the bed with her hands tightly bound with rope strung on the edge of the bed, in a deplorable state of illness and neglect."

After untying his elderly mother and bringing her some water, which she could request only "by gesture because her mouth was injured," the columnist set off for the nurses' office to "clarify the situation." The woman responsible for the wing dismissed his complaints, declaring, "you don't understand anything . . . your mother leaves the sanatorium and torments us because we have to run after her."[115]

At this, the columnist was beside himself. He demanded to know: "How is it possible for my sick mother to go out of the sanatorium when she can't even leave her bed without help?" He wondered how his mother is supposed to receive basic care, such as a drink of water, and asked rhetorically, "How is it possible to express what you want if you cannot speak, and your hands are bound?" The columnist claimed that in the sanatorium, the nurses had enacted a "constitution" in order "to impose their total control over all patients." He pointed out the irony of this situation: "You see the nurse, who represents everything in humanity that is related to kindness and understanding, you see she shouts at and insults the patients . . . she scolds and slaps them as though the sanatorium is a prison and not a sanctuary for the sick." For this reporter, the solution to patient abuse was Kuwaitization of the nursing staff. He cited a local proverb, "Nothing can scratch an itch in your own skin like your own nail." The meaning, he believed, was that "our sanatoriums, especially the women's ones, are in desperate need of Kuwaiti nurses who are able to be understanding and kind with the female patients without arrogance."[116] In gendering nurses' labor as based in "kindness and understanding," he concluded that Kuwaiti women are best suited to care for sick Kuwaitis. He reasoned that because Kuwaiti women came from the same community, they would feel an emotional bond as caregivers, in stark contrast to the foreign workers who neglected patients like his mother.

Another patient's narrative suggests that the behavior of the nurses differed depending on the patient's class, revealing that all was not equal in the state's health-care system, even for Kuwaiti citizens. Following an ear operation, a nineteen-year-old girl spent nine months in and out of the hospital. She claimed that "in the public wing patients are treated like prisoners by the nurses. . . . I won't forget when a blind patient remained screaming all night asking for the sister's help. She heard her and didn't do her duty." In the private wing, in contrast, "the nurse is at your service." The woman reporter, Mufida Hilmi, decided to verify these claims by visiting the public wing of the hospital. Amid "patients and the ringing bells and the hustle and bustle," the nurse "appeared, her clothes the clothes of an angel, and her features the features of a devil." On seeing the visitors, the nurse "released a string of impolite words." But most alarming of all, Hilmi "witnessed a young man standing in the doorway of her private room." Hilmi described her thoughts as she walked away: "If this is her treatment of visitors and journalists, then how does she behave towards patients who are powerless?"[117]

Such implications of sexual misconduct and accusations of neglecting and abusing patients were serious indeed for a professional group that garnered credibility by enacting the feminine ideals of self-sacrifice and caregiving. They also reveal that in the 1960s, Kuwaitis were articulating a vision of medical care in the local media, and they were prepared to complain when state facilities and health-care professionals did not live up to their expectations. But the gendered standards of care were in flux, and nurses also used the press to speak back to unhappy patients and difficult hospital visitors.

In 1967, the same year that the reporter found that his mother was being abused in the sanatorium, a nurse who identified herself as "Safiyya from al-Ahmadi" wrote an open response to a Kuwaiti woman's previous complaint against the nurses in *Usrati*, a Kuwaiti women's publication.[118] "My dear Khaldiya lady," she wrote (identifying the woman by her Kuwaiti neighborhood), your previous letter contained "false accusations against nurses . . . that crossed boundaries and human values." Safiyya reminded the woman, "The nurse is a human, my dear lady, and not a stone—she feels and she gets angry." Safiyya also sought to clarify the nature of the relationship between a nurse and the hospital's patients and visitors. She wrote: "The nurse, my dear, is not a 'maid' as some imagine her to be. Rather, she is a human who has her dignity and her feelings." Where the investigative reporter to the rural clinic believed that single women should be removed from remote nursing posts, and the distressed son saw that the solution to nurse-patient relations was for nurses to be Kuwaitis rather than foreigners, Safiyya had a different remedy in mind. Safiyya suggested that what the disgruntled woman needed was to gain perspective on the nurse's working conditions. She declared, "How I wished you were in the place of the nurse you described in your letter, to see with your own eyes how the nurse suffers from exhaustion, oppression, and the harassment of some patients." Finally, Safiyya scolded the woman, and by extension, other women who might similarly complain rather than take action. She defended nurses by circling back to the idea that women contribute to the national project by becoming nurses: "The nation needs her labor more than it needs . . . these empty words." Safiyya suggested that it was the nurses in the hospitals (whether they were Kuwaiti citizens or not), rather than this woman writing incendiary letters from home, who were advancing the national interest.[119]

The (Failed) Kuwaitization of Nursing

The question of whether nurses were "angels of mercy" or fallen women in morally compromising situations came to a head in the state's efforts to produce Kuwaiti citizen nurses. In 1965, one journalist described the first generation of Kuwaiti women nurses as "the story of a long, bitter struggle against traditions."[120] The Ministry of Health and the Ministry of Education joined together to open a nursing institute in Kuwait in 1962. The government also opened a school for training nurses' assistants in 1964. By the 1969–1970 school year, eighty-six women students would graduate from the nursing institute. Forty-nine of them specialized in childbirth and women's diseases. Some of the women had gone abroad at the state's expense to continue their studies.[121] The Ministry of Health proclaimed that the institute "follows in its organization the highest level of education reached by the finest nations in the world." It emphasized a patient-centered approach that focused on "caring for [the patient] during his illness so that he can recover his health and lead a normal life."[122] The state's desire to recruit nurses locally materialized in nurses' salaries: in 1965, foreign nurses in Kuwait made fifty-one dinars per month; Kuwaiti nurses were paid eighty-seven dinars.[123]

For Jamila Fadil Khoury, the presence of Kuwaiti women on the nursing staff was "a benefit for all female nurses." She explained the cultural shift somewhat quixotically in 1965: "The Kuwaiti citizen has come to believe that the profession of the female nurse is a noble and honorable profession, like the soldier who carries a weapon, defending his country with courage and honor." In one of her interviews, Khoury "smiled and looked at a picture in front of her of the first group of girls in the nursing institute of Kuwait," and she described the girls as "youthful vanguards" and "a picture of our own lives. A picture of the reality of every girl raised living in a bigoted environment."[124] For Khoury, the production of Kuwaiti women nurses was the culmination of a career in which she sought to normalize Arab women's professionalization as nurses. As a government employee, Khoury was likely making an argument for how she *hoped* society would view Kuwaiti nurses rather than representing current realities.

Relative to the total quantity of nurses working in Kuwait, the numbers of Kuwaiti nurses remained small. Nevertheless, the press praised "the role played by the Kuwaiti girl" in this field as "a wonderful patriotic act."[125] In 1968, once a graduate of Kuwait's nursing institute passed exams in biology, chemistry, Arabic, and English, she could enroll for further study in Egypt. Mufida Hilmi interviewed some of these women, whom she called angels "on the way to the top," in the office of the dean of Kuwait's nursing institute. 'A'isha Salih, twenty years old, had joined the nursing institute at age fifteen. We learn that "her entry into the institute was a story of struggle with the family," especially with her uncle who "adamantly opposed that his niece become a nurse" even though he worked in the Ministry of Health. But 'A'isha was enamored of the idea of becoming a nurse after "the dean of the nursing institute visited the schools and held lectures highlighting the importance of the institute." 'A'isha enlisted doctors and health-care workers to convince her uncle, and eventually "she got what she wanted."[126] This narrative emphasizes 'A'isha's role as an agent of change within her family as she convinces them that nursing is, in fact, a respectable profession for a Kuwaiti woman.

Even as Kuwaiti women were praised for serving the nation as nurses, they also faced specific constraints. One of them revealed that "it is forbidden for the Kuwaiti nurse to work in the men's ward." In other words, foreign women were subjected to greater risk to their reputations in the workplace. Moreover, the nurses' choices of specialization emphasized their purity but also minimized the likelihood of their encounters with men: ʿAʾisha worked with children "because sick children need tenderness and care." Another Kuwaiti nurse, ʿAwataf al-Qattan, claimed that her happiest memory of work was "entering the delivery room and receiving the first child in my hands—I feel I have contributed to the reception of a new life." But al-Qattan also declared that "if marriage comes and it stands between me and the profession then I refuse marriage, for our country needs our services." Delivering and caring for the nation's children allowed this Kuwaiti nurse to fulfill her national role while avoiding contact with potentially threatening male patients. When Layla ʿAli was asked whether Kuwaiti nurses faced problems, she replied: "Never. We, the Kuwaiti girls, have a message that must be performed to meet the needs of the country in this field. Every profession has its troubles, but can be overcome with patience and level headedness."[127]

Despite the optimism expressed by some of the first Kuwaiti nurses, by the early 1970s, not only were attempts to Kuwaitize nursing failing, but also the Ministry of Health was struggling to recruit nurses from other Arab countries. In the midst of a wider "reverse migration" of Arab workers out of the Gulf in 1973, the minister of health toured the Arab world in an effort to address Kuwait's persistent nursing shortage.[128] The ministry projected that Kuwait would need three thousand additional nurses by 1977, but in Egypt, the minister of health could secure only thirty nurses. He also came up short in Lebanon, Syria, and Jordan. Meanwhile, in Kuwait, the nursing institute that the ministry had opened in the 1960s had produced 320 graduates, but only 38 of them were actually at work in Kuwaiti health institutions.[129] In the early twentieth-century United States, "white Southerners tended to associate nursing with black women's low-status servant work and shied away from the profession."[130] Similarly in Kuwait, because the state did not respond to its failure to recruit Kuwaiti, and even Arab nurses, by improving their professional status, the nursing profession failed to gain prestige and respectability.[131]

In 1973, flush with oil wealth, the Ministry of Health's response to the shortfall was to send a delegation, headed by Jamila Fadil Khoury, to

Bombay. Like the British Empire in an earlier era, Kuwait turned to South Asian labor as a cost-cutting measure. No longer promoting pan-Arab development through the recruitment of Arab women nurses, in Bombay, Khoury planned to hire 540 nurses for government hospitals and clinics, "despite some problems that usually occur due to the fact that the Indian women do not know Arabic."[132] The ministry hoped that the nurses would be tempted by a salary that offered as much as 50 percent more than what they earned in India. This shift to Indian labor in the wake of failing to recruit Kuwaiti women to the nursing profession also represented part of a global pattern in which "Kerala nurses emerged as 'the' Indian nurse migrant" during the 1970s.[133] By the 1980s, nurses would constitute the majority of skilled Indian labor in the Gulf region, joining a population of colleagues from around the world.[134]

Nurses in the Public Sphere

In the 1960s, Kuwait's residents scrutinized the presence of professional and frequently unmarried women who had migrated from other Arab countries to work as nurses. The press served as a platform to criticize nurses' morality, their commitment to their profession, and their treatment of patients. Jamila Fadil Khoury articulated this uneasy dynamic between nurses and the Kuwaiti press: "The nurse works in an atmosphere of physical and psychological exhaustion, carrying huge responsibilities—people's lives. What is most needed is society's encouragement, not destructive criticism."[135] Another nurse, writing anonymously, presented the problem more directly. She stated that "the press attacks nurses for any slight mistake that one of them may make. The patients grumble if a nurse enters any department and the usual smile is not painted on her lips."[136] Such remarks reveal that nurses themselves were well aware of their manifold responsibilities of managing day-to-day health-care operations and navigating the gendered expectations of women caregivers. The tension between the reliance on poorly compensated and carefully surveilled women workers for powering health care and the lofty promises of the welfare system resulted in an erasure of noncitizen women from histories of state building. In recovering nurses' voices and experiences through a close reading of the local press, this chapter has sought to place women workers at the center of social history in postwar Kuwait.

Arab nurses like Jamila Fadil Khoury in 1960s Kuwait envisioned medical projects through the conjoined frameworks of development and modernization. The next chapter, however, challenges the linearity of the standardization of biomedicine through state institutions by examining the resurgence of *al-ṭibb al-shaʿbī* (folk medicine) in the 1990s and early 2000s as a form of nativist nostalgia. Despite the massive investment in biomedical infrastructure and personnel, nonstate cultures of health did not disappear with the emergence of state medicine. In the late twentieth and early twenty-first centuries, nostalgia for the pre-oil period and nativism in the face of a large noncitizen population prompted citizens of the Gulf region to articulate an alternative history of medicine that emphasized folk medicine as an indigenous tradition.

CHAPTER 6

FOLK MEDICINE

IN HIS 2012 BOOK on Qatari healers, the local historian Khalifa al-Sayyid Mohammad Salih al-Maliki describes a time when one of his informants fled the state hospital in favor of a folk healer. When Mohammad al-Karani felt a searing pain in his stomach, al-Maliki recounts, his brother Ahmad rushed him to Doha's central hospital. The hospital's doctors examined him, discovered that his appendix was inflamed, and prepared Mohammad for surgery. But victims from an accident flooded the emergency room just moments before the procedure, and the doctors departed to care for the new patients. At that, Ahmad, Mohammad's brother, declared, "Enough [*khalāṣ*]! Get dressed, we'll go home, and I'll bring 'Abd al-Rahman Mazmun to you." They left the hospital, and Mazmun came to examine Mohammad in his house. The healer requested a bowl of water and then "went to a place no one could see." When he returned, he commanded Mohammad: "Drink this water! For in it is your medicine and God will heal you!" Mohammad drank the water, curing his appendicitis and relieving his pain.[1]

Writing from the early twenty-first century, al-Maliki evokes an ambiguous temporality in which modern hospitals and folk medicine coexist. Typical of his narrative style, al-Maliki does not date this vignette of healing precisely, although he tells us that Mazmun worked from the 1930s until his death in the 1970s. Doha's first hospital opened in 1947, so Mohammad's medical emergency probably occurred in the 1960s or 1970s, although al-Maliki conducted his oral histories decades later.[2] In al-Maliki's account,

Mohammad and his brother Ahmad experience the trip to Doha's state hospital as alienating and impersonal. The doctors, nameless professionals and probably (like the nurses discussed in chapter 5) noncitizen employees, diagnosed, or perhaps misdiagnosed, the ailment and prepared the procedure. But when a more pressing emergency called them away, they abandoned Mohammad, who was undressed and on the verge of an invasive surgery. Unwilling to wait, the brothers returned home and summoned a known Qatari healer, 'Abd al-Rahman Mazmun. Al-Maliki leaves the mechanisms that made Mazmun's treatment effective unexplained, but the vanishing pain offers ample proof of its success. The brothers in this narrative eschewed the progression from the disorder of acute pain to the neat resolution of diagnosis and scientific cure offered by modern medicine. Instead, with an air of triumph, al-Maliki suggests that it is better to seek healing from someone in your own community who will cure you in your home than to receive treatment from expatriate surgeons in an impersonal institution who might abandon you at your most vulnerable moment.

This narrative of fluid health seeking between hospital and home reminds us that people in Arabia did not necessarily experience medical modernization as a linear transition from traditional to modern practices; nor, in the late twentieth and early twenty-first centuries, did they always view modern medicine as beneficial. Indeed, even when offered up-to-date services, people sometimes turned to folk practices. Locally produced Arabic-language histories of healing from the late twentieth and early twenty-first centuries reveal that nostalgic discussions of *al-ṭibb al-sha'bī* (folk medicine) emerged as an alternative to state-driven medical projects. The category of *al-ṭibb al-sha'bī* as it is used to describe medical practices in this region generally includes cautery (*al-kayy*), cupping (*al-ḥijāma*; expanding blood vessels by using cups to create suction on the skin), prescribing herbal medicines, setting broken bones (*al-tajbīr*), attending to women's and children's health and midwifery (see chapter 3), and religious healing rituals such as reading the Qur'an over a patient (*al-ruqya*).

Through a socially situated discursive analysis of two texts, this chapter illustrates how the collecting and recording of memories of *al-ṭibb al-sha'bī* is a politicized act that seeks to delineate who is included and excluded in the modern Gulf nation. First, ʿAbd Allah ʿAli al-Tabur's 1996 book *Al-Tibb al-Shaʿbi fi al-Imarat al-ʿArabiyya al-Muttahida* (Folk medicine in the United Arab Emirates) draws on interviews, research, and his own knowledge and observations to describe medical practices in Emirati history.[3] In his discussion of the presence of magical practices in the region's past, al-Tabur registers his disapproval and, ultimately, he sanitizes the historical landscape by displacing magical practices from elite male society onto women and enslaved people. The second section explores the oral history that opens this chapter. Al-Maliki's 2012 study *Jawab Kull Saʾil ʿind Muʿalijin Qatar al-Awaʾil* (Answer for every questioner from the early healers of Qatar) portrays the healers who practiced *al-ṭibb al-shaʿbī* in Qatar over the course of the twentieth century with reverence and embellishes their personal qualities to the point of saintliness. In his biographies of male and female healers, their acts of caring for members of the national community constitute strong evidence of their virtuous status, whereas noncitizen populations remain invisible. Although the two texts differ in their valuation of traditional medical practice, both represent *al-ṭibb al-shaʿbī* as an indigenously Arab counterpoint to the hypermodern lifestyles, demographic insecurities, urban spaces, and biomedical facilities of the post-oil Gulf states.

Approaching *al-ṭibb al-shaʿbī* as a discourse and a cultural project of the late twentieth and early twenty-first centuries reminds us not to think of biomedicine as a narrative of progress in which scientifically proven formulas continuously displace existing cultures of health. Instead, local health practices persist, change over time, and assume heightened political significance in an age of ethnic nationalism and demographic angst. As I have shown in previous chapters, medicalization in the Gulf was not characterized by the collision of fully formed and mutually exclusive spheres of indigenous and Western medicine. Rather, it unfolded contingently as healers and health seekers creatively drew from hybrid and fluctuating assemblages of practices and ideologies.

In contrast to representing a complex medical heritage that incorporated multiple traditions, these texts prioritize cultural authenticity over scientific or technical innovation. The authors suggest that *al-ṭibb al-shaʿbī* has survived the ruptures of the oil economy unchanged, enduring as a repository of the nation. Although they do not discount the benefits of modern medicine, many interlocuters in these texts express a sense of alienation resulting from institutionalized and bureaucratized care. As in this chapter's opening vignette, when Mohammad and his brother flee the hospital and its expatriate staff for the safety of their home and the comfort of a known healer, hegemonic modern medicine emerges as a foil for *al-ṭibb al-shaʿbī*.

Yet even as the two texts contribute to the larger project of politicizing heritage, tensions emerge in the oral histories of *al-ṭibb al-shaʿbī* that constitute the authors' repositories of data. On the one hand, the authors seek to demonstrate that the folk healers of the pre-oil community had valuable skills and genealogical authenticity, and performed important therapeutic acts. On the other hand, the narratives also reveal points of conflict and hierarchies of belonging in the national community. While the motivation to explore *al-ṭibb al-shaʿbī* is rooted in nativist politics, the grassroots methodology of oral history unsettles the idealized image of the past by uncovering contentious accounts of enslaved people, marginalized women, and magic.

Al-Ṭibb Al-Shaʿbī and the Politics of Heritage

Following the large-scale expansion of state medicine around the Gulf in the mid-twentieth century, measurable health outcomes drastically improved. As in other parts of the world, life expectancies became higher and child mortality rates lower; however, unlike residents of other regions, many people in the Gulf, especially those with the privileges of citizenship, came to enjoy free access to state-of-the-art health care.[4] Although epidemic and infectious diseases continue to pose a major threat to the global population, the predominant health challenges of many Gulf residents (in step with those of other developed countries) shifted toward concerns like diabetes, obesity, and heart disease. But even as overall health outcomes improved, nostalgia for *al-ṭibb al-shaʿbī* permeated local discourse and historical memory, and, decades after medical modernization, a media-driven cultural nostalgia for folk medicine registered an enthusiastic following in the late twentieth century.

A comparison to the politicization of indigenous medical systems in India as essentialist repositories of culture reveals how medical nostalgia in the Gulf connects to a global narrative. Like folk medicine in the Gulf, India's curative landscape is not a holdover from an authentic, precolonial past, but the result of unpredictable patterns of exchange and mutual influence, mediated by class, caste, and gender, as well as by colonial imbalances of power. Projit Bihari Mukharji, for example, traces how Ayurvedic physicians of late nineteenth- and early twentieth-century Bengal braided together strands of knowledge from multiple traditions, creating new meanings and altering the terms of cultural exchange.[5] In the postcolonial era, the cultural meanings of India's indigenous medical systems have come to reflect the violence and politics of nationalism. As Richard Weiss has pointed out, professional differences between traditional medical practitioners "closely parallel the political divisions that developed with Indian nationalism. Hindu/Muslim tensions are reflected in ayurveda/unani formulations, while an emergent Tamil revivalism has characterized siddha medicine as absolutely distinct from ayurveda."[6] Politicians have co-opted such affiliations between medicine and religion. A government representative of India declared in 2016, for example, that doctors who advised patients against ayurvedic medicines are "anti-nationals."[7] In 2017, the Hindu nationalist prime minister Narendra Modi inaugurated the first All India Institute of Ayurveda in Delhi, and he has encouraged private investment in Ayurveda-inspired research.[8] While sectarianism is a persistent political concern in the Gulf, religious politics are not mapped onto indigenous medicine as starkly as they are in South Asia. Instead, carefully policed binaries of citizen and noncitizen and indigenous Arab and foreigner (I discuss these categories subsequently) find their medical cultural expression in nostalgic formulations of *al-ṭibb al-shaʿbī* that assume an Islamic but also autochthonous orientation.

My examination of *al-ṭibb al-shaʿbī* joins a robust scholarship that has traced how late twentieth- and early twenty-first-century Gulf states sought to bolster their legitimacy through efforts to preserve local heritage (*turāth*). As Amal Sachedina writes, heritage projects eliminate "alternative histories by substantiating a homogenous national territorial community while directing its efforts to recalibrate the relationship between past and present."⁹ In a pioneering critique of how Gulf heritage projects depoliticize history, Ahmed Kanna argues that the Emirati state represents itself as the guardian of "ethno-nationally inflected values" and claims to protect "the citizenry from the threats posed" by what many perceive as the cultural danger of demographic imbalance between citizens and noncitizens.¹⁰ He explains how nativist heritage discourse emerged as central to state building in the late twentieth century by way of effacing earlier contested histories and political possibilities: "mid-twentieth-century nationalist discourses of self-determination," in which a range of political movements offered alternative futures to Gulf autocracy, "transformed into late twentieth and early twenty-first century discourses of economic autochthony and ethno-nationalism."¹¹ Building on Kanna's work, Farah Al-Nakib further traces how recent heritage projects seek to erase the political legacy of mid-twentieth-century movements. She writes, "The exaggerated contrast between the composed antiquated tableaus of the pre-oil past and the contemporary Gulf city's hypermodern skyline projects a smooth, linear, teleological narrative of progress, a jump from then to now that serves to emphasize the magnitude and magnificence of the present. But this narrative leaves something crucial out: at least three or four decades of what happened in between the pre-oil past and the 'globalized' present."¹² Al-Nakib reminds us that in the period following World War II, far from clinging to a vanishing past, local people deliberately and enthusiastically sought to transform their built environments, politics, and ways of life. By rebranding the pre-oil past as a source of nostalgia, heritage projects of the late twentieth and early twenty-first centuries expunge and depoliticize histories of local people who creatively "embraced new ways of being modern."¹³

Discussions of *al-ṭibb al-shaʿbī* in the late twentieth- and early twenty-first-century Arabian Peninsula emerge out of two coexisting narratives of national heritage. In the first narrative, recent accounts of *al-ṭibb al-shaʿbī* emphasize the category of Gulf Arab culture as spatially, ethnically, religiously, and nationally unified in ways that differentiate the citizen population from noncitizen residents. That is, cultural productions of medical nostalgia operate as one thread in a vast assemblage that maintains the citizen-noncitizen binary and, by extension, discursively flattens hierarchies among citizens. Citizens who enjoy privileged access to state resources, including health care, benefit from efforts to highlight the cultural unity of the Gulf Arab population across time and within national space. Meanwhile, the faces of expatriate residents, including those who provide labor and expertise in modern biomedical institutions (such as the hospital workers in this chapter's opening vignette or the noncitizen nurses discussed in chapter 5), remain nameless and external to the community in these accounts. In the second narrative, the acts of praising and practicing *al-ṭibb al-shaʿbī* in contemporary Gulf states occur in reaction to the institutionalized nature of modern biomedicine. As I unpack in the following sections, al-Tabur's and al-Maliki's texts represent *al-ṭibb al-shaʿbī* as an intrinsically social and communal experience. They highlight the personal relationship between the healer and the patient, in contrast to the alienating bureaucracies that the texts allude to as characteristic of modern medicine. Such accounts draw on oral histories to displace the primacy of scientific progress in valuing the medical experience.

Most translations of *al-ṭibb al-shaʿbī* miss the contextual nuance of this phrase.[14] *Al-ṭibb*, which means "medical treatment," "medicine," or "medical science," can refer to modern biomedicine, but it also has a rich linguistic history in relation to traditional forms of healing, as well as humoral medicine as discussed in classical Arabic-language medical texts. *Shaʿbī* is the adjective form of *al-shaʿb*, which can mean "people," "folk," or "nation."[15] In reference to mid-twentieth-century Arab nationalist parlance, *al-shaʿb* has been translated as "the people," meaning, in one example, "a social group formed by Iraq's geography, natural traditions, and history."[16] In a political context, it also can refer to the "masses," or even the totality of the nation as represented in the now famous cry of the 2011 revolutions, "al-shaʿb yurīd isqāṭ al-niẓām!" ("the people want the overthrow of the regime").

Shaʿbī also is frequently denoted as "folk," as in folk literature or folk music. Similar to *folk* in English, *shaʿbī* has taken on distinct class and cultural connotations. The category of *shaʿbī* music in Egypt exemplifies these dynamics. Ted Swedenburg locates the origins of *shaʿbī* music in the *ashwa'iyyat*, "unplanned settlements that teem with the poor, working and lower middle classes" where around half of Cairo's population reside.[17] He explains, "*Sha'bī* music, rooted in the *'ashwa'iyyat* as well as the traditional popular quarters of Cairo, has long been derided as unsophisticated at best by Egypt's educated elites."[18] *Sha'bī* music emerged in the 1970s, and Daniel J. Gilman translates the term idiomatically as "working-class music."[19] He writes, "Although it is highly stigmatized among the *haute bourgeoisie*, who consider the musical genre part of a low-taste culture, a great many Cairenes listen to *sha'bi* at least once in a while," and appreciate its "potential for bawdiness" and "the possibility of commenting directly on social matters."[20] In Egypt, the central socioeconomic tensions are between a small percentage of Egyptian elites, who control most of the country's resources and live in increasingly isolated residential and commercial developments, and the vast majority of the population of citizens, who dwell in poverty, are neglected by the state, and suffer from unreliable or nonexistent basic infrastructure, education, and health services. In this cultural setting, *sha'bī* has come to signify the difference between westernized and privileged elites and lower-class—but culturally authentic—"people" (*al-sha'b*). In contrast, in the late twentieth- and early twenty-first-century Arabian Peninsula, *sha'bī* has dramatically different cultural connotations given discomfort with demographic conditions in which Arabic-speaking citizens are in the minority and the working and lower classes are, in many cases, noncitizens. In this context, discussions of *al-ṭibb al-sha'bī* reflect ongoing politically and ideologically charged efforts to rebrand local culture as remnants of an authentic and pure nativist past.

Al-Tabur and al-Maliki employ the category of healer broadly to include not only anyone who practiced *al-ṭibb al-sha'bī* but also individuals who are remembered as indigenous Arab members of the protonation (with some revealing exceptions, which I discuss later in this chapter). In the Arabian Peninsula, as Mandana E. Limbert argues, "Arabness" has a meaning beyond a presumption of shared identity based on language. Instead, "the term 'Arab' has referred primarily to a person who is from Arabia and who is patrigenealogically *not* a servant (a descendent of a slave)."[21] Arabness is inherited through the father. Cultural values, manners, and behavior are associated with "good" Arabness, but phenotypic variation is less indicative given long histories of marriage and concubinage between Arab men and partners around the Indian Ocean world, particularly East Africa.[22] But Limbert further notes that a focus on "Arabness" as geographically tied to the Arabian Peninsula has "reoriented identification away from the Indian Ocean."[23] To be a folk healer and the subject of these nostalgic renditions is, first, to exemplify idealized behavior in the form of service and commitment to the geographically delineated national community and, second, to be recognized as genealogically part of that community. *Sha'bī* healers embody and safeguard proper Muslim values and preserve the hierarchies of the social order. Furthermore, representations of their authority in the past reflect gendered values of the present. The most revered male healers are depicted as wise elites who combined political status with medical acumen, whereas women healers generally confined their skills to domestic or interpersonal tasks such as midwifery, children's health, or Qur'an reading. Finally, when folk medical traditions as reported in oral histories fall short of the standards of "good Arabness" in the present, unsavory practices are ascribed to women and lower-status or enslaved people rather than to the community's leading men.

The somewhat vague temporality of Gulf society "before oil" is generally when nationalist accounts locate mythologized cultural and communal identities. The exact date that oil was discovered varies by state: in Bahrain in 1932; in Saudi Arabia, Kuwait, and Qatar in the late 1930s; and in the regions that became the United Arab Emirates and Oman in the late 1950s and 1960s. Despite this wide time frame, the scramble for oil and the anticipation of its discovery deeply implicated the politics and social fabric of the entire region during the mid-twentieth century. In the contemporary Gulf, notions of time are inseparable from the wealth and environmental destruction of the oil economy. Limbert explains how interlocuters in Oman conceptualized a "problem of time" in which the present was "sandwiched between the rapidity of change from the past and the threat to the depletion of oil in the future."[24] With increasing urgency, other scholarship predicts that as a result of climate change, Gulf cities could become too hot for human habitation in the coming decades.[25]

Al-ṭibb al-shaʿbī occupies a dual temporality in these textual accounts. In the first temporality, it signifies the medical practices of the local Arab community (represented as the national community) in the period before oil wealth. The second temporality depends on the fact that biomedicine had achieved such a degree of prominence following several decades of national development in the late twentieth-century Gulf that it came to permeate state-society relations through the privilege of universal care for citizens and, to some extent, other Gulf residents. Local people could enjoy the privilege of nostalgia for a time of lesser overall health but—in their rendition—greater communal unity and cultural purity. In this conceptualization, *al-ṭibb al-shaʿbī* becomes an immutable cultural artifact as well as a foil to biomedicine as an alienating and overly institutionalized experience. Its practitioners transcend the temporal break of pre- and post-oil by continuing to provide and to memorialize *al-ṭibb al-shaʿbī* despite the prevalence of state-provided biomedicine.

Finally, an important methodological point in grappling with these texts is that the nationalist use of *al-ṭibb al-shaʿbī* as a marker of authentic culture makes it particularly difficult to tease out change over time in local medical practices. The textual representations of *al-ṭibb al-shaʿbī* examined here draw heavily on oral interviews the authors conducted with Gulf citizens, whereas noncitizen residents remain outside their narrative scope.[26] A belief in or desire for the continuity of cultural traits despite the transformations brought by the oil economy and the wish to "preserve" these cultures have been important motivations to conduct oral histories for scholars who draw on nationalist framings of history.

Displacing Magical Medicine onto Enslaved People and Women

ʿAbd Allah ʿAli al-Tabur grapples with the recurring theme of healing practices infused with magic in his oral histories on *al-ṭibb al-shaʿbī* in the Emirates. In his chapter "The Magical Recipes" (*al-waṣfāt al-siḥriyya*), he reconciles contemporary discomfort with practices that might appear unsavory or even un-Islamic by suggesting that magical practices, while undeniably present in the Emirates of the past, represent external corruptions of authentic national history. Yet in identifying magical healing practices among enslaved people and women, al-Tabur introduces uncomfortable social tensions into the idealized historical landscape. On the one hand, al-Tabur's depiction of those who engaged in magical medicine expresses his repudiation of these practices and his desire to demonstrate that magic was never part of mainstream or respectable Emirati folk culture. On the other hand, the fact that he includes this chapter on magical treatments in his book on *al-ṭibb al-shaʿbī* demonstrates how suppressed histories of enslavement reemerge in oral histories when local researchers are committed to representing their interlocuters' narratives. Al-Tabur's methodology of integrating a range of local voices into his analysis opens the door to a nuanced depiction of the Emirates' sociomedical past that incorporates social conflicts and exclusions.

Born in Ras Al Khaimah in 1964, al-Tabur graduated from United Arab Emirates University in 1986. He is a researcher and author whose publications demonstrate a long-standing interest in Emirati history and culture.[27] In al-Tabur's introduction, he describes how increasing national attention to *al-ṭibb al-shaʿbī* in the context of wider projects to preserve Emirati heritage (*turāth*) sparked his interest in this field. As early as 1985, he started conducting interviews with practitioners of *al-ṭibb al-shaʿbī*, "as well as with elderly people who hold knowledge of traditional treatments."[28] Although he locates his study in a global trend of preserving heritage, al-Tabur's primary audience is the group of Emirati nationals seeking to answer the call of Shaykh Zayed bin Sultan Al Nahyan (ruler of Abu Dhabi from 1966 to 2004; first president of the United Arab Emirates, from 1971 to 2004) to actively embrace their cultural history.

The Emirates, like other Gulf states, pursued large-scale biomedical projects in the mid-twentieth century. Al Maktum hospital in Dubai opened in 1949; a hospital at Ras Al Khaimah opened in 1963; and clinics, touring doctors, and a 1967 smallpox vaccination campaign further expanded the scope of care.[29] As in other Gulf cities, such institutions were central to the modernizing project. In the 1950s, for example, Al Maktum hospital "signaled Dubai as a legitimate place of welfare and safety."[30] But by the 1980s and 1990s, with biomedical care firmly established and state efforts to capture a depoliticized version of the pre-oil past underway, al-Tabur could look back at *al-ṭibb al-shaʿbī* with nostalgia. He places his research in the wider heritage project, writing, "In our time heritage is considered an established field, it has so many faculty and patrons and journals that it is difficult for us to mention them all here . . . they focus on protecting and preserving heritage as the cultural legacy of peoples and the creative history of nations."[31] Al-Tabur emphasizes state efforts to preserve heritage in the Emirates, and attributes this project to the ruling Shaykh. He explains, "The state of the Emirates assumed this responsibility, especially after the call of His Highness Shaykh Zayed bin Sultan Al Nahyan, head of the state, for the importance of returning to the heritage of forefathers in our contemporary lives, for he who doesn't have a past, doesn't have a present."[32] In this rendition, the act of preserving *al-ṭibb al-shaʿbī* is a top-down initiative that emphasizes the citizen-noncitizen binary by defining heritage genealogically. Al-Tabur places his own research within this larger national project.

For al-Tabur, postwar Emirati modernization does not represent a rupture between the modern state and Islamic heritage. Instead, he identifies the medical history of the contemporary Emirates as a continuation of the larger legacy of Islamic civilization. He divides his study into three sections: first, the development of the history of medicine in the Islamic world from ancient times through the Abbasid period; second, medicine in the Emirates, including discussions of the appearance of *al-ṭibb al-shaʿbī*, proverbs and sayings on *al-ṭibb al-shaʿbī*, and old methods of treatment; and third, diseases and their treatment in *al-ṭibb al-shaʿbī*, including religious methods and the use of magic.[33] The book also contains pictures of herbs traditionally used for medicine and a list of some of the famous healers of the Emirates. This list includes the name, region, and healing skills of 128 male healers and 59 women, divided by gender.[34]

Yet even in the category of *al-ṭibb al-shaʿbī* in the Emirates of the past, tensions over social status, gender, and religious orthodoxy surround some methods of healing. In his chapter on magical medicine, magic and its practitioners represent a threat to respectable members of the community. Al-Tabur resolves the tension between his derision of magical medicine and its recurrence among his informants by rendering magic as marginal to mainstream society. He sorts the participants in magic in Emirati society of the past into several categories. The first group are people who performed *zār* ceremonies. The term *zār* refers both to jinn who possess humans and to the healing rituals that are intended to placate those jinn, who in turn allow their human hosts to live a normal life. Magicians make up the second group. Al-Tabur describes the magicians' activities as harmful and claims that they practiced their arts "far from society" and "in secret."[35] The third group comprised those who carried out what he deems to have been benign magical activities like providing charms to be placed around the neck to protect the wearer from danger and illness. The final group were the seekers of these supernatural services, or "the victims who were easy prey . . . to the first three categories, and they were ignorant fools and women who did not find adequate protection from the man and the family."[36] He says, "Some commoners and simpletons among the people returned to magical explanations for some sicknesses like madness, mental illness, impotence, and paranoia."[37] Practitioners of magical medicine, in his depiction, were ignorant at best and crooked swindlers at worst. Al-Tabur contends that the local people who sought such care were naive victims.

Al-Tabur attempts to reconcile an image of Emirati society as appropriately Islamic according to late twentieth-century standards with the reality that practices that he condemns as magic appear frequently in his sources. He writes, "*Al-ṭibb al-shaʿbī* in the Emirates is connected to Islamic medicine. Islamic medicine has a general concept of creation and life and death . . . it includes all the expertise of Muslim peoples and Arab and Persian doctors, and it is far away from mysteries, magic, and sorcery."[38] Importantly, magical medicine predates Islam, which implies a connection between Emiratis who practice magical medicine and the period of pre-Islamic ignorance (*jāhiliyya*). He explains the pre-Islamic history of the practices: "The first to use the talisman and dances . . . in treating sicknesses and lesions were the Arab Semites . . . and in *al-jāhiliyya* the Arabs believed in jinn and demons as being both harmful and beneficial."[39] As Ana Vinea writes, jinn are "an uncontested part of Islamic cosmology," but their "empirical manifestations . . . particularly their ability to possess humans has been disputed and remains an unsettled question within the

Islamic tradition."⁴⁰ For al-Tabur, although he does not deny the reality of jinn, he associates belief in their meddling in human affairs with the time of ignorance before Islam. By locating magical medicine in a pre-Islamic time frame, he employs a temporality that dissociates the practices from Islam and a scripturalist modernity.

After noting the historical precedence of magical medicine in the pre-Islamic era, al-Tabur addresses how magic appears in the Islamic tradition. He raises both the presence of jinn in the Qur'an and the Prophet's denunciation of magical medicine, but he carefully avoids putting the two in conflict. Al-Tabur quotes Surat al-Jinn (Qur'an 72.6), "And there were men from mankind who sought refuge in men from the jinn, so they [only] increased them in burden,"⁴¹ and the hadith, "Punish the magician with the sword's blow."⁴² He explains the meaning: "When Islam came it invalidated [magic], and emphasized that it should not be practiced because it devastated human intellect and distanced the human being from his Creator."⁴³

Al-Tabur establishes, first, that magical medicine is an ancient and widespread phenomenon and, second, that Islam condemns those practices. For al-Tabur, Islam represents a historic break in medical practice in that the Islamic tradition reoriented Muslims away from magic and toward "human intellect." His narrative thus uses Islamic sources to prove that magical medicine predates Islam. Islam, in this account, reformed human society by forbidding such activities, thus opening the way for truly scientific medical discoveries. He distinguishes between the existence of jinn and magical practices that were condemned by the Prophet. In this reading, believing in jinn is not itself an act of magic, but ceremonies and behaviors that are performed in reaction to a belief in the presence of jinn or other supernatural forces are not acceptable.

For the purposes of reading al-Tabur's discussion of magic as a lens onto local historical experiences, one striking aspect of al-Tabur's discussion of *zār* is that he addresses the prevalence and practice of slavery in Emirati and Gulf history with unusual candor. In the early 1950s, there were an estimated two thousand enslaved people in the Trucial States and Buraimi.⁴⁴ As Matthew Hopper notes, however, state-sponsored museums, publications, and scholarship, consistently practice "deliberate omissions, sanitized accounts, and convenient (if awkward) editing" when it comes to the history of slavery in the region.⁴⁵ Amal Sachedina refers to the legacy of the slave trade in Oman as a "residue" that challenges state-driven attempts to present the national community as a "homogenous entity." For Omanis, she writes, "slavery's ongoing legacy has been conditioned by the clash between two different senses of time and historicity—the first being a supratribal national history solidified by heritage discourse and practice and, the second, a past anchored to ancestral lineage and genealogy."⁴⁶ The stigma of descent from enslaved people continues to manifest in the politics of selecting marriage partners.⁴⁷

In contrast to patterns of silencing, for al-Tabur it becomes necessary to engage with the history of enslavement in his discussion of the heritage of magic. He states that "Emirati society—like other Arab Gulf societies—practiced the slave trade, and this trade depended on buying negroes [*al-zanūj*] who were brought from Africa."⁴⁸ Al-Tabur does not downplay the fact that slavery touched the lives of most Gulf residents: "Selling and buying servants was a social practice of the Gulf population until recently. No house in the Emirates was without slaves who served the head of the family and his children without compensation except for food and accommodation."⁴⁹ Finally, his discussion is also significant in that it elides the fact that many enslaved people in the region were *not* of African descent.⁵⁰

What is it about *zār* and its prevalence in accounts of *al-ṭibb al-shaʿbī* in the Gulf that makes al-Tabur—who otherwise sees himself as contributing to a state-driven national project of heritage preservation—acknowledge the history of enslaved people of African descent in this region so unequivocally? *Zār*, according to al-Tabur's own definition, is a form of magical medicine and therefore does not cast the Emirati community in a favorable light. However, by frequently alluding to his information as having been reported to him by Emirati elders, he tacitly acknowledges that the ceremony is part of Emirati traditions of *al-ṭibb al-shaʿbī*. *Zār* practitioners historically have been found in the Horn of Africa, sub-Saharan East Africa, and Egypt, as well as in the Arabian Peninsula, given the long-standing interconnectivities of the Indian Ocean and Red Sea regions.⁵¹ Referring to nineteenth-century Egypt, Ehud Toledano suggests that *zār* was an expression of cultural hybridity as it "formed an integral part of the enslaved culture that came into contact with the vernacular forms of Islam practiced along the road into Ottoman territory."[52] *Zār* and jinn derive from separate cultural traditions, but they were "often superimposed upon one another";[53] for example, Benjamin Reilly indicates that in Khaybar (an oasis in what is now Saudi Arabia), African traditions of *zār* "spirits" were "Islamized into *jinn*."[54] Religious authorities affiliated with both the late Ottoman Empire and the twentieth-century Wahhabi movement in the Arabian Peninsula condemned *zār* as un-Islamic.[55] Moreover, antagonism toward *zār* was starkly racialized and gendered. As Taylor M. Moore demonstrates, at the turn of the twentieth century in Egypt, elite men feared that "uneducated and gullible Egyptian women were [for *zār* practitioners] most susceptible victims."[56] Moore reveals that their antipathy toward *zār* stemmed from anxiety regarding intimate spaces shared with domestic workers who were recently enslaved Sudanese and Abyssinians as well as working-class and peasant migrants to urban centers.

By displacing *zār* from the Emirati or Gulf Arab cultural core, al-Tabur resolves the tension that arises from recognizing *zār* as an aspect of Emirati heritage while simultaneously acknowledging its unorthodoxy. In the Arabian Peninsula, although many people who practiced *zār* probably believed they were doing so as faithful Muslims, some religious authorities censured their activities.[57] Al-Tabur emphasizes, first, that *zār* entered the Gulf region by way of outside (African and non-Arab) cultural influences and, second, that the practice was sustained by the activities of socially marginal groups—that is, enslaved people and women. He declares, "I believe that African communities in the Arab Gulf were the first to introduce *zār* to Gulf society."[58] Al-Tabur cites other scholars who condemn these rituals. He quotes one 1986 study that was published in Abu Dhabi: "The *zār* is a demon from the jinn." Al-Tabur elaborates on this statement, this jinn "is a *kāfir*—and he loves dancing and singing and animal sacrifice and wearing silk and golden rings."[59] In al-Tabur's construction, the jinn is real, but because he is a troublemaker, he is causing Muslims to perform *zār*, which leads them to practice medicine and seek healing by slaughtering an animal and asking the patient to drink the blood, eating a black chicken, or burning eggs in an abandoned place—acts that modern Muslims frown on or forbid.

Al-Tabur locates himself squarely on the side of orthodoxy, declaring, "These actions are an example of idol worship."[60] Even though he admits that "*zār* is a widespread heretical innovation in the Arab Gulf region and in the traditional Emirates among some people," he maintains that religious scholars and official agents did their utmost "to fight these practices."[61] After establishing that the respectable guardians of the social order were opposed to such activities, he again locates their origins in Africa, outside of the Gulf region itself, quoting another scholar who stated: "The people of the Emirates denounce whoever believes in *zār* or its effects, for it is the slaves who [practice *zār*], and he who has no morals. Fear the amirs [rulers], for when they hear of someone who has performed the *zār* he is punished with beating and imprisonment."[62] By including this quote, al-Tabur conjures an image of the elites of the past sternly protecting their people from these dangerous practices that had been disseminated by outsiders.

One reason enslaved people continued to practice *zār* rituals, according to al-Tabur, was "due to the social oppression they experienced" and also to relieve "the daily pressures that they were exposed to."[63] Women likewise are associated with *zār*, and in this context al-Tabur portrays women as being, like enslaved people, downtrodden and socially marginalized, and therefore not integral to established orthodox opinions. Although al-Tabur acknowledges that men also led *zār* circles in this region, he echoes other scholarship on *zār* cults when he suggests that women were especially susceptible to the appeal of *zār* due to their social weakness, noting that "the woman in traditional society suffered from persecution and at the hands of men as well as from his arrogance and control over her."[64] He posits that the oppressive gendered conditions produced "a type of psychological and social burden, which resulted in the woman performing some rituals and practices that helped her to find some relief, so she resorted to the *zār* dance."[65] Although al-Tabur offers an excuse for women by blaming their supposedly downtrodden gendered position, he also presents these women as counter to mainstream culture, as evidenced by their reliance on the *zār* simply because their lack of status gave them no better options.

Significantly, al-Tabur's criticism of *zār* does not focus on whether it is medically effective. Like other nationalist-oriented accounts, for al-Tabur, the purpose of addressing *al-ṭibb al-shaʿbī* is not primarily to recreate its scientific efficacy, epidemiological understandings, or medical logic. Rather, he constructs *al-ṭibb al-shaʿbī* as part of heritage. In this context, the fact that *zār* is condemned by Muslim elites is more relevant than questions of its capacity to cure health complaints. Al-Tabur attributes *zār* practices to the agency of enslaved people and women. Yet his interlocuters, whom he refers to as "elderly people in the Emirates," seem to represent a wider swath of Emirati society than these categories might suggest.[66] By locating the origins of *zār*, a major example in his category of magical medicine, outside of Emirati genealogical and geographic boundaries, he renders it inauthentic to Emirati heritage despite its persistence in popular discourse and its presence in recorded memories of the Emirates' past.

Healing as Commitment to the Nation

Khalifa al-Sayyid Mohammad Salih al-Maliki's *Jawab Kull Saʾil ʿind Muʿalijin Qatar al-Awaʾil* (Answer for every questioner from the early healers of Qatar) combines oral histories with the author's personal knowledge and opinions on Qatari folk medicine and culture to produce a hagiographic and nostalgic representation of medical history. Although the text maintains a narrative tension in the contrast between modern biomedicine and *al-ṭibb al-shaʿbī*, al-Maliki does not presume a clear temporal binary between pre- and post-oil Qatar. That is, he does not identify a break in time when Qatari society switched from *shaʿbī* healers to biomedical doctors and institutions. Instead, al-Maliki assumes that *al-ṭibb al-shaʿbī*, as a manifestation of Qatari Arab culture, has persisted intact throughout the decades of change since the mid-twentieth-century discovery of oil. The first half of his text contains the biographies of eighty-seven male healers, and the second half describes eighty-three female healers. According to al-Maliki, the healers practiced "from the beginning of the last century until the last third" of the twentieth century.[67] By not locating these healers clearly in time and by separating them by gender, the text posits that the cultural elements they bring to medicine—living as members of the community, behaving as normatively gendered Muslims, and performing acts of healing out of commitment to the community rather than for professional advancement—persist as the essence of ethnic nationalism in the periods both predating and following state oil revenues.

Al-Maliki was born in Doha in 1947, and his publications have focused on describing and preserving Qatari *sha'bī* culture, heritage, and traditions. Al-Maliki worked for oil companies from 1963 to 1979, so he is among the generation of Qataris who witnessed the development of the oil industry in his country. A prolific purveyor of culture, al-Maliki also has written for local theater, television, and newspapers.[68] In their focus on categorizing and inscribing Qatari *sha'bī* heritage, al-Maliki's works demonstrate his desire to remind Qatari citizens of their distinct culture and identity. He depicts the Qatari community as timeless, rooted in national geographical space, and existing apart from the temporary expatriate population.

Even though he encountered opposition and other research pitfalls, al-Maliki informs us, he persevered in his study of *al-ṭibb al-sha'bī* to preserve the life stories of Qatari healers and their place in Qatari national heritage. Writing in a hagiographic mode, al-Maliki opens his book, "Thank God for my success in gathering this modest number for this constellation from the male and female healers from the fathers and the mothers."[69] By elevating the importance of these healers and identifying them as mothers and fathers of the nation, he also highlights his own commitment and service to the Qatari national community in the act of carrying out this research. He draws attention to challenges he encountered: "I passed through abnormal conditions while I was gathering these personalities; some people still held back."[70] Despite these obstacles, al-Maliki reassures the reader: "My determination to move forward and to achieve this wish, which I consider a reward from God Almighty, [persists]. I aim to immortalize the memory of these people and to collect them in a single book, serving as a reference for male and female researchers from this generation and from coming generations."[71]

Through the act of collecting and preserving these biographies, al-Maliki asserts his commitment to the national community. Moreover, he presents his efforts as a continuation of the labors of the healers themselves, who expressed their devotion to this same community through their work as healers using whatever means were available to them. Al-Maliki frames the role of healer in an Islamic context, claiming that these healers were following the Qurʾan and the Prophet by performing their work for other Qataris. He writes, "Our blessed Prophet—prayers upon him—says: 'There is no disease that God has created for which He has not also created the treatment, some people know this treatment while others do not.'" In quoting this hadith, al-Maliki emphasizes the idea that seeking to heal is a religious duty, so the act of pursuing curative treatments renders the people collected in this book exemplary Muslims.[72] Notably, al-Maliki does not dwell on whether these methods were medically effective. Rather, the important point is that the individuals were committed to healing fellow Qataris, thereby fulfilling their religious and patriotic duties in a praiseworthy manner.

Al-Maliki's evident goal was to collect the names of as many individual healers as possible, to preserve their memories for future researchers, and to integrate them into the Qatari national narrative by drawing on the cultural authority of the Islamic *ṭabaqāt*. This biographical genre reflects the practice of early Muslim scholars to establish their community's claim to the Prophetic legacy and then to document "the transmission of that legacy from one generation of practitioners to the next."[73] In the medieval Islamic world, *ṭabaqāt* works listed the generations of members of a particular class, or genre, of people, such as caliphs, hadith scholars, jurists, physicians, grammarians, or poets. By listing the names of indigenous healers and categorizing them according to their skills, geography, and gender, al-Maliki constructs a genre of people who garner authority simultaneously from their containment within national space and their location in Islamic traditions of the transmission of knowledge.

His research combines his own personal experiences as a Qatari and his interviews with fellow Qataris, including the healers themselves and people who had known them or heard about them. Because he does not provide citations within the biographies or even a list of interviews or sources, all of the information is heavily filtered through al-Maliki's own perspective and his ideological objective to present the history of *al-ṭibb al-shaʿbī* in Qatar through an ethno-nationalist hagiographic narrative. He describes his methodology: "My journey in gathering this number of personalities took a lot of time. I visited throughout this period many people. Among them were those who have passed away and those who are still living. I searched for their names, those who treated the people in those past days, through any available method, but some among them forgot his past and some among them even refused to mention a single name and some others wouldn't speak openly to me to mention whom they knew or their time or what he heard about them."[74]

It is interesting that he seems to have encountered some opposition among his interview subjects, but it remains ambiguous whether this was out of personal animosity, hostility to his project, or simply the author's embellishment of challenges in an attempt to highlight his perseverance while conducting research. Nevertheless, al-Maliki must have collected a significant number of interviews (although he does not specify how many). He describes his subjects: "Some of them I knew personally, and I knew of their ability in healing the people, whereas others I knew of through my research and tracing their biographies of this or that male or female healer. And I am sure that there are still names and individuals whom I was unable to connect with nor was I able to find their biographies."[75] He relied on his personal and family connections in Qatar, establishing his authority by emphasizing the idea that the book is written from within the Qatari community and primarily for an audience of contemporaries as well as imagined future Qataris.

Al-Maliki's biography of the healer Shaykh 'Abd al-'Aziz bin Ahmad Al Ahmad Al Thani (significantly, a member of the Qatari ruling family) illustrates al-Maliki's ideological argument, narrative style, and methodology. He immediately frames such healers in terms of their place within the Muslim community: "By the grace of the high and almighty God on us we find our teachers, guides, Imams, and *sha'bī* healers of different methods and paths of their treatments."[76] Having established the religious communal boundaries, al-Maliki further constructs the world of these healers in terms of their inclusion in the nascent national Qatari community: "From us and in us from our family, our kind, and our country, just as He made doctors and healers from the poor, He made doctors and healers from the rich;

and He also made doctors and healers from the rulers and the shaykhs."⁷⁷ What all the healers—rich, poor, elite, and nonelite—have in common is that they come from within this established community, although they can be from any social group. Al-Maliki writes, "In addition to their ongoing charitable contributions, morality, generosity, and modesty . . . they freely volunteer to treat the people with the best of their knowledge."⁷⁸ Especially when a skilled healer is also an elite man, his status emphasizes the fact that he is practicing healing only to serve his community generously and charitably rather than for the sake of salary, reward, or professional recognition. Although elite healers earn praise for their noblesse oblige, poor healers are credited for their generosity to the community despite their own lack of resources.

Al-Maliki's introduction to his discussion of Shaykh ʿAbd al-ʿAziz bin Ahmad Al Ahmad Al Thani emphasizes how healers in general practiced their skills out of commitment to the nascent nation and religious duty. Turning to the subject of this particular biography, al-Maliki remarks that ʿAbd al-ʿAziz was known for cautery and offers a firsthand account of ʿAbd al-ʿAziz's healing skills. Cautery "requires strength and determination," and although ʿAbd al-ʿAziz was "of a slender body he was strong and severe."⁷⁹ Moreover, ʿAbd al-ʿAziz, according to al-Maliki, was the first to take charge of security in the 1930s and 1940s in Doha, and in that role "he was known for his strictness and lack of leniency with law-breakers."⁸⁰ In fact, Al-Maliki experienced ʿAbd al-ʿAziz's healing expertise personally, and he recounts the following story about his own childhood:

> My father al-Sayyid Mohammad (God rest his soul) told me that when I was a small child, I became sick and none of the known healers in the neighborhood at that time could find the treatment. As my father was one of the merchants in al-Suq Al-Dakhili (what is now known as Souq Waqif) he took me with him to the suq intending to give me a change, thinking that entertainment was better than remaining bedridden at home. And while I was sleeping in my father's shop His Excellency Shaykh ʿAbd al-ʿAziz bin Ahmad Al Thani greeted my father then asked him about me. My father (God rest his soul) told him that

I was sick, and of the inability of the healers to reach a cure, and that now I was under the care of God. The shaykh said, I want to examine him. So he carefully took my body then said to my father "Bring him to the blacksmith for your son is infected with a disease of the seventh and the seventh is an area of the upper back and he needs cautery by fire." The blacksmiths at that time were a part of the suq and weren't far from my father's shop, so my father took me, and there they put a number of irons in the iron oven, then I was cauterized with three irons on my back. My father said to me, they cauterized you with three irons, but you didn't feel it because you were nearly unconscious. After that they took me to the house and after three days God healed me from this ailment.[81]

Al-Maliki's father suppressed his anxiety over seeing his son have hot irons put on his back. His trust in the shaykh's healing methods signifies his participation in this form of community authority, as well as his deference to the status of the shaykh as a ruling elite.

Shaykh 'Abd al-'Aziz was not a professional healer in the sense that he earned a living by practicing medicine; rather, his expertise in cautery signifies his general wisdom and desire to serve his community, even those who were his social inferiors. Indeed, the shaykh encountered the patient by accident when he greeted a merchant acquaintance in the marketplace. This concern for a young boy demonstrates, in al-Maliki's rendering, the shaykh's social commitment and enforces the idea that all the members of the community were connected. Notably lacking from the account is a consideration of 'Abd al-'Aziz's scientific or medical thought process, the symptoms of the illness, or why the shaykh's prescription of cautery resulted in success. These details, al-Maliki implies, are left to the grace of God. Instead, al-Maliki emphasizes that 'Abd al-'Aziz's interest in healing reflected his general piety, charity, and determination to serve other Qataris. Although the tale is unusual in including the author's firsthand account of the healer, al-Maliki neatly diverts the reader to the moral message of authority and communal responsibility, rather than verification by third party, eyewitnesses, or other medical practitioners. The other narratives likewise emphasize the piety and commitment of various healers rather than the details of their medical process.

Al-Maliki's text argues that *sha ʿbī* healers are a noteworthy aspect of Qatari nationalist heritage, important to today's citizens because these stories remind them of the cohesive community of the past. Yet al-Maliki also reveals an underlying defensiveness about the persistent relevance of the traditional healers. Absent in al-Maliki's biographies are the British or missionary medical institutions that were also present in the region throughout the twentieth century. Not far from Qatar, the American mission hospital in Bahrain opened at the turn of the twentieth century (see chapter 2); it attracted patients from throughout the Gulf and continues to operate today. Because al-Maliki seems to have collected these oral histories in the early 2000s, the older healers would have worked contemporaneously with early biomedical institutions in Qatar or its surroundings. In the 1930s, thousands of Qataris migrated to Bahrain and other neighboring regions to search for employment following the 1937 attempt by Bahrain to press territorial claims over Zubarah by imposing an embargo.[82] Many of the migrant Qataris would have been exposed to American missionary and British medicine. Instead of exploring interactions between folk healers and emerging medical institutions, the author chooses to ignore them.

Echoing al-Tabur, al-Maliki also connects Muslim identity to the cultural heritage of *al-ṭibb al-shaʿbī* by emphasizing that good Muslims of the Qatari national past condemned magical medical practices. He recounts the following story in his biography of ʿAbd Allah bin Salih al-Yafʿi: "Once some youths came to him wanting him to perform some magic for them. As soon as he knew the story and understood their demands, he went to the door of the house and closed it. Then he brought a stick intending to hit these youths. No options were left for them except to flee saving their skins and moaning about the bad luck that this man had brought to them."[83] This sketch reveals that part of what was admirable about the healers of Qatar was that they policed the boundaries between medicine that was proper in an Islamic setting and magical medicine that defied Islam. In other words, the healers are deserving of inclusion in the nationalist canon because they encouraged the Qatari community to maintain the standards set by Islamic medicine rather than the medicine of the *jāhiliyya* period as condemned by Islam and the Prophet. These healers, in al-Maliki's account, often turned to prophetic and Islamic medical techniques like reading Qur'an, but the anecdote reassures the modern reader that they firmly condemned magic.

Like al-Tabur, al-Maliki discusses jinn and *zār*, but rather than criticizing the ritual, he includes a *zār* practitioner among his list of exemplary healers. In a long preamble to the healer Bediyyu bin Farhan, al-Maliki describes how jinn differ in their preferences of spaces to inhabit. He writes, "Some of them love clean places, while some of them love deserted, unclean places like ruins or cemeteries."[84] When jinn caused people to have seizures and convulsions, al-Maliki explains, Bediyyu bin Farhan might be called to perform *zār*. He had a special musical troupe for the ceremony, and he was known for his ability to identify what the jinn demanded in exchange for leaving the human host in peace. In contrast to al-Tabur's efforts to connect enslaved people of African descent and women to *zār*, al-Maliki makes no reference to Bediyyu bin Farhan's relative social status, and we are left to wonder whether he was of African descent, as was common for *zār* practitioners and musicians in the region.[85] Instead, al-Maliki elides potential social tensions and histories of enslavement by listing Bediyyu bin Farhan among the national fathers who engaged in healing without questioning his curative methods.

For al-Maliki, the purpose of preserving *al-ṭibb al-shaʿbī* is to emphasize that the characteristics of piety and commitment to caring for one another is a common thread that connects Qatari healers of the past and the present. In this narrative world, the impersonal institutionalization of modern medicine contrasts with the *shaʿbī* healers who knew your family and would come to your home to offer treatment. Al-Maliki emphasizes the communal benefits of sacrifice for the good of your neighbor, but he is not interested in discussing the medical or scientific milieus these healers participated in. He seems to accept as established fact the efficacy of modern medicine. In one of the rare instances when he addresses modern medicine, he states, "By the grace of God [the patient] is healed by the presence of modern hospitals and competent doctors, whereas in the past there was no alternative to them but *shaʿbī* healers."⁸⁶ His goal is neither to discount nor to praise the benefits of modern medicine, but rather to highlight the cultural unity of the Arab population of Qatar and its historical continuity as exemplified by practitioners of *al-ṭibb al-shaʿbī*.

Medical Nostalgia

Renewed interest in *al-ṭibb al-shaʿbī* opens a potential rendering of health history that challenges top-down teleological narratives of medical science. In the late twentieth- and early twenty-first-century Gulf, the resurgence of interest in *al-ṭibb al-shaʿbī* occurred as an expression of cultural nostalgia and contrived traditions that posit a distinctly nativist Arabian Peninsula. State and state-sympathetic agents have turned to oral histories to create politically palatable memories and prehistories for the nation-states of the oil economy, matching a contemporary nostalgia for imagined pre-oil unity. Indeed, along with radically restructuring every aspect of social and economic life and politics in the Gulf states, the oil economy also transformed historical subjectivities by tying collective memory to the nation-state. Memory is essentially social, and every social group—families, religious communities, tribes, and nations—has a collective memory.⁸⁷ Autobiographical memories are lost unless they are periodically socially reinforced, a process that may occur in the construction of oral histories gathered for the formulation of a nationalist historiography. Such projects draw on a sense of a vanishing past embodied by an elderly generation who carry exclusive knowledge of authentic regional heritage. Indeed, the National Archives of the United Arab Emirates describes its oral history initiative as contributing to national identity: "Oral history monitors historical events and lifestyles in the past to preserve the material and moral characteristics of the UAE society for future generations."⁸⁸ In Doha, Msheireb Museums seek to re-create life in predevelopment downtown Doha by including video recordings of "oral histories of personal memories of this former commercial neighborhood."⁸⁹ One nonstate initiative is that of Texas A&M University Qatar, whose student-produced oral history project aimed "to preserve the history of daily life of Qatar's past for future generations of Qatar's residents."⁹⁰

Across the Gulf petro-states, narratives of history engage with ambiguous future temporalities in which projects of development and modernity can only be achieved through state agency. This process must remain in motion but never reach completion for the recently established states of the Gulf Cooperation Council to maintain their legitimacy through a continuously reproduced and repackaged discourse of improvement. In the case of health and medicine, supporters of the nativist narrative, through their politicized reprocessing of oral history, frame *al-ṭibb al-shaʿbī* as a manifestation of national culture, and thus present the nation-state itself as the vehicle for preserving cultural practices that are delimited by rigid categories of national spaces and citizen populations. Yet historical methods invite us to move beyond imagined realities and discursive constructions. By focusing on folk medicine practitioners as bearers of cultural heritage who remain untouched by modern transformations rather than as contingent historical actors, nativist accounts of *al-ṭibb al-shaʿbī* render the early introduction of medical institutions by American missionaries, British officials, and local health professionals and consumers irrelevant to the development of medicine and public health in the region.[91] As I have shown, medicine was not an inevitable consequence of an externally imposed modernity. Instead, the variegated desires and efforts of heterogeneous and mobile communities fashioned dynamic histories of health in the modern Gulf and Arabian Peninsula.

CONCLUSION

THE RESILIENT EVERYDAY

LEADING UP TO Qatar's formal independence from Britain in 1971, state health officials dispatched a trusted midwife, Maryam ʿAbd al-Malik, to encourage local women to enroll in the government's new nurses' training institute.[1] The institute was managed by international staff from the World Health Organization (WHO), and it sought to teach Qataris to work as nurses. A renowned midwife, ʿAbd al-Malik was "regarded as the mother of most of Qatar's youth, from east to west and from south to north."[2] What allowed her "fame and reputation" for delivering babies to extend across Qatar was the fact that "she lived in a time of opening and communications," so she could reach troubled mothers in labor quickly by car.[3] As further testament to her skill, "even the maternity hospital used to seek her help and listen to her advice . . . she was offered a job more than once, but she refused."[4] Unwilling to limit herself to the hospital's institutional confines, she insisted on traveling to women's homes, where she expertly massaged fetuses into position and oversaw difficult births. Nevertheless, when the WHO staff sought her help, ʿAbd al-Malik dutifully visited young women in their homes to convince their families of the respectability of working as a nurse even as she herself continued to decline job offers from the nascent state hospital.

On the threshold of formal independence, modernizing Qataris and international health experts relied on ʿAbd al-Malik's local acclaim as a mobile midwife to entice young Qatari women to don the nurse's white uniform and join the workforce of the fledgling state health institutions. In recruiting international experts and constructing centralized hospitals, Qatar's rulers enthusiastically joined the global cohort of decolonizing elites who embraced scientific medicine and its gendered professionalization as a yardstick of modernity and a tool of statecraft. For her part, 'Abd al-Malik helped to advance this agenda among local people despite her personal insistence on delivering babies in the intimacy of the home.

This book has attempted to foreground the mutually constitutive and sometimes paradoxical relationship between a vision of health care that was, as Maryam 'Abd al-Malik saw it, a local and personalized project, and the arrival of biomedicine and sanitation as tools of state power. In exploring the modernization and globalization of this region before oil and during the transition to the oil-dominated economy, one of my major interventions has been to emphasize the roles of overlooked individuals and communities in these processes. Indeed, it was my concern for locating the voices of nonelites that first led me to the conjoined topics of health, medicine, and disease. The construction of state-driven health care and the ensuing formulations of new categories of territories and populations was, as 'Abd al-Malik's career exemplifies, a process that involved actors from across the social spectrum. Everyday people were deeply involved in envisioning, challenging, and putting into practice profoundly transformative health systems.

The entry of the imperial state into quotidian life in the Persian Gulf and Arabian Peninsula corresponded with the global repercussions of the bacteriological revolution and dramatically accelerated communications through steam and rail. Framing this study as regional, rather than national, history points to both environmental and political currents: the Gulf and its Arabian hinterland functioned as a unified epidemiological and medical zone due to the intense interconnectivities of its littorals, itinerant populations, and shared historical experiences of empire and global capitalism. The institutionalization of health and medicine from the late nineteenth century created extraordinary new opportunities for negotiating hierarchies between emerging states and diverse societies.

Similarly, our understanding of the relationship between British India and the Gulf expands when we observe the frictions and disagreements between Gulf Political Agencies and the Government of India as their public health policies and experts constructed flows of technologies and scientific knowledge. But Gulf health care resisted a top-down, Eurocentric, and imperial-driven vision of modern medicine, and it quietly maintained its own character and practice even as it assessed and admitted outside innovations. Indeed, far from remaining removed from modern processes, the residents of port cities and their hinterlands engaged with and influenced global developments in sanitation, disease control, and gendered medical labor. Indigenous elites shaped the institutions that emerged out of the bacteriological revolution to suit their own agendas. Local healers wove biomedical innovations into long-standing cultures and health-seeking practices. Patients journeyed far to reach mission hospitals, choosing to benefit from medical services while resisting or ignoring Christian proselytizing. Malaria and trachoma shifted from seasonally rhythmic facts of life to objects of preventive interventions and medical experimentation. Countless social interactions and scientific translations across the region forged a new health system and set the stage for the emergent biopolitical regimes of the oil states.

Gulf historiography that centers tribes, shaykhs, and oil in accounts of empire and state building does not recognize the roles of individuals who lived beyond the gaze of elite decision makers, even as they experienced modern transformations throughout the region. However, disease and its companion, contagion, posed a risk to the imperial project and thus made their way into imperial records, even when passing through the most marginalized populations. An enslaved boy in a shaykh's garden who contracted malaria might appear in the imperial archive that would otherwise have ignored him because of the recognition that his ailment risked transmission to more valued bodies. Women who angrily approached the political agent in Manama in response to proposals to restructure their water supply were able to change the course of town planning.[5] And infants and the elderly appeared in medical records as they arrived at mission hospitals and Aramco clinics hoping to salvage eyesight threatened by trachoma or cataracts.

A strength of medical and health history is how well these topics facilitate the conceptual intertwining of the material and the ideological. The medicalization of health is material in that it draws on specific technologies and practices to transform, often at the biological and chemical level, the individual body. But it is just as ideological, in that medicalization is accompanied by assumptions about modernity and cultural superiority. The missionaries offer an exemplary demonstration of this dynamic in their unironic conflation of biomedicine and Christ as Savior. Gulf populations proved adept at navigating the ideological and the material in the medical sphere as they sought out hospital services.

What does it mean for a historian to access nonelite subjectivity in records that have largely been produced by members of a dominant or privileged class? How should historians understand "experience"? Through the lens of medical and disease histories, scholars can access the material and lived experiences of subalterns and reconstruct the ideological limitations and possibilities of the worlds they inhabited. The subaltern may not always be granted her voice or have the privilege of framing events in her own words, but she does get sick, becomes an object of study, dodges quarantine, gives birth, carries bacteria, and struggles to preserve her child's eyesight. She lives in a political environment and makes choices about her health. Even when we are not privy to how such actors understood and conceptualized their movement through health systems, historians can reconstruct certain processes endured by their bodies. We can ask at which points physical practices and biological conditions would have been something new, or when they would have occurred with altered social or political significance. Having to pause in time and space at quarantine stations, for example, dramatically altered what it was like to voyage between Karachi and Muscat. The act of traveling several days or even weeks to visit a hospital, which we can document as an active choice by many people of Arabia and the Gulf, likewise represented a significant transformation in the voluntary use of institutions and the conceptualizing of health and sickness. Accessing the experiences of groups that generally have been left out of our historical considerations of the region helps us to reconstruct the movement between the material and ideological in the medicalization of health.

Did the oil industry mark a dramatic rupture from or an intensified continuity with the power structures and class dynamics of the pre-oil period? The answer is, of course, both. The trachoma experiments and the experiences of migrant Arab nurses demonstrate how the onset of oil resulted in a dramatic transformation in the target of spaces and populations of public health as the oil industry sought to ensure healthy workers and as health care emerged as integral to the Gulf welfare state. But the resilience of folk medicine and its reemergence as a national heritage project reveals the cultural and medical reverberations of the pre-oil period in the late twentieth- and early twenty-first-century Gulf. When I refer to the hegemony of biomedicine, what I mean is that the state, and the dominant citizen classes whose interests it represents, have naturalized the tenets of biomedicine as a universalizing system of values. They have turned to modern technologies and institutions to target specific health conditions. This project is a continuation of imperial medicine of the nineteenth and twentieth centuries, whose practitioners assumed that the causative processes they traced from microscope to ailing body overruled and negated any preexisting health imaginaries, especially those of non-European peoples. But I attempted to capture a counternarrative to this passing of the biomedical baton from empire to nation-state in my examination of *al-ṭibb al-sha'bī*. It is precisely the confluence of Gulf demographics, hierarchies of citizenship and noncitizenship, and biomedical hegemony that has created the conditions for the nostalgic repurposing of *al-ṭibb al-sha'bī* as an element of ethno-national heritage.

Finally, it is worth reiterating that I do not take national borders and communities as predetermined frameworks; indeed, a major goal of my analysis has been to show how public health and medicine contributed to the process of reifying the people who inhabited or passed through this region into categorical population groups that could be counted and classified by the intertwined measurements of race, religion, class, health status, and disease risk. By incorporating local voices and integrating a wide range of archival genres, I also have emphasized that overwhelming state biopolitical power was not an inevitable outcome of these developments; on the contrary, local communities and individuals were central to processes of negotiating and managing the evolving relationship between health and politics. The above story of midwife Maryam 'Abd al-Malik, who managed her career on her own terms, is just one reminder of how practitioners and patients alike can slip among frameworks and offer us subjectivities not always found in official narratives.

NOTES

Introduction

1. Atmaram Sadashiva Grandin Jayakar (1844–1911) earned a degree in medicine and surgery in India and then passed the Indian Medical Service exam at the Royal Victoria Hospital in Southampton, England. During his twenty-seven years in Muscat, he worked under twelve different political agents, spent a period as acting agent, and served as the personal physician to Sultan Turki bin Saʿid (r. 1871–1888). In addition to his medical writings, he produced studies of Omani proverbs and sent specimens of local wildlife to the British Museum, which resulted in some local species being named in his honor. Mark Hobbs, "A Polymath in Muscat," *Untold Lives* (blog), British Library, 28 August 2014, https://blogs.bl.uk/untoldlives/2014/08/a-polymath-in-muscat.html. See also Charlie Sammut, "The Life of Dr Jayakar: A British Agency Surgeon in Muscat," Anglo-Omani Society, 14 May 2020, https://www.ao-soc.org/news/aos/podcast-transcript-cs; Charlie Sammut, "Medicine and Politics at the Edge of Empire: Surgeon Lt Col Atmaram Sadashiva Grandin Jayakar," Anglo-Omani Society, 18 May 2022, YouTube video, 1:00:52, https://www.youtube.com/watch?v=YRC8-j_MjWk.

2. India Office Records (hereafter IOR) V/23/77, no. 379, "Administration Report on the Persian Gulf Political Residency and Maskat Political Agency for 1899/1900," 23.

3. IOR V/23/77, 23.

4. IOR V/23/77, 25.

5. IOR V/23/77, 23. Cholera, the hallmark pandemic calamity of the nineteenth century, was no stranger to Arabia and the Persian Gulf. Arabia's Gulf coast was vulnerable to epidemic invasions by way of land communications with the Hijaz as well as by sea. The most common periodization of cholera pandemics is as follows: 1817–1824 (first), 1829–1851 (second), 1852–1859 (third), 1860–1875 (fourth), 1881–1895 (fifth), 1899–1923 (sixth), 1960– (seventh). See Christopher Hamlin, *Cholera: The Biography* (Oxford: Oxford University Press, 2009), 4.

6. Historically, *Oman* referred to the interior region, as distinct from the coast. For a succinct description of Oman's geography, see Thomas F. McDow, *Buying Time: Debt and Mobility in the Western Indian Ocean* (Athens: Ohio University Press, 2018), 28–29.

7. IOR V/23/29, no. 138, "Report on the Administration of the Persian Gulf Political Residency and Muscat Political Agency for the Years 1876–77," 96. British-backed coastal rulers had long been subject to resistance from the interior, where people viewed the sultanate as illegitimate due to its dependance on British imperial power. Expressions of opposition to the sultan had punctuated the years leading up to the cholera epidemic. In 1896, for example, a British agent penned a strikingly forthright assessment of the situation: "The authority of the Sultan is quite rotten beyond Muscat and Mattrah where our gunboats protect him. . . . Yet the fiction of keeping the Sultan's rule is to us as useful as keeping off Foreign Powers from some 600 miles of coast. But how long can we keep the fiction going, when the Sultan is afraid to go 10 miles from his capital?" Quoted in Briton Cooper Busch, *Britain and the Persian Gulf, 1894–1914* (Berkeley: University of California Press, 1967), 59–60.

8. IOR V/23/77, no. 379, "Administration Report on the Persian Gulf Political Residency," 31.

9. J. C. Wilkinson, *Water and Tribal Settlement in South-East Arabia: A Study of the Aflāj of Oman* (Oxford: Oxford University Press, 1977).

10. "Cholera—*Vibrio cholerae* Infection," Centers for Disease Control and Prevention, https://www.cdc.gov/cholera/general/index.html.

11. IOR V/23/77, no. 379, "Administration Report on the Persian Gulf Political Residency," 31.

12. Sultan bin Mubarak bin Hamad al-Shaybani, *Al-Tawaʿ in fi al-Dhakira al-ʿUmaniyya* (Muscat: Mahboub, 2021), 69–70. Following the 1856 death of Sultan Sayyid Saʿid al Bu-Saʿidi and the ensuing competition between his sons, in 1861 the British separated Zanzibar from Muscat and Oman. The British established a protectorate over Zanzibar in 1890.

13. IOR V/23/77, no. 379, "Administration Report on the Persian Gulf Political Residency," 31.

14. In his encyclopedic *Gazetteer of the Persian Gulf,* Lorimer estimated that the population of the sultanate (excluding Dhofar) was around five hundred thousand at the beginning of the twentieth century, although Wilkinson believed that number was too high. See Wilkinson, *Water and Tribal Settlement,* 5. On Lorimer's *Gazetteer* as an imperial project, see Nelida Fuccaro, "Knowledge at the Service of the British Empire: The Gazetteer of the Persian Gulf, Oman, and Central Arabia," in *Borders and the Changing Boundaries of Knowledge,* ed. Inga

Brandell, Marie Carlson, and Önver A. Çetrez, Transactions 22 (Istanbul: Swedish Research Institute in Istanbul, 2015), 17–34.

15. IOR V/23/77, no. 379, "Administration Report on the Persian Gulf Political Residency," 25. Population estimates for Muscat and Muttrah in the nineteenth and early twentieth centuries fluctuate, but Jayakar's numbers are close to other contemporary figures. For a helpful list of population estimates, see Willem Floor, *Muscat: City, Society & Trade* (Washington, DC: Mage Publishers, 2015), 69–70.

16. IOR V/23/77, no. 379, "Administration Report on the Persian Gulf Political Residency," 26.

17. Oman had the largest Indian presence in the Gulf from the 1750s to the 1950s, concentrated in Muscat and Muttrah. James Onley, "Indian Communities in the Persian Gulf, c. 1500–1947," in *The Persian Gulf in Modern Times: People, Ports, and History*, ed. Lawrence G. Potter (New York: Palgrave Macmillan, 2014), 242. See also Calvin H. Allen Jr., "The Indian Merchant Community of Masqat," *Bulletin of the School of Oriental and African Studies* 44, no. 1 (1981): 39–53. On Oman's Khoja, or Lawatiyya, community, see Marc Valeri, "High Visibility, Low Profile: The Shiʻa in Oman under Sultan Qaboos," *International Journal of Middle East Studies* 42, no. 2 (2010): 251–268.

18. IOR V/23/77, no. 379, "Administration Report on the Persian Gulf Political Residency," 26. By the end of the nineteenth century, Muscat's Indians constituted a privileged class, enjoying extensive landholdings and, more often than not, status as protected subjects of the British Empire. The Indian community's protected status was also expressed in relatively greater trust in Jayakar, possibly enhanced by the fact that he was also an Indian British subject.

19. IOR V/23/77, no. 379, "Administration Report on the Persian Gulf Political Residency," 26.

20. The British reported that, "so far as is known with the exception of one or two suspicious cases reported, there was no spread of [plague] to the interior as was the case with cholera." The water system described offers a likely explanation of this distinction between the interior's greater susceptibility to cholera than plague. IOR V/23/77, no. 379, "Administration Report on the Persian Gulf Political Residency," 20.

21. IOR V/23/77, 20. See also Robert Geran Landen, *Oman since 1856: Disruptive Modernization in a Traditional Arab Society* (Princeton, NJ: Princeton University Press, 1967), 154–155.

22. My regional framework is in dialogue with Lawrence G. Potter's assertion that "what is needed is a new historical approach in which the unit of study is the Persian Gulf in its entirety." Lawrence G. Potter, introduction to *The Persian Gulf in History*, ed. Lawrence G. Potter (New York: Palgrave Macmillan, 2009), 4.

Potter's work on the Gulf region has exemplified a regional approach. See also Lawrence G. Potter, ed., *The Persian Gulf in Modern Times: People, Ports, and History* (New York: Palgrave Macmillan, 2014); and Lawrence G. Potter, *Society in the Persian Gulf: Before and after Oil* (Doha: Georgetown University in Qatar, Center for International and Regional Studies, 2017). Another recent study that embraces a regional approach is Laleh Khalili, *Sinews of War and Trade: Shipping and Capitalism in the Arabian Peninsula* (London: Verso, 2020). Khalili usefully incorporates Aden and the Suez Canal into histories of Arabian ports in her examination of regional patterns of integration into global networks of capitalism.

23. In her study of the Ottoman experience of plague in the early modern Mediterranean, for example, Nükhet Varlık presents the Mediterranean world "as a unified disease zone, with shared epidemiological experiences, as well as a common heritage of medical traditions." Nükhet Varlık, *Plague and Empire in the Early Modern Mediterranean World: The Ottoman Experience, 1347–1600* (New York: Cambridge University Press, 2015), 3. For the interwar period, Samuel Dolbee demonstrates how ideas of disease, climate, and race played a constitutive role in consolidating borders between post-Ottoman states. Samuel Dolbee, "Borders, Disease, and Territoriality in the Post-Ottoman Middle East," in *Regimes of Mobility: Borders and State Formation in the Middle East, 1918–1946*, ed. Jordi Tejel and Ramazan Hakkı Öztan (Edinburgh: Edinburgh University Press, 2022), 205–227. Other work also takes up the Arabian Peninsula and Persian Gulf regions as interconnected spaces of disease. Sabri Ateş demonstrates how corpse traffic converged with nineteenth-century cholera epidemics along the Ottoman-Iranian frontier. Amir A. Afkhami offers an overview of how pandemic cholera shaped modern Iran. From the perspective of Arabia's Red Sea Coast and in the contact zone of Ottoman and British imperial rivalries, Michael Christopher Low integrates the Ottoman experience into the globally significant history of environment, disease, and mobility surrounding the Hajj. Sabri Ateş, "Bones of Contention: Corpse Traffic and Ottoman-Iranian Rivalry in Nineteenth-Century Iraq," *Comparative Studies of South Asia, Africa, and the Middle East* 30, no. 3 (2010): 512–532; Amir A. Afkhami, *A Modern Contagion: Imperialism and Public Health in Iran's Age of Cholera* (Baltimore: Johns Hopkins University Press, 2019); Michael Christopher Low, *Imperial Mecca: Ottoman Arabia and the Indian Ocean Hajj* (New York: Columbia University Press, 2020).

24. Henri Lefebvre, *The Production of Space*, trans. Donald Nicholson-Smith (Oxford, UK: Blackwell, 1991), 23.

25. Here I draw from Johannes Fabian's discussion of the denial of coevalness. Johannes Fabian, *Time and the Other: How Anthropology Makes Its Object* (New York: Columbia University Press, 1983), 37.

26. Nelida Fuccaro's pioneering work on Bahrain laid the groundwork for a historical critique of Gulf exceptionalism. Nelida Fuccaro, *Histories of City and State in the Persian Gulf: Manama since 1800* (Cambridge: Cambridge University Press, 2009). For a more recent discussion, see Ahmed Kanna, Amélie Le Renard, and Neha Vora, *Beyond Exception: New Interpretations of the Arabian Peninsula* (Ithaca, NY: Cornell University Press, 2020).

27. For a cogent critique of this trend, see Alex Boodrookas and Arang Keshavarzian, "The Forever Frontier of Urbanism: Historicizing Persian Gulf Cities," *International Journal of Urban and Regional Research* 43, no. 1 (2019): 14–29.

28. Frederick F. Anscombe, *The Ottoman Gulf: The Creation of Kuwait, Saudi Arabia, and Qatar* (New York: Columbia University Press, 1997); Fuccaro, *Histories of City and State*; Farah Al-Nakib, *Kuwait Transformed: A History of Oil and Urban Life* (Stanford, CA: Stanford University Press, 2016); Omar H. AlShehabi, *Contested Modernity: Sectarianism, Nationalism, and Colonialism in Bahrain* (London: Oneworld Academic, 2019); Marc Owen Jones, *Political Repression in Bahrain* (New York: Cambridge University Press, 2020).

29. Matthew S. Hopper, *Slaves of One Master: Globalization and Slavery in Arabia in the Age of Empire* (New Haven, CT: Yale University Press, 2015); Johan Mathew, *Margins of the Market: Trafficking and Capitalism across the Arabian Sea* (Oakland: University of California Press, 2016); Fahad Ahmad Bishara, *A Sea of Debt: Law and Economic Life in the Western Indian Ocean, 1780–1950* (Cambridge: Cambridge University Press, 2017). Bishara succinctly makes the case for an oceanic history of the Gulf in "The Many Voyages of *Fateh Al-Khayr*: Unfurling the Gulf in the Age of Oceanic History," *International Journal of Middle East Studies* 52, no. 3 (2020): 397–412.

30. As Maryam Alsada asks, if "men are the established actors in pearl trade activities," then "where were all the women?" Maryam Mohamed Abdulla Ebrahim Alsada, "The Lives of Girls and Women in Bahrain and Qatar: Dress, Marriage, Health and Education in the Pearl Fishing and Early Oil Era" (PhD diss., University College London, 2022), 8. Haya al-Mughni offers a similar observation in *Women in Kuwait: The Politics of Gender*, rev. ed. (London: Saqi Books, 2001), 44. For an important intervention that challenges the idea that women were not active participants in Indian Ocean mobilities, see Scott Reese, "The Myth of Immobility: Women and Travel in the British Imperial Indian Ocean," *Journal of World History* 33, no. 2 (June 2022): 301–320.

31. Helen Mary Rizzo, *Islam, Democracy, and the Status of Women: The Case of Kuwait* (New York: Routledge, 2005); Khalid M. Al-Azri, *Social and Gender Inequality in Oman: The Power of Religious and Political Tradition* (New York: Routledge, 2013); Alessandra L. González, *Islamic Feminism in Kuwait: The Politics*

and Paradoxes (New York: Palgrave Macmillan, 2013); Madawi Al-Rasheed, *A Most Masculine State: Gender, Politics, and Religion in Saudi Arabia* (Cambridge: Cambridge University Press, 2013); Meshal Al-Sabah, *Gender and Politics in Kuwait: Women and Political Participation in the Gulf* (London: I. B. Tauris, 2013).

32. James Onley, *The Arabian Frontier of the British Raj: Merchants, Rulers, and the British in the Nineteenth-Century Gulf* (Oxford: Oxford University Press, 2007), 66.

33. Onley, *Arabian Frontier of the British Raj*, 69.

34. Michel Foucault, *Security, Territory, Population: Lectures at the Collège de France, 1977–78*, ed. Michel Senellart, François Ewald, and Alessandro Fontana, trans. Graham Burchell (New York: Palgrave Macmillan, 2007).

35. Allan Megill, "The Reception of Foucault by Historians," *Journal of the History of Ideas* 48, no. 1 (1987): 132.

36. David Scott, "Colonial Governmentality," *Social Text*, no. 43 (1995): 193.

37. To cite some illustrative examples, Afsaneh Najmabadi is critical of "a reductive Foucauldian concept of 'the techniques of domination'" in her excavation of plural subjectivities of sexuality in contemporary Iran. Afsaneh Najmabadi, *Professing Selves: Transsexuality and Same-Sex Desire in Contemporary Iran* (Durham, NC: Duke University Press, 2014), 2. Omar Dewachi's notion of ungovernable life in Iraq interfaces with biopolitics and governmentality and finds "the entire state to be a margin in which the constellations of historically situated regimes of knowledge and power are continuously confronting their own limits." Omar Dewachi, *Ungovernable Life: Mandatory Medicine and Statecraft in Iraq* (Stanford, CA: Stanford University Press, 2017), 176. Khaled Fahmy argues that in Egypt, the Ottoman government "never developed a policy that could be interpreted as signaling an understanding of what Foucault called 'the problem of the population'"; instead, Fahmy emphasizes the role of everyday Egyptians in forging a distinctly modern relationship between law and medicine in the nineteenth century. Khaled Fahmy, *In Quest of Justice: Islamic Law and Forensic Medicine in Modern Egypt* (Oakland: University of California Press, 2018), 51.

38. Joelle M. Abi-Rached, *'Aṣfūriyyeh: A History of Madness, Modernity, and War in the Middle East* (Cambridge: Massachusetts Institute of Technology Press, 2020), 15, 16.

39. Abi-Rached, *'Aṣfūriyyeh*, 16–17.

40. Helen Tilley, "Medical Cultures, Therapeutic Properties, and Laws in Global History," in "Therapeutic Properties: Global Medical Cultures, Knowledge, and Law," ed. Helen Tilley, special issue, *Osiris* 36 (2021): 6.

41. By "biomedicine," or scientific medicine, I mean medicine that seeks to apply the biological sciences to the diagnosis, treatment, and prevention of disease. For an overview of scientific medicine and public health from the nineteenth through

the first half of the twentieth centuries, see Roy Porter, *The Greatest Benefit to Mankind: A Medical History of Humanity from Antiquity to the Present* (London: Fontana Press, 1999), 304–461.

42. Here I take inspiration from Asef Bayat's concept of social nonmovements. Asef Bayat, *Life as Politics: How Ordinary People Change the Middle East* (Stanford, CA: Stanford University Press, 2010, 2013).

Chapter 1

1. Johan Mathew examines this incident from the perspective of maritime regulation and formal and informal trade and travel. Johan Mathew, *Margins of the Market: Trafficking and Capitalism across the Arabian Sea* (Oakland: University of California Press, 2016), 50–51.

2. Fahad Ahmad Bishara, "'No Country but the Ocean': Reading International Law from the Deck of an Indian Ocean Dhow, ca. 1900," *Comparative Studies in Society and History* 60, no. 2 (2018): 339. According to Matthew Hopper, as late as 1900 "at least one thousand enslaved Africans were still annually imported to the Omani port of Sur." Matthew S. Hopper, *Slaves of One Master: Globalization and Slavery in Arabia in the Age of Empire* (New Haven, CT: Yale University Press, 2015), 147.

3. IOR R/15/1/403, File 35/85 I A 8, Muscat: French Flag Question, "Statement of the Quarantine Superintendent of His Highness the Sultan of Muscat Regarding Flight of Five Sooris from Quarantine on the Night of April 9th 1903."

4. IOR R/15/1/403, "Statement of the Quarantine Superintendent."

5. Mathew, *Margins of the Market*, 50–51.

6. The Permanent Court of Arbitration at The Hague ruled against the practice in 1904. Matthew S. Hopper, "Imperialism and the Dilemma of Slavery in Eastern Arabia and the Gulf, 1873–1939," *Itinerario* 30, no. 3 (2006): 83–84. See also Hideaki Suzuki, *Slave Trade Profiteers in the Western Indian Ocean: Suppression and Resistance in the Nineteenth Century* (Gewerbestrasse, Switzerland: Palgrave Macmillan, 2017), 167–187; and Guillemette Crouzet, *Inventing the Middle East: Britain and the Persian Gulf in the Age of Global Imperialism* (Montreal: McGill-Queen's University Press, 2022), 178–182. For a discussion of this incident in the context of "flags of convenience" in Arabia, see Laleh Khalili, *Sinews of War and Trade: Shipping and Capitalism in the Arabian Peninsula* (London: Verso, 2020), 236–237.

7. Abdel Razzaq Takriti, *Monsoon Revolution: Republicans, Sultans, and Empires in Oman, 1965–1976* (Oxford: Oxford University Press, 2013), 10–24.

8. IOR R/15/1/403, File 35/85 I A 8, Muscat: French Flag Question, "Sultan Seyyid Faisal bin Turki to French Consul," 12 April 1903.

9. IOR R/15/1/403, "Sultan Seyyid."

10. For an account of the Gulf as a political frontier and buffer zone in relation to British India, see Crouzet, *Inventing the Middle East*.

11. A large body of work focuses on sanitary concerns and the hajj. See, e.g., John Baldry, "The Ottoman Quarantine Station on Kamaran Island 1882–1914," *Studies in History of Medicine* 2, nos. 1–2 (March–June 1978): 3–138; S. J. Watts, "From Rapid Change to Stasis: Official Responses to Cholera in British-Ruled India and Egypt: 1860 to c. 1921," *Journal of World History* 12, no. 2 (Fall 2001): 321–374; Michael Christopher Low, "Empire and the Hajj: Pilgrims, Plagues, and Pan-Islam under British Surveillance, 1865–1908," *International Journal of Middle East Studies* 40, no. 2 (2008): 269–290; Valeska Huber, *Channelling Mobilities: Migration and Globalisation in the Suez Canal Region and Beyond, 1869–1914* (Cambridge: Cambridge University Press, 2013); Eric Tagliacozzo, "Hajj in the Time of Cholera: Pilgrim Ships and Contagion from Southeast Asia to the Red Sea," in *Global Muslims in the Age of Steam and Print*, ed. James L. Gelvin and Nile Green (Berkeley: University of California Press, 2013), 103–120; Gülden Sariyildiz and Oya Dağlar Macar, "Cholera, Pilgrimage, and International Politics of Sanitation: The Quarantine Station on the Island of Kamaran," in *Plague and Contagion in the Islamic Mediterranean*, ed. Nükhet Varlık (Kalamazoo, MI: Arc Humanities Press, 2017), 243–273; Ulrike Freitag, *A History of Jeddah: The Gate to Mecca in the Nineteenth and Twentieth Centuries* (New York: Cambridge University Press, 2020), 261–267; Michael Christopher Low, *Imperial Mecca: Ottoman Arabia and the Indian Ocean Hajj* (New York: Columbia University Press, 2020). For a discussion of Ottoman and Egyptian quarantines, plague, and empire in the 1830s and 1840s, see Vladimir Hamed-Troyansky, "Ottoman and Egyptian Quarantines and European Debates on Plague in the 1830s–1840s," *Past and Present* 253, no. 1 (November 2021): 235–270.

12. Theodore Thomson, *Report by Dr. Theodore Thomson on the Sanitary Requirements of Certain Places in or near the Persian Gulf, &.*, printed for the use of the Foreign Office, October 1906, London School of Hygiene & Tropical Medicine Library & Archives Service, https://archive.org/details/b21359118, 3. This report also appears in FO 881/8780 and FO 368/37 Public Record Office (PRO).

13. Tagliacozzo, "Hajj in the Time of Cholera," 105.

14. Watts, "From Rapid Change to Stasis," 338–339.

15. Saurabh Mishra, "Incarceration and Resistance in a Red Sea Lazaretto, 1880–1930," in *Quarantine: Local & Global Histories*, ed. Alison Bashford (London: Palgrave, 2016), 56.

16. Baldry, "The Ottoman Quarantine Station," 33. Eight thousand pilgrims passed through Kamaran in 1882. By 1886, 15,031 pilgrims arrived for quarantine,

and 9,500 Indians, although the camp was built to hold only 3,000. See Baldry, "Ottoman Quarantine Station," 38.

17. Radhika Singha, "Passport, Ticket, and India-Rubber Stamp: 'The Problem of the Pauper Pilgrim' in Colonial India c. 1882–1925," in *The Limits of British Colonial Control in South Asia: Spaces of Disorder in the Indian Ocean Region*, ed. Ashwini Tambe and Harald Fischer-Tiné (New York: Routledge, 2009), 54.

18. The El Tor lazaretto opened in 1877. Liat Kozma and Diane Samuels, "Beyond Borders: The Egyptian 1947 Epidemic as a Regional and International Crisis," *British Journal of Middle Eastern Studies* (2017): 4, https://doi.org/10.1080/13530194.2017.1370999. Valeska Huber analyzes El Tor as a mechanism for preventing and controlling pilgrims' movements. Huber, *Channelling Mobilities*, 226–231.

19. John G. Lang, "The Quarantine Camp at El Tor," *Public Health Reports (1896–1970)* 17, no. 20 (1902): 1157.

20. Aytuğ Arslan and Hasan Ali Polat, "Travel from Europe to Istanbul in the 19th Century and the Quarantine of Çanakkale," *Journal of Transport & Health* 4 (2017): 13.

21. Khalid Al-Jarallah, *Tarikh al-Khadamat al-Sihhiyya fi al-Kuwayt* (Kuwait: Markaz al-Buhuth wa-l-Dirasat al-Kuwaytiyya, 1996), 23.

22. Mark Harrison, *Contagion: How Commerce has Spread Disease* (New Haven, CT: Yale University Press, 2012), 159–166.

23. Stephanie Jones, "British India Steamers and the Trade of the Persian Gulf, 1862–1914," *Great Circle* 7, no. 1 (1985): 27. Steamer traffic on the Tigris and Euphrates rivers started in the 1830s. See Omar Dewachi, *Ungovernable Life: Mandatory Medicine and Statecraft in Iraq* (Stanford, CA: Stanford University Press, 2017), 33.

24. IOR L/P&S/18/B394: "Quarantine Control in the Persian Gulf," 9 August 1928.

25. Willem Floor, *Public Health in Qajar Iran* (Odenton, MD: Mage Publishers, 2004), 210–212.

26. Lorimer, *Gazetteer*, "Sanitary Regulations and Arrangements of Turkey in the Persian Gulf, 1896–1907," 2546.

27. Frédéric Borel, *Étude d'hygiene Internationale: Choléra et peste dans le pèlerinage musulman, 1860–1903* (Paris: Libraires de l'Académie de Médecine, 1904), https://archive.org/details/b21354315.

28. Borel, 63.

29. Borel, 63.

30. One exception is that during the 1899–1900 cholera epidemic in Oman, the British civil surgeon Atmaram Sadashiva Grandin Jayakar tried to establish a "camp

of detention" outside of Muttrah, "but the watch kept there was so ineffective that instances of persons supposed to be detained there, having found their way into the town often came to my notice." IOR V/23/77, no. 379, "Administration Report on the Persian Gulf Political Residency and Maskat Political Agency for 1899/1900," 30. For fascinating accounts of journeys by foot or camel from southern Arabia to Mecca, see Janet C. E. Watson, "Travel to Mecca from Southern Oman in the Pre-Motorized Period," in *The Hajj: Collected Essays*, ed. Venetia Porter and Liana Saif (London: British Museum Press, 2013), 96–99.

31. Borel, *Choléra et peste dans le pèlerinage musulman*, 184.

32. For an apt warning not "to confuse an appreciation of contagion *qua* contagiousness with one explanation of its mechanics," see Vivian Nutton, "The Seeds of Disease: An Explanation of Contagion and Infection from the Greeks to the Renaissance," *Medical History* 27 (1983): 1.

33. David Arnold, "The Indian Ocean as a Disease Zone, 1500–1950," *South Asia: Journal of South Asian Studies* 14, no. 2 (1991): 1–21; and Monica H. Green and Lori Jones, "The Evolution and Spread of Major Human Diseases in the Indian Ocean World, in *Disease Dispersion and Impact in the Indian Ocean World*, ed. Gwyn Campbell and Eva-Maria Knoll (London: Palgrave Macmillan, 2020), 25–57.

34. Ahmad Mustafa Abu-Hakima, *Tarikh al-Kuwayt al-Hadith, 1750–1965* (Kuwait: N.p., 1984), 73.

35. Al-Jarallah, *Tarikh al-Khadamat al-Sihhiyya fi al-Kuwayt*, 31.

36. Abu-Hakima, *Tarikh al-Kuwayt*, 74.

37. Abu-Hakima, 75.

38. IOR V/23/37, no. 171, "Report on the Administration of the Persian Gulf Residency and Muscat Political Agency for the Year 1879–80," 19–20.

39. Paul Harrison, *The Arab at Home* (New York: Thomas Y. Crowell Co., 1924), 310. Eleanor Abdella Doumato also discusses Harrison's description of this procedure in *Getting God's Ear: Women, Islam, and Healing in Saudi Arabia and the Gulf* (New York: Columbia University Press, 2000), 201–202.

40. Harrison, *Arab at Home*, 310.

41. Behnaz A. Mirzai, *A History of Slavery and Emancipation in Iran, 1800–1929* (Austin: University of Texas Press, 2017), 60.

42. IOR R/15/6/65, File XXXVIII/5, "Report on Sur, by Major G.P. Murphy, I.A. P.A., Muscat," 10 October 1928, 13.

43. 'Abd Allah 'Ali al-Tabur, *Al-Tibb al-Sha'bi fi al-Imarat al-'Arabiyya al-Muttahida* (Dubai: Markaz al-Khalij li-l-Kutub, 1998), 144–145.

44. *Al-'azl* also can refer to coitus interruptus.

45. Al-Tabur, *Al-Tibb al-Sha'bi fi al-Imarat al-'Arabiyya al-Muttahida*, 145. For a discussion of the history of leprosy in Iran, see Willem Floor, "Qal'eh-ye Mehran Khan: The First Leprosarium in Iran," *Iranian Studies* 53, nos. 1–2 (2020): 9–41.

46. Al-Jarallah, *Tarikh al-Khadamat al-Sihhiyya fi al-Kuwayt*, 21. There is even reference to ideological quarantine in Arabia. David Commins writes that in the late nineteenth and early twentieth centuries the Ikhwan "would quarantine anyone who travelled to Kuwait," which they considered a "land of infidelity." David Commins, *The Wahhabi Mission and Saudi Arabia* (London: I. B. Tauris, 2006), 83.

47. Amir A. Afkhami, *A Modern Contagion: Imperialism and Public Health in Iran's Age of Cholera* (Baltimore: Johns Hopkins University Press, 2019), 17.

48. See Ahmad al-Bishr, *Maqalat 'an al-Kuwayt* (Kuwait: Maktabat al-Amal, 1966), 37; Muhammad bin Ibrahim al-Shaybani, *Al-Amrad al-Fattaka fi Tarikh al-Kuwayt: al-Ta'un, al-Judariyy, al-Influwanza* (Kuwait: Markaz al-Makhtutat wa-l-Turath wa-l-Watha'iq, 2017), 10.

49. Al-Bishr, *Maqalat 'an al-Kuwayt*, 37–38, quoting 'Uthman bin 'Abd Allah bin Bashr, *'Unwan al-Majd fi Tarikh Najd*, pt. 1, 229.

50. Al-Jarallah, *Tarikh al-Khadamat al-Sihhiyya fi al-Kuwayt*, 31. Unfortunately, I have not been able to locate contemporary accounts of the symptoms presented in nineteenth-century incidences of plague, and it is difficult to confirm if the *al-ṭā'un* referred to in the Arabic literature was in fact the infectious disease caused by the bacterium *Yersinia pestis*. However, it is telling that 'Uthman bin 'Abd Allah bin Bashr referred to the 1820 incident as *al-wabā'*, a general term for epidemic, while 1831 is referred to as the year of *al-ṭā'un*, specifically meaning plague. In the Ottoman context, Varlık points out that *ṭā'un* and *wabā'* could be "used almost interchangeably for emphasis or stylistic purposes," but scholars writing in Arabic after the fourteenth-century Black Death did distinguish the two. See Nükhet Varlık, *Plague and Empire in the Early Modern Mediterranean World: The Ottoman Experience, 1347–1600* (New York: Cambridge University Press, 2015), 11.

51. J. R. Wellsted, *Travels to the City of the Caliphs along the Shores of the Persian Gulf and the Mediterranean* (London: Henry Colburn, 1840), 1:280. See also James Onley, *The Arabian Frontier of the British Raj: Merchants, Rulers, and the British in the Nineteenth-Century Gulf* (Oxford: Oxford University Press, 2007), 307.

52. Monica H. Green and Lori Jones remind us that camels are highly effective transmitters of plague. Green and Jones, "Evolution and Spread of Major Human Diseases in the Indian Ocean World," 46.

53. 'Uthman bin Bashr al-Najdi, referenced in al-Jarallah, *Tarikh al-Khadamat al-Sihhiyya fi al-Kuwayt*, 32.

54. Mohammad Ma'yyid 'Abd Allah al-'Azmi, "Al-Maqabir wa-l-Shawahid al-Qabriyya fi al-Kuwayt: Masdar li-Darrasa ba'd Jawanib al-Tarikh al-Ijtima'iyy al-Kuwayti khilal al-Qarnayn" (master's thesis, Al-Bayt University, 2016), 105; al-Jarallah, *Tarikh al-Khadamat al-Sihhiyya fi al-Kuwayt*, 33.

55. When cholera struck Alexandria in 1865 following the return of pilgrims from Mecca, for example, "almost overnight, tens of thousands of the city's residents, especially from its foreign communities, put to sea." Daniel A. Stolz, "The Voyage of the *Samannud*: Pilgrimage, Cholera, and Empire on an Ottoman-Egyptian Steamship Journey in 1865–66," *International Journal of Turkish Studies* 23, nos. 1–2 (2017): 7.

56. Al-'Azmi, "Al-Maqabir wa-l-Shawahid al-Qabriyya fi al-Kuwayt," 105.

57. Yusif al-Qina'i, *Safahat min Tarikh al-Kuwayt* (Kuwait: Matba'at Hukumat al-Kuwayt, 1968), 58.

58. Al-'Azmi is referencing 'Abd Allah Khalid al-Hatim. Al-'Azmi, "Al-Maqabir wa-l-Shawahid al-Qabriyya fi al-Kuwayt," 105.

59. Al-'Azmi, 106.

60. Cited in al-Shaybani, *Al-Amrad al-Fattaka fi Tarikh al-Kuwayt*, 15.

61. Mary Douglas, *Purity and Danger: An Analysis of Concepts of Pollution and Taboo* (1966; repr., London: Routledge, 2000), 30. For a discussion of how Douglas's work informs the study of ritual in Islam, see A. Kevin Reinhart, "Impurity/No Danger," *History of Religions* 30, no. 1 (1990): 1–24.

62. Al-Salimi was part of a transregional Ibadi renaissance, or *nahḍa*, that drew together scholars from North Africa, Zanzibar, and Oman. Printing presses, such as the one Sultan Barghash bin Sa'id of Zanzibar (r. 1870–1888) established in 1879, circulated their ideas among far-flung Muslims. Al-Salimi's teacher, Saleh bin 'Ali al-Harthi, had been a student of Sa'id bin Khalfan al-Khalili, an Ibadi jurist who defied the British when he played an instrumental role in overthrowing the sultan in Muscat and establishing an Ibadi Imamate there between 1868 and 1871. Al-Salimi's historical writings praised his predecessors' Imamate, exhibited his contempt for the British and the sultans of the al-Busa'idi family, and expressed his opposition to Christian institutions like missionary schools. Barghash also had established a steamship to carry pilgrims from Oman and East Africa, which would have given Omanis firsthand exposure to the convergence of the global sanitary regime on the Hajj; al-Salimi himself undertook the trip to Mecca in 1905/6. John C. Wilkinson, *The Imamate Tradition of Oman* (Cambridge: Cambridge University Press, 1987), 243–245; Amal N. Ghazal, *Islamic Reform and Arab Nationalism: Expanding the Crescent from the Mediterranean to the Indian Ocean (1880s–1930s)* (London: Routledge, 2010), 20–36, 136 n. 50; Fahad Ahmad Bishara, *A Sea of Debt: Law and Economic Life in the Western Indian Ocean, 1780–1950* (Cambridge: Cambridge University Press, 2017), 107–115, 193–197.

63. As Bishara points out in reference to al-Khalili, published fatwas have undergone layers of editing and abridging, so unfortunately the dates of the questions and the names of the questioners are omitted. Bishara, *A Sea of Debt*, 86n13.

64. ʿAbdullah bin Humayd al-Salimi, *Jawabat al-Imam al-Salimi*, ed. ʿAbdullah bin Muhammad bin ʿAbdullah al-Salimi and ʿAbd al-Sattar Abu Ghuddah (Muscat: Maktabat al-Imam al-Salimi, 2010), 2:120.

65. The word used here, *al-ṭaʿn*, might also mean "stabbing," so the question could refer to "the days of the stabbing." The spelling is different from the usual word for plague, *al-ṭāʿun*, but given the description of local people's fear of the body it seems likely that *al-ṭaʿn* refers to disease.

66. The local term for Oman's expansive network of engineered underground water channels, *aflāj* (sing. *falaj*), comes from an Arabic root meaning to split or to divide.

67. Al-Salimi, *Jawabat*, 2:125–126.

68. Saʿid bin Khalfan al-Khalili, *Ajwibat al-Muhaqqiq al-Khalili* (Muscat: Maktabat Al-Jil Al-Waʿid, 2010), 6:310.

69. Hopper, *Slaves of One Master*, 121.

70. Harrison, *Arab at Home*, 309.

71. W. Norman Leak, "Medicine and the Traditions," *Neglected Arabia*, no. 125 (April–June 1923): 4, quoted in Doumato, *Getting God's Ear*, 208. Doumato elaborates on this procedure's wide use: "Jaundice was treated by cauterizing fingers and toes, ordinary stomach ache by burning the skin over the pain, and malaria by cauterizing the abdomen" (207–208).

72. Tony Judt, *The Memory Chalet* (New York: Penguin Books, 2010), 69.

73. J. C. Wilkinson, *Water and Tribal Settlement in South-East Arabia: A Study of the Aflāj of Oman* (Oxford: Oxford University Press, 1977), 21.

74. Lorimer, *Gazetteer*, "Preventive Measures in Bahrain," 2553.

75. Lorimer, *Gazetteer*, "Preventive Measures in the ʿOmān Sultanate, 1896–1907," 2551. IOR R/15/1/403, 'File 35/85 I A 8. Muscat: French Flag Question,' "Statement of the Quarantine Superintendent of His Highness the Sultan of Muscat Regarding Flight of Five Sooris from Quarantine on the Night of April 9th 1903."

76. Lorimer, *Gazetteer*, "Preventive Measures in Bahrain," 2553.

77. National Archives of India (hereafter NAI) Foreign Department, Establishment A. Nos. 36–39, "Quarantine Arrangements at Bahrein," October 1910.

78. A similar process occurred in Qing China during the 1910–1911 epidemic of pneumonic plague in Manchuria. See Sean Hsiang-lin Lei, *Neither Donkey nor Horse: Medicine in the Struggle over China's Modernity* (Chicago: University of Chicago Press, 2014), 21–44.

79. IOR V/23/82, no. 412, "Administration Report on the Persian Gulf Political Residency and Maskat Political Agency for 1903–1904," 1; Lucy M. Patterson, "Nine Months Medical Work at Bahrein," *Neglected Arabia* 52 (October–December 1904): 8.

80. IOR R/15/1/710, "Administration Reports 1905–1910," 1907–1908, 18.

81. IOR R/15/1/711, "Administration Report of the Persian Gulf Political Residency for the Years 1911–1914," 1911, 94.

82. IOR R/15/1/713, "Administration Reports 1920–1924," 1924, 62. The estimates of numbers of plague deaths are suspiciously alike. It is likely that observers drew from established categories of epidemics and then inserted a round number into each case.

83. IOR R/15/1/710, "Administration Reports 1905–1910," 1905–1906, 18.

84. On regional circulations of trade, see Hala Fattah, *The Politics of Regional Trade in Iraq, Arabia, and the Gulf 1745–1900* (Albany: State University of New York Press, 1997). Fattah argues that regional patterns of trade persisted until the 1860s, "when European trade finally managed to subsume regional operations into the wider context of the world economy." This periodization corresponds to the emergence of quarantine stations around the Gulf. Fattah, *Politics of Regional Trade*, 1.

85. Cornelia Dalenberg, *Sharifa* (Grand Rapids, MI: Eerdmans Publishing, 1983), 15.

86. Onley, *Arabian Frontier of the British Raj*, 37.

87. Bishara, *Sea of Debt*, 115–116.

88. Thomson, "Sanitary Requirements," 8.

89. Lawrence G. Potter, introduction to *The Persian Gulf in History*, ed. Lawrence G. Potter (New York: Palgrave Macmillan, 2009), 5.

90. Onley, *Arabian Frontier of the British Raj*, 46.

91. Afkhami, *Modern Contagion*, 89.

92. Afkhami, 102–105.

93. Afkhami, 100.

94. Thomson, "Sanitary Requirements," 17.

95. Thomson, 17.

96. Varlık, *Plague and Empire in the Early Modern Mediterranean World*, 177–178.

97. Bishara, *Sea of Debt*, 30.

98. Reidar Visser, *Basra, the Failed Gulf State: Separatism and Nationalism in Southern Iraq* (London: Global Book Marketing, 2005), 19; Isacar A. Bolaños, "The Ottomans during the Global Crises of Cholera and Plague: The View from Iraq and the Gulf," *International Journal of Middle East Studies* 51, no. 4 (2019): 603–604.

99. Thomson, "Sanitary Requirements," 18.

100. National Archives of the United Kingdom (hereafter NAUK), Major P. E. Cox, Political Resident in the Persian Gulf to Sir Lewis Dame, Secretary to the Government of India in the Foreign Department, 7 January 1906, FO 368/37 PRO; Thomson, "Sanitary Requirements," 15.

101. Frederick F. Anscombe, *The Ottoman Gulf: The Creation of Kuwait, Saudi Arabia, and Qatar* (New York: Columbia University Press, 1997), 91–112.

102. Visser, *Basra, the Failed Gulf State*, 34.

103. Talal Sa'd al-Rumaydi, *al-Kuwayt wa-l-Khalij al-'Arabi fi al-Salnama al-'Uthmaniyya* (Kuwait: N.p., 2009), 122.

104. Al-Rumaydi, 124.

105. Al-Rumaydi, 122.

106. China was presumed to be the source of the third global plague pandemic, which is typically dated from around 1894 to 1950 and claimed at least fifteen million lives. On the origins of the third pandemic, see Carol Benedict, *Bubonic Plague in Nineteenth-Century China* (Stanford, CA: Stanford University Press, 1996). On the global diffusion of the third pandemic, see Myron Echenberg, *Plague Ports: The Global Urban Impact of Bubonic Plague* (New York: New York University Press, 2007).

107. Al-Rumaydi, *al-Kuwayt wa-al-Khalij al-'Arabi fi al-Salnama al-'Uthmaniyya*, 123.

108. Khaled Albateni, "The Arabian Mission's Effect on Kuwaiti Society, 1910–1967" (PhD diss., Indiana University, 2014), 62–63.

109. Captain S. G. Knox to Major P. Z. Cole, 12 September 1904, IOR L/PS/10/47/1, File 1855/1904 Pt. 1 "Koweit:- H.M. Govt and Political Agent at Koweit (Representations from Turkish Govt & Temporary Withdrawal of Agent)."

110. Thomson, "Sanitary Requirements," 13.

111. Thomson, 13.

112. Echenberg, *Plague Ports*, 12.

113. Mark Gamsa, "The Epidemic of Pneumonic Plague in Manchuria 1910–1911," *Past and Present* 190 (2006): 167.

114. Christos Lynteris, "Skilled Natives, Inept Coolies: Marmot Hunting and the Great Manchurian Pneumonic Plague (1910–1911)," *History and Anthropology* 24, no. 3 (2013): 305.

Chapter 2

1. NAUK: FO 1016/103, "Translated purport of the address delivered by His Highness the Sultan of Muscat at the meeting for the construction of a new Hospital dated the 14th Moharram 1327" (6 February 1909).

2. NAUK: FO 1016/103, Holland, I.C.S. Political Agent Muscat to Political Resident in the Persian Gulf, Bushire, 15 April 1909, "Muscat Hospital."

3. IOR L/PS/10/27/4, "P. 6. 733/1904. Muscat:- Hospital," Captain Norman Scott to R. E. Holland, 28 December 1908.

4. IOR L/PS/10/27/4, "P. 6. 733/1904. Muscat:- Hospital," "The Muscat Hospital," R. E. Holland, 21 January 1909.

5. NAUK: FO 1016/103, Holland, I.C.S. Political Agent Muscat to Political Resident in the Persian Gulf, Bushire, 15 April 1909, "Muscat Hospital."

6. NAUK: FO 1016/103, "Translated purport of the address delivered by His Highness the Sultan of Muscat at the meeting for the construction of a new Hospital dated the 14th Moharram 1327" (6 February 1909).

7. NAUK: FO 1016/103, "Translated purport of the address delivered by His Highness the Sultan of Muscat at the meeting for the construction of a new Hospital dated the 14th Moharram 1327" (6 February 1909).

8. NAUK: FO 1016/103, Madhouji Jivandas, for the Bhatia Mahajan, to Holland, Political Agent, 5 February 1909, "Muscat Hospital."

9. NAUK: FO 1016/103 "Muscat Hospital," translated purport of a letter dated the 13th Moharram 1327 (5 February 1909), from the Agha Khani residents of Muscat and Mutrah, to the Political Agent, Muscat. Until the 1860s, most Khojas (Muslim Indian merchants from Gujarat and later Bombay) in the Gulf were Agha Khani. In the 1860s, around half of the Agha Khani population in the Gulf converted to Ithna'ashari (Twelver) Shi'ism in the wake of a schism with the Agha Khan, and most of those who had converted lived in Oman. The wording of this donation letter seems to reflect the reality that Oman's Agha Khani community was small and had fallen on hard times. See James Onley, "Indian Communities in the Persian Gulf, c. 1500–1947," in *The Persian Gulf in Modern Times: People, Ports, and History*, ed. Lawrence G. Potter (New York: Palgrave Macmillan, 2014), 243–244.

10. NAUK: FO 1016/103 "Muscat Hospital," 6 February 1909, from Memon Abdul Latif Isani Kutchi, representative of the Memon Community of Muscat and Mutrah, to the Political Agent, Muscat. A Sunni community from Sindh, Kutch, and Gujarat and tracing their origins to Rajasthan, the Memons were one of the smallest merchant communities in the Gulf. They were reportedly forced out of Muscat by the Khojas in the late nineteenth century. Onley, "Indian Communities in the Persian Gulf," 244–245. It would appear that the three remaining members were still appealed to for a hospital contribution.

11. NAUK: FO 1016/103 "Muscat Hospital" "List of Donors to the New Hospital."

12. IOR L/PS/10/27/4, "P. 6. 733/1904. Muscat:- Hospital," Captain Norman Scott to R. E. Holland, 28 December 1908.

13. NAUK: FO 1016/103, Madhauji Jivandas for the Bhatia Mahajan to Mr. R. E. Holland, Political Agent & H.B.M's Consul, Muscat (5 February 1909).

14. Nile Green, *Bombay Islam: The Religious Economy of the West Indian Ocean, 1840–1915* (Cambridge: Cambridge University Press, 2011), 24.

15. NAUK: FO 1016/103, Major P. Z. Cox, Political Resident in the Persian Gulf, to S. H. Butler, Secretary to the Government of India in the Foreign Department, Simla (2 May 1909).

16. Fatma Hassan Al-Sayegh, "American Women Missionaries in the Gulf: Agents for Cultural Change," *Islam and Christian-Muslim Relations* 9, no. 3 (1998): 339.

17. Catherine S. Woodward, "The Discourse and Experience of the Arabian Mission's Medical Missionaries: Part I 1920–39," *Middle Eastern Studies* 47, no. 5 (2011): 779.

18. Hilal al-Hajri, "Through Evangelizing Eyes: American Missionaries to Oman," *Proceedings of the Seminar for Arabian Studies Held at the British Museum, London 22 to 24 July 2010* 41 (2011): 124. In discussing how various outsiders used it "to gain entry into the region," Nasser Hammad Al-Azri describes biomedicine as "a Trojan Horse of Arabia." See Nasser Hammad Al-Azri, "Sent to Explore, Conquer and Heal: History of the Evolution of Biomedicine in Oman during the 19th Century," *Sultan Qaboos University Medical Journal* 11, no. 2 (2011): 189.

19. Beth Baron, *The Orphan Scandal: Christian Missionaries and the Rise of the Muslim Brotherhood* (Stanford, CA: Stanford University Press, 2014), 36.

20. Khaled Albateni, "The Arabian Mission's Effect on Kuwaiti Society, 1910–1967" (PhD diss., Indiana University, 2014), 20.

21. Albateni, 27.

22. Albateni, 29.

23. Albateni, 40. Although the hospital was not officially dedicated and opened until 1903, the missionaries started operating their medical services in the building as early as October 1902. See Marion Wells Thoms, "Women Patients," *Neglected Arabia* 44 (October–December 1902): 18.

24. Rev. John Van Ess, "The Annual Meeting," *Neglected Arabia* 45 (January–March 1903): 3–4.

25. S. J. Thoms, "The Hospital at Bahrein," *Neglected Arabia* 44 (October–December 1902):13.

26. IOR R/15/2/960, "V M Hospital Building," Assistant Political Agent, Bahrein, to Political Resident in the Persian Gulf, Bushire, 16 November 1901.

27. IOR R/15/2/960, "V M Hospital Building," Assistant Surgeon to Political Agent, Bahrein, 13 July 1905.

28. Albateni, "Arabian Mission's Effect on Kuwaiti Society," 55.

29. Albateni, 50, 62–63.

30. IOR L/PS/10/47/1, "File 1855/1904 Pt I 'Koweit:- H.M. Govt and Political Agent at Koweit (Representations from Turkish Govt & Temporary Withdrawal of Agent)," Shaykh Mubarak to Captain S. G. Knox, 13 September 1904.

31. IOR R/15/6/504, "Administration Report on the Persian Gulf Political Residency and Maskat Political Agency for 1904–1905," 159.

32. IOR L/PS/10/47/1, "File 1855/1904 Pt 1 'Koweit:- H.M. Govt and Political Agent at Koweit (Representations from Turkish Govt & Temporary Withdrawal of Agent)," Captain S. G. Knox to Major P. Z. Cox, 6 September 1904.

33. Khalid al-Jarallah, *Tarikh al-Khadamat al-Sihhiyya fi al-Kuwayt* (Kuwait: Markaz al-Buhuth wa-l-Dirasat al-Kuwaytiyya, 1996), 57.

34. The total population in Kuwait territory in 1901 was estimated to be about eighty-nine thousand. See IOR L/PS/20/153, "Koweit [Kuwait]. A report compiled in the Intelligence Branch, Quarter Master General's Department," 1903, 18.

35. Albateni, "Arabian Mission's Effect on Kuwaiti Society," 63–64.

36. Albateni, 64.

37. Albateni, 2.

38. 'Abd Allah Khalid al-Hatim, *Min Huna Bada'at al-Kuwayt* (Damascus: Al-Matba'a al-'Umumiyya, 1962), 104.

39. Al-Hatim, *Min Huna Bada'at al-Kuwayt*, 104–105; Yusif Shihab, *Al-Kuwayt 'Abra al-Tarikh* (Kuwait: N.p., 1989), 289.

40. IOR R/15/6/504, "Administration Report on the Persian Gulf Political Residency and Maskat Political Agency for 1904–1905, 159.

41. IOR R/15/6/504, "Administration Report on the Persian Gulf Political Residency and Maskat Political Agency for 1904–1905," 159.

42. Al-Jarallah, *Tarikh al-Khadamat al-Sihhiyya fi al-Kuwayt*, 110.

43. Rasim Rushdi, *Kuwayt wa-Kuwaytiyyun: Dirasat fi Madi al-Kuwayt wa-Hadiriha* (Beirut: Matba'at al-Rahbaniyah al-Lubnaniyah, 1955), 79, paraphrased in al-Jarallah, *Tarikh al-Khadamat al-Sihhiyya fi al-Kuwayt*, 21.

44. Al-Jarallah, *Tarikh al-Khadamat al-Sihhiyya fi al-Kuwayt*, 21.

45. C. Stanley G. Mylrea, "The Enemy at the Gates," *Neglected Araba* 117 (April–June 1921): 6.

46. Kamal Fahmy, "Salt Atresia in Arabia," *Australian and New Zealand Journal of Obstetrics and Gynaecology* 5, no. 2 (1965): 103.

47. IOR L/PS/10/27/3, "P. 5. 733/1904. Muscat:- American Dispensary," R. E. Holland to Political Resident in the Persian Gulf, 3 April 1909.

48. Al-Azri, "History of the Evolution of Biomedicine in Oman during the 19th Century," 193.

49. IOR L/PS/10/27/3, "P. 5. 733/1904. Muscat:- American Dispensary," J. A. Ray, American Consul to Seyyid Faisul bin Turki, Sultan of Oman, 15 November 1909.

50. IOR L/PS/10/27/3, "P. 5. 733/1904. Muscat:- American Dispensary," R. E. Holland to Political Resident in the Persian Gulf, 23 November 1909.

51. IOR L/PS/10/27/3, "P. 5. 733/1904. Muscat:- American Dispensary," R. E. Holland to Political Resident in the Persian Gulf, 23 November 1909.

52. IOR L/PS/10/27/3, "P. 5. 733/1904. Muscat:- American Dispensary," R. E. Holland to Political Resident in the Persian Gulf, 23 November 1909.

53. Al-Sayegh, "American Women Missionaries in the Gulf," 339.

54. Amy E. Zwemer, "The Ups and Downs of Work for the Women," *Neglected Arabia* 47 (July–September 1903): 8.

55. S. J. Thoms, "Bahrein," *Neglected Arabia* 37 (January-March 1901): 7.

56. Amy E. Zwemer, "Lay-Preaching in the Women's Dispensary," *Neglected Arabia* 43 (July–September 1902): 8.

57. Mrs. S. M. Zwemer, "Work for Women," *Neglected Arabia* 37 (January–March 1901): 9.

58. Thoms, "Women Patients," 18.

59. Thoms, 18.

60. Eleanor T. Calverley, *My Arabian Days and Nights: A Medical Missionary in Old Kuwait* (New York: Thomas Y. Crowell Company, 1958), 20.

61. Calverley, *My Arabian Days and Nights*, 102.

62. IOR R/15/1/710, "Administration Reports 1905–1910," 1910, 76.

63. NAI: Foreign Department, February 1902, Nos. 3–6, "Increase to the Medical Establishment at Maskat."

64. Sharon J. Thoms, "Opening Work at Bahrein: A Shark Bite," *Neglected Arabia* 35 (July–September 1900): 6.

65. Thoms, "A Shark Bite," 6.

66. Thoms, 6.

67. Thoms, 6.

68. Thoms, 6.

69. Thoms, "Women Patients," 19.

70. Thoms, 19.

71. Marion Wells Thoms, "Bahrein Station," *Neglected Arabia* 36 (October–December 1900): 8. The missionaries do not mention that Ibn Sina's *Canon of Medicine* had greatly advanced approaches to the diagnosis and management of cataracts centuries before modern biomedical surgical techniques.

72. Thoms, "Women Patients," 19.

73. Thoms, 19.

74. Thoms, 20.

75. Zwemer, "Ups and Downs of Work for the Women," 7.

76. Zwemer, 7.

77. Zwemer, 7.
78. Zwemer, 7–8.
79. Zwemer, 8.
80. Zwemer, 8.
81. Zwemer, 9.
82. Zwemer, 8. More recent research on the effects of temperature on the transmission of *Y. pestis* by the flea shows that, in contrast to Amy Zwemer's belief that the plague germs died in the heat, the issue was that transmission efficiencies of fleas begin to decline at twenty-seven degrees Celsius, coinciding with declining median bacterial loads and lower survival and feeding rates in fleas at high temperatures. See Anna M. Schotthoefer et al., "Effects of Temperature on the Transmission of *Yersinia Pestis* by the Flea, *Xenopsylla Cheopis*, in the Late Phase Period," *Parasites & Vectors* 4, no. 191 (2011): https://doi.org/10.1186/1756-3305-4-191.
83. S. M. Zwemer, "Bahrein," *Neglected Arabia* 35 (July–September 1900): 5.
84. Lucy M. Patterson, "Two Weeks at the Hospital," *Neglected Arabia* 50 (April–June 1904): 10.
85. This discussion draws from Laura Frances Goffman, "A Jar of Shaykhs' Teeth: Medicine, Politics, and the Fragments of History in Kuwait," *International Journal of Middle East Studies* 53, no. 4 (November 2021): 589–603.
86. Albateni, "Arabian Mission's Effect on Kuwaiti Society," 84.
87. Talal Al-Rashoud, "Modern Education and Arab Nationalism in Kuwait, 1911–1961" (PhD diss., SOAS University of London, 2016), 45.
88. Leor Halevi, *Modern Things on Trial: Islam's Global and Material Reformation in the Age of Rida, 1865–1935* (New York: Columbia University Press, 2019), 99.
89. Suliman Al-Atiqi, "The Origins of Kuwaiti Nationalism: Rashid Rida's Influence on Kuwaiti National Identity," *Arab Studies Journal* 23, no. 1 (Fall 2015): 81.
90. Edwin E. Calverley, "Evangelistic Activities at Kuweit," *Neglected Arabia* no. 92 (January–March 1915): 8.
91. Al-Atiqi, "Origins of Kuwaiti Nationalism," 93.
92. Albateni, "Arabian Mission's Effect on Kuwaiti Society," 99; IOR R/15/1/711, "Administration Report of the Persian Gulf Political Residency for the Years 1911–1914," 1913, 127.
93. Khalid al-Jarallah, *Dawakhana: Dirasa Tawthiqiyya fi Tarikh al-Kuwayt al-Sihhi min Khilal Dafatir 'Abd al-Ilah al-Qina'i* (Kuwait: Markaz al-Buhuth wa-l-Dirasat al-Kuwaytiyya, 2005), 18–19.
94. Calverley, "Evangelistic Activities at Kuweit," 9.
95. Shihab, *Al-Kuwayt 'Abra al-Tarikh*, 287.
96. Al-Jarallah, *Tarikh al-Khadamat al-Sihhiyya fi al-Kuwayt*, 118.

97. Mylrea, "Enemy at the Gates," 6.
98. "Da'ira al-Sihha al-'Amma," *Al-Kuwayt al-Yawm* 11 (19 February 1955): 6–7; Al-Jarallah, *Tarikh al-Khadamat al-Sihhiyya fi al-Kuwayt*, 156.
99. IOR R/15/2/132, "File 9/5 Bahrain Reforms. Reforms in Pearling and Boat Registration," Political Resident, Persian Gulf to Foreign, Delhi, 13 March 1924.
100. Al-Hatim, *Min Huna Bada'at al-Kuwayt*, 107.
101. IOR R/15/2/1825, "File A/2 Slave Trade. Correspondence with Bushire regarding Slaves and Their Manumission Certificates and Applications," "Statement of Slave Suwailim bin Faraj Aged about 25 Years Recorded in the Political Agency, Bahrain," 18 October 1934.

Chapter 3

1. Sabika Al Najjar and Fawzeya Matar, *Al-Mar'a al-Bahrayniyya fi al-Qarn al-'Ishrin: Marhalat Ma Qabl al-Istiqlal 1900–1970* (Ottawa: Masaa Publishing and Distribution, 2017), 191–192.
2. According to Maryam Alsada, women purchased salt that was imported from Persia to prepare the salt suppositories. Maryam Mohamed Abdulla Ebrahim Alsada, "The Lives of Girls and Women in Bahrain and Qatar: Dress, Marriage, Health and Education in the Pearl Fishing and Early Oil Era" (PhD diss., University College London, 2022), 208.
3. Hibba Abugideiri, "A Labor of Love: Making Space for Midwives in Gulf History," in *Gulf Women*, ed. Amira El-Azhary Sonbol (Syracuse, NY: Syracuse University Press, 2012), 180.
4. Eleanor Abdella Doumato, *Getting God's Ear: Women, Islam, and Healing in Saudi Arabia and the Gulf* (New York: Columbia University Press, 2000), 187.
5. Avner Giladi, *Muslim Midwives: The Craft of Birthing in the Premodern Middle East* (Cambridge: Cambridge University Press, 2014), 161.
6. While physically absent from the scene of birth, men's influence may have been related to their financial role. In the premodern period, as Avner Giladi describes, Muslim jurists "debated the question of who should hire and pay for the midwife: the mother- or the father-to-be?" Opinions varied, with Shafi'is charging the husband, Hanafis making the one who called the midwife responsible for her wages when she was summoned well in advance, and Malikis determining that the husband became financially responsible only when "it became clear that the midwife's help was essential for the well-being of the infant, and, moreover, that the mother could not manage without her." In short, Giladi concludes that "men—husbands, potential fathers—while excluded from the childbirth scene were nevertheless indirectly involved by selecting a midwife and paying for her services." Giladi, *Muslim Midwives*, 133–134.

7. Catherine S. Woodward, "The Discourse and Experiences of the Arabian Mission's Medical Missionaries: Part II 1939–1960," *Middle Eastern Studies* 47, no. 6 (2011): 887.

8. Eleanor T. Calverley, *My Arabian Days and Nights* (New York: Thomas Y. Crowell Co., 1958), 88–90.

9. M. N. Tiffany, "Women's Medical Work in Bahrain," *Neglected Arabia* 154 (July–September, 1930): 8.

10. Cornelia Dalenberg, "Unforgetable [sic] Patients," *Arabia Calling* 217 (Summer 1949): 13. Khaled Fahmy describes a parallel use of the "metaphors of light and darkness" in his critique of how some Egyptian historiography has addressed Egypt's relationship with Europe in the pursuit of modernization in science, medicine, and other fields after Bonaparte's 1798 invasion. Khaled Fahmy, *In Quest of Justice: Islamic Law and Forensic Medicine in Modern Egypt* (Oakland: University of California Press, 2018), 9. Whereas Egyptian historiography has contrasted the "dark" Ottoman period with the "light" brought by Europe, the missionaries in the Gulf presented their medical institutionalization as a process of enlightenment that contrasted a backward, Islamic society with their modernizing Christianity.

11. Cornelia Dalenberg, "From Shadowed Thresholds, Dark with Fear: A Village Woman's Story," *Arabia Calling* 225 (Autumn 1951): 14.

12. Woodward, "Discourse: Part II," 902.

13. Quoted in Woodward, 901.

14. "Appendix to Kuwait Report," ARC 59729, British Petroleum Archive (hereafter BP).

15. Quoted in Woodward, "Discourse: Part II," 901.

16. Quoted in Woodward, 902.

17. Exceptionally, many iterations later, the American Mission Hospital in Bahrain continues to treat patients.

18. Beth Baron, *The Orphan Scandal: Christian Missionaries and the Rise of the Muslim Brotherhood* (Stanford, CA: Stanford University Press, 2014), 41.

19. Arabian Gulf Digital Archives (hereafter AGDA), FCO 8/685, 1967–1986, R. G. Smedley, "Closure of US Mission Hospital," 29 July 1967.

20. These articles progressively cite each other, demonstrating that they are in conversation: A. E. Kingston, "The Vaginal Atresia of Arabia," *BJOG: An International Journal of Obstetrics and Gynaecology* 64, no. 6 (December 1957): 836–839; Kathleen Frith, "Vaginal Atresia of Arabia: Four Cases," *BJOG: An International Journal of Obstetrics and Gynaecology* 67, no. 1 (February 1960): 82–85; Ismail El Guindi, "Vaginal Atresia in Saudi Arabia," *BJOG: An International Journal of Obstetrics and Gynaecology* 69, no. 6 (December 1962): 996–998; Kamal Fahmy, "Cervical and Vaginal Atresia due to Packing the Vagina with Salt

after Labor," *American Journal of Obstetrics and Gynecology* 84, no. 11 (1962): 1466–1469; Betty M. L. Underhill, "Salt-Induced Vaginal Stenosis of Arabia," *BJOG: An International Journal of Obstetrics and Gynaecology* 71, no. 2 (1964): 293–298; Kamal Fahmy, "Salt Atresia in Arabia," *Australian and New Zealand Journal of Obstetrics and Gynaecology* 5, no. 2 (1965): 103–112. Missionary doctors also had published in scientific journals based on their work in Arabia. See, e.g., C. Stanley G. Mylrea, "A Case of Snake Bite in Kuwait, Arabia," *Transactions of the Royal Society of Tropical Medicine and Hygiene* 21, no. 5 (February 1928): 426, reproduced in Khalid al-Jarallah, *Sihhat al-Kuwayt: Qira'a fi Watha'iq Kuwaytiyya wa Ajnabiyya* (Kuwait: Markaz al-Buhuth wa-l-Dirasat al-Kuwaytiyya, 2019), 100.

21. El Guindi, "Vaginal Atresia in Saudi Arabia," 996.

22. El Guindi, 996.

23. Doumato, *Getting God's Ear*, 189; Abugideiri, "Labor of Love," 189; Catherine S. Woodward, "The Discourse and Experience of the Arabian Mission's Medical Missionaries: Part I, 1920–39" *Middle Eastern Studies* 47, no. 5 (2011): 795.

24. Ida Paterson Storm, "Touring Troubles, "*Arabia Calling*, no. 218 (Autumn–Winter 1949–1950): 7.

25. Doumato, *Getting God's Ear*, 190.

26. Sayyid 'Ali al-Sayyid Baqir al-'Awwami, *Al-Haraka al-Wataniyya Sharq al-Sa'udiyya 1373–1393 h/ 1953–1973 m*, 2 vols. (2011), 1:44. Toby Matthiesen notes that the memoirs were published posthumously. See Toby Matthiesen, "The Cold War and the Communist Party of Saudi Arabia, 1975–1991," *Journal of Cold War Studies* 22, no.3 (Summer 2020): 33n6.

27. Al-'Awwami, *Al-Haraka al-Wataniyya Sharq al-Sa'udiyya*, 1:44.

28. Fahmy, "Salt Atresia in Arabia," 103.

29. Viewing women patients' body parts with an emphasis on their sexuality was hardly particular to doctors working in this region. As Barron H. Lerner notes of breast cancer exams in the postwar United States, the fact that "x-rays and other images of women's bodies, while purportedly obtained for medical purposes," provided observers with "visual and even sexual pleasure" infused efforts to make breast cancer curable with "sexual and political tensions." Barron H. Lerner, *The Breast Cancer Wars: Hope, Fear, and the Pursuit of a Cure in Twentieth-Century America* (Oxford: Oxford University Press, 2003), 56–57.

30. Omar H. AlShehabi, *Contested Modernity: Sectarianism, Nationalism, and Colonialism in Bahrain* (London: Oneworld Academic, 2019), 202; Nelida Fuccaro, *Histories of City and State in the Persian Gulf: Manama since 1800* (Cambridge: Cambridge University Press, 2009), 116.

31. Charles Belgrave, *Personal Column* (London: Hutchinson & Co., 1960), 90.

32. Belgrave, 91.

33. Kingston, "Vaginal Atresia of Arabia," 836–837.
34. Frith, "Vaginal Atresia of Arabia," 82.
35. Underhill, "Salt-Induced Vaginal Stenosis of Arabia," 293.
36. Fahmy, "Salt Atresia in Arabia," 103.
37. Quoted in Norman E. Himes, *Medical History of Contraception* (1936; rpt., New York: Schocken Books, 1970), 139. Himes adds in a footnote, "Ordinary modern table salt is an excellent spermicide. An 8 per cent solution kills sperms rapidly. As used in our time five tablespoonfuls are dissolved in a quart of water; or half a teaspoonful to a vaginal bulbful." I am grateful to Leslie Reagan for this reference.
38. Fahmy, "Salt Atresia in Arabia," 103.
39. Frith, "Vaginal Atresia of Arabia," 82–83.
40. Frith, 83.
41. Frith, 84.
42. Underhill, "Salt-Induced Vaginal Stenosis of Arabia," 295.
43. Frith, "Vaginal Atresia of Arabia," 84.
44. Fahmy, "Cervical and Vaginal Atresia," 1468.
45. Underhill, "Salt-Induced Vaginal Stenosis of Arabia," 293.
46. Fahmy, "Salt Atresia in Arabia," 111.
47. Frith, "Vaginal Atresia of Arabia," 85.
48. Nabil Subhi Hanna, *Al-Tibb al-Shaʿbi fi al-Khalij* (Doha: Markaz al-Turath al-Shaʿbi li Majlis al-Taʿaun li Duwal al-Khalīj al-ʿArabī, 1998), 9.
49. Hanna, *Al-Tibb al-Shaʿbi fi al-Khalij*, 9.
50. Hanna, 17.
51. Hanna, 20.
52. Hanna, 22. The list of field researchers includes four women and five men (7).
53. Hanna, 27.
54. Mahmoud Sinan, *Tarikh Qatar al-ʿAmm* (Baghdad, Iraq: Al-Maʿaref Press, 1966), 224–225.
55. Hanna, *Al-Tibb al-Shaʿbi fi al-Khalij*, 26–27.
56. Sara Scalenghe points out that the discrete categories "the disabled" and "disability" are products of modern Europe and did not appear in the Arab world until the twentieth century. The current Arabic translations of "disability" (*iʿāqa*) and "disabled" (*muʿawwaq* and *maʿūq*) derive from the Arabic verb *ʿāqa*, "to hinder" or "to hamper." Sara Scalenghe, *Disability in the Ottoman Arab World, 1500–1800* (New York: Cambridge University Press, 2014), 1.
57. Hanna, *Al-Tibb al-Shaʿbi fi al-Khalij*, 205.
58. Hanna, 365.
59. Hanna, 28. Abugideiri describes a similar process of acquiring obstetrical knowledge from elders: "To become a midwife, a girl learned the trade from a senior

woman in the tribe, typically her mother or grandmother . . . Thus, midwifery was a trade that was passed on generationally." Abugideiri, "Labor of Love," 181.

60. Hanna, *Al-Tibb al-Shaʿbi fi al-Khalij*, 22.

61. Marcia C. Inhorn, *Quest for Conception: Gender, Infertility, and Egyptian Medical Traditions* (Philadelphia: University of Pennsylvania Press, 1994), 3.

62. Storm, "Touring Troubles," 6.

63. Al-ʿAwwami, *Al-Haraka al-Wataniyya Sharq al-Saʿudiyya*, 1:72n20.

64. Hanna, *Al-Tibb al-Shaʿbi fi al-Khalij*, 365.

65. Hanna, 366.

66. Hanna, 368.

67. Hanna, 406.

68. Hanna, 371.

69. Hanna, 389.

70. Hanna, 389–390.

71. Hanna, 395.

72. Hanna, 396.

73. Hanna, 397. This need for water access during home births may have been one of the reasons women in Bahrain were so alarmed by the proposal to fill in house wells for the sake of malaria control in 1940. See Laura Frances Goffman, "Malaria and Empire in Bahrain, 1931–1947," *Gulf Studies Monographic Series* 7 (2020): 1–30.

74. Hanna, *Al-Tibb al-Shaʿbi fi al-Khalij*, 396.

75. Sarah Laskow, "How the Plastic Bag Became So Popular," *The Atlantic*, October 10, 2014, https://www.theatlantic.com/technology/archive/2014/10/how-the-plastic-bag-became-so-popular/381065/.

76. There are some exceptions when men do play a role. For example, Hanna mentions that sometimes it might be the husband's job to go and summon the other women when his wife started labor. Hanna, *Al-Tibb al-Shaʿbi fi al-Khalij*, 398.

77. Hanna, 401.

78. Hanna, 402.

79. Hanna, 404.

80. Hanna, 397.

81. Abeer Abu Saud, *Qatari Women Past and Present* (Essex, UK: Longman Group, 1984), 111.

82. Mai Ahmad Zaki Yamani, "Birth and Behaviour in a Hospital in Saudi Arabia," *Bulletin (British Society for Middle Eastern Studies)* 13, no. 2 (1986): 169.

83. Hanna, *Al-Tibb al-Shaʿbi fi al-Khalij*, 406.

84. Hanna, 405.

85. Hanna, 206.

Chapter 4

1. Later the organization's name would change to the Arabian Gulf Medical Society. See the interview with Armand P. Gelpi, an oral history conducted in 1996 by Carole Hicke, in "Health and Disease in Saudi Arabia: Oral History Transcript: The Aramco Experience, 1940s-1990s/1998," Regional Oral History Office, Bancroft Library, University of California, Berkeley (hereafter "Health and Disease in Saudi Arabia"), 64.

2. Robert Vitalis, *America's Kingdom: Mythmaking on the Saudi Oil Frontier* (Stanford, CA: Stanford University Press, 2007).

3. "Health and Disease in Saudi Arabia," 50.

4. Helen Lackner, *A House Built on Sand: A Political Economy of Saudi Arabia* (London: Ithaca Press, 1978), 96–97; Vitalis, *America's Kingdom*, 149–153; Alexei Vassiliev, *The History of Saudi Arabia* (London: Saqi Books, 2000), 686–689. Population estimates of al-Hasa at the beginning of the 1950s varied between 150,000 and 250,000. See Toby Craig Jones, *Desert Kingdom: How Oil and Water Forged Modern Saudi Arabia* (Cambridge, MA: Harvard University Press, 2010), 269n24.

5. Scholarship on labor and opposition movements in mid-twentieth-century Eastern Province has long offered an important counternarrative to official Saudi and Aramco histories. Classic studies from the 1970s include Fred Halliday, *Arabia without Sultans* (Middlesex, UK: Penguin Books, 1974), and Lackner, *A House Built on Sand*. More recently, the authoritative account of Aramco and the labor movement is Vitalis, *America's Kingdom*. Toby Jones integrates a critical environmental lens, while Toby Matthiesen offers an account of the Shi'i experience. See Jones, *Desert Kingdom*; Toby Matthiesen, *The Other Saudis: Shiism, Dissent and Sectarianism* (Cambridge: Cambridge University Press, 2015). Useful articles include John Chalcraft, "Migration and Popular Protest in the Arabian Peninsula and the Gulf in the 1950s and 1960s," *International Labor and Working-Class History* 79, no. 1 (Spring 2011): 28–47; Toby Matthiesen, "Migration, Minorities, and Radical Networks: Labour Movements and Opposition Groups in Saudi Arabia, 1950–1975," *International Review of Social History* 59, 3 (Autumn 2014): 473–504; Claudia Ghrawi, "Structural and Physical Violence in Saudi Arabian Oil Towns, 1953–56," in *Urban Violence in the Middle East: Changing Cityscapes in the Transition from Empire to Nation State*, ed. Ulrike Freitag, Nelida Fuccaro, Claudia Ghrawi, and Nora Lafi (New York: Berghahn Books, 2015), 243–264; Claudia Ghrawi, "A Tamed Urban Revolution: Saudi Arabia's Oil Conurbation and the 1967 Riots," in *Violence and the City in the Modern Middle East*, ed. Nelida Fuccaro, (Stanford, CA: Stanford University Press, 2016), 109–126; Rosie Bsheer, "A Counter-Revolutionary State: Popular Movements and the Making of Saudi Arabia," *Past and Present* 238 (November 2018): 233–277.

6. John C. Snyder, "Trachoma Project: A Written Account," in "Health and Disease in Saudi Arabia," 246.

7. Snyder, 247.

8. Chad H. Parker, *Making the Desert Modern: Americans, Arabs, and Oil on the Saudi Frontier, 1933–1973* (Amherst: University of Massachusetts Press, 2015), 86.

9. Allan M. Brandt, "Polio, Politics, Publicity, and Duplicity: Ethical Aspects in the Development of the Salk Vaccine," *International Journal of Health Services* 8, no. 2 (1978): 258.

10. On the Tuskegee syphilis study, see, e.g., Allan M. Brandt, "Racism and Research: The Case of the Tuskegee Syphilis Study," *Hastings Center Report* 6, no. 8 (1978): 21–29; James H. Jones, *Bad Blood: The Tuskegee Syphilis Experiment*, new and expanded ed. (New York: Free Press, 1993); Susan M. Reverby, ed., *Tuskegee's Truths: Rethinking the Tuskegee Syphilis Study* (Chapel Hill: University of North Carolina Press, 2012); and Susan M. Reverby, *Examining Tuskegee: The Infamous Syphilis Study and Its Legacy* (Chapel Hill: University of North Carolina Press, 2009). Melissa Graboyes provides a helpful overview of scholarship on experimental global medical research. See Melissa Graboyes, *The Experiment Must Continue: Medical Research and Ethics in East Africa, 1940–2014* (Athens: Ohio University Press, 2015), 210–218.

11. This was the same year that over a million young children in the United States participated in the field trial of the Salk polio vaccine. Paul Meier, "The Biggest Public Health Experiment Ever: The 1954 Field Trial of the Salk Poliomyelitis Vaccine," in *Statistics: A Guide to the Unknown*, ed. Judith M. Tanur et al. (San Francisco: Holden-Day, 1972), 2–13.

12. F. F. Tang, H. Chang, Y. Huang, and K. Wang, "Studies on the Etiology of Trachoma with Special Reference to Isolation of the Virus in Chick Embryo," *Chinese Medical Journal* 75 (1957): 429–447.

13. Interview with Dorothy McComb, in "Health and Disease in Saudi Arabia," 305.

14. Interview with Elinor Nichols, in "Health and Disease in Saudi Arabia," 269–270.

15. Lorania K. Francis, "U.S. Hospital Oasis of Health for Arabs: Medical Science Defeats Tide of Ancient Diseases in Oil Area," *Los Angeles Times*, April 2, 1951.

16. Samuel S. Stratton, Country Director, Technical Cooperation Administration, 4 November 1952; Saudi Arabia, Background—Health Conditions; Health & Sanitation; Subject Files, 1950–54; Record Group 469: Records of US Foreign Assistance Agencies, 1948–1961.

17. Madawi Al-Rasheed, *A History of Saudi Arabia*, 2nd ed. (London: Cambridge University Press, 2010), 89–92.

18. Vitalis, *America's Kingdom*. Other scholars have also shifted attention from Aramco to the Saudi state as a mid-twentieth-century modernizing force. As Pascal Ménoret states, "modernization succeeded because, in the 1960s, state revenues doubled, economic activity increased and an endogenous industry gradually took shape around the production of consumer goods and construction materials." Pascal Ménoret, *The Saudi Enigma: A History* (London: Zed Books, 2005), 100. Fred Halliday summarized the matter with his typical bluntness: "The rise in oil revenues in the 1960s and 1970s enabled even the most wasteful regime to initiate development of some kind." Halliday, *Arabia without Sultans*, 63.

19. For example, in 1968 Eastern Province only had 15 percent of the hospitals and 10 percent of the physicians of the Ministry of Health. Al-Awaji contextualizes these figures by noting that Aramco employees in Eastern Province "may benefit from [the company's] health services." See Ibrahim Mohamed Al-Awaji, "Bureaucracy and Society in Saudi Arabia" (PhD diss., University of Virginia, 1971), 240, 241.

20. Matthiesen, *The Other Saudis*, 73; Jones, *Desert Kingdom*, 145–150.

21. Crown Prince Faisal rivaled his brother for leadership, and Faisal eventually overthrew Saʿud in 1964. Bsheer, "Counter-Revolutionary State," 240.

22. David Commins, *The Gulf States: A Modern History* (London: I. B. Tauris, 2012), 136.

23. Khalid al-Jarallah, *Tarikh al-Khadamat al-Sihhiyya fi al-Kuwayt* (Kuwait: Markaz al-Buhuth wa-l-Dirasat al-Kuwaytiyya, 1996), 111.

24. C. Stanley G. Mylrea, *Kuwait before Oil*, unpublished, written between 1945 and 1951 (Kuwait: Center for Research and Studies on Kuwait), 67–68, 71.

25. Vassiliev, *History of Saudi Arabia*, 505. Three of Ibn Saʿud's sons and one of his wives died in the pandemic. See also Paul L. Armerding, *Doctors for the Kingdom: The Work of the American Mission Hospitals in the Kingdom of Saudi Arabia 1913–1955* (Grand Rapids, MI: William B. Eerdmans Publishing, 2003), 147.

26. ʿAbd al-ʿAziz Rifaʿi and Sayyid Ahmad Yunis, *Binaʾ al-Dawla al-ʿArabiyya al-Saʿudiyya fi al-ʿAsr al-Hadith wa-l-Muʿasir 1902–1953* (Cairo: Al-Maktaba al-ʿAlamiyya, 1978), 156.

27. Sayyid ʿAli al-Sayyid Baqir al-ʿAwwami, *Al-Haraka al-Wataniyya Sharq al-Saʿudiyya 1373–1393 h/ 1953–1973 m*, 2 vols. (2011), 1:70.

28. Quote attributed to Al-Hajiri is from Mulligan Papers; *Biographies of New Members of the Council of Ministers*, Dhahran, Saudi Arabia, 6 November 1962, "Dr. Yusuf Yaʿqub Al-Hajiri, Minister of Health," box 2, folder 4, Mulligan Papers.

29. ʿAbd Allah al-Saliʿ, *Al-Khadamat al-Sihhiyya bi Madinat Mecca al-Mukarrama* (Mecca: Umm Al-Qura University, 1983), 29.

30. Laura Frances Goffman, "Popular Politics and Epidemics in Eastern Arabia," *Labor: Studies in Working-Class History* 20, no. 2 (2023): 74–94.

31. David Harvey, *Spaces of Hope* (Berkeley: University of California Press, 2000), 106.

32. Richard H. Daggy and R. C. Page, "Aramco's Preventive Medicine Program," *Medical Bulletin* 16 (1956): 196.

33. Daggy and Page, 204.

34. The most common malaria plasmodia in the Arabian Peninsula were *Plasmodium falciparum* (the most lethal strain) and *Plasmodium vivax*. See Benjamin Reilly, *Slavery, Agriculture, and Malaria in the Arabian Peninsula* (Athens: Ohio University Press, 2015), ch. 4; Richard H. Daggy, "Malaria in Oases of Eastern Saudi Arabia," *American Journal of Tropical Medicine and Hygiene* 8 (1959): 235. On Aramco's malaria-related initiatives, see Jones, *Desert Kingdom*, 91–137; Parker, *Making the Desert Modern*, 74–90; Reilly, *Slavery, Agriculture, and Malaria in the Arabian Peninsula*, 113–115; Laura Frances Goffman, "Medical Frontiers: Health, Empire, and Society in the Gulf and Arabian Peninsula, 1862–1959" (PhD diss., Georgetown University, 2019), ch. 4.

35. Jones, *Desert Kingdom*, 97.

36. On housing, see Parker, *Making the Desert Modern*, 79. On the date economy, see Jones, *Desert Kingdom*, 109–110.

37. Health—Sanitation; Health and Sanitation—Long Term Program Budget, Activity Authorization; Subject Files, 1950–54; Record Group 469: Records of US Foreign Assistance Agencies, 1948–1961, National Archives at College Park, MD.

38. Reilly, *Slavery, Agriculture, and Malaria*, 114.

39. Daggy, "Malaria in Oases of Eastern Saudi Arabia," 285.

40. Matthiesen, *The Other Saudis*, 74. The decrease in Saudi workers is especially striking given that Arab oil executives were emphasizing the need to expand local workforces during the same period. See Alex Cobb Boodrookas, "The Making of a Migrant Working Class: Contesting Citizenship in Kuwait and the Persian Gulf, 1925–1975" (PhD diss., New York University, 2020), ch. 6.

41. James L. A. Webb Jr., *Humanity's Burden: A Global History of Malaria* (Cambridge: Cambridge University Press, 2009), 160.

42. Daggy, "Malaria in Oases of Eastern Saudi Arabia," 266.

43. Parker, *Making the Desert Modern*, 75.

44. Cornelia Dalenberg, *Sharifa* (Grand Rapids, MI: Wm. B. Eerdmans Publishing, 1983), 33.

45. During his first year in Eastern Province, Roger Nichols explored the fly-trachoma relationship by collecting ten thousand flies from around the region. Interview with Elinor Nichols, "Health and Disease in Saudi Arabia," 266.

46. Dalenberg, *Sharifa*, 33–34.

47. "Trachoma," World Health Organization, 9 May 2021, https://www.who.int/news-room/fact-sheets/detail/trachoma; "Hygiene-Related Diseases: Trachoma,"

Centers for Disease Control and Prevention, US Department of Health and Human Services, https://www.cdc.gov/healthywater/hygiene/disease/trachoma.html.

48. For a discussion of the prevalence of blind and partially blind *ulema* in Arabia, largely prompted by the inability of these individuals to work in other trades, see Guido Steinberg, "Ecology, Knowledge, and Trade in Central Arabia (*Najd*) during the Nineteenth and Early Twentieth Centuries," in *Counter-Narratives: History, Contemporary Society, and Politics in Saudi Arabia and Yemen*, ed. Madawi Al-Rasheed and Robert Vitalis (New York: Palgrave Macmillan, 2004), 86–87. The Saudi genealogist and historian Hamad al-Jasir (1909–2000), whose "sickly frame and partial blindness made him unfit for work in the village's date plantations," offers a notable illustration of this pattern. Nadav Samin, *Of Sand or Soil: Genealogy & Tribal Belonging in Saudi Arabia* (Princeton, NJ: Princeton University Press, 2015), 24. Sara Scalenghe also notes the prevalence of trachoma across the Ottoman Arab world. In addition to the frequency of blindness, she argues that favorable depictions of blind people in the Islamic tradition meant that it "enjoyed the most privileged place in the hierarchy of cultural meanings ascribed to physical impairments in the Arab-Islamic world." Sara Scalenghe, *Disability in the Ottoman Arab World, 1500–1800* (New York: Cambridge University Press, 2014), 53.

49. Charles Belgrave, *Personal Column* (London: Hutchinson & Co., 1960), 91.

50. Hasan al-ʿAwwami, "Nuʾarkhum fi 'al-labbania' wa yarhhabun bina fi 'al-wadi,'" 7 February 2021, https://www.sobranews.com/sobra/108836. Sayyid ʿAli al-Sayyid Baqir al-ʿAwwami also references the prevalence of *"al-tarākhūmā"* in the region. See al-ʿAwwami, *Al-Haraka al-Wataniyya Sharq al-Saʿudiyya*, 43.

51. Henny Harald Hansen, *Investigations in a Shīʿa Village in Bahrain* (Copenhagen: National Museum of Denmark, 1967), 129.

52. Al-ʿAwwami, *al-Haraka al-Wataniyya Sharq al-Saʿudiyya*, 43.

53. Al-ʿAwwami, 43.

54. Al-ʿAwwami, 71.

55. Health—Sanitation; Health and Sanitation—Long Term Program Budget, Activity Authorization; Subject Files, 1950–54; Record Group 469: Records of US Foreign Assistance Agencies, 1948–1961, National Archives at College Park, MD.

56. Parker, *Making the Desert Modern*, 62, quoting Armand P. Gelpi.

57. Interview with Julius W. Taylor, "Health and Disease in Saudi Arabia," 200.

58. Interview with Taylor, 201.

59. Interview with Taylor, 204.

60. Interview with Taylor, 232. As a point of comparison, based on her 1960 ethnographic work in the Shiʿi village of Sār in Bahrain, Danish anthropologist Henny Harold Hansen observed that the body of a local man who had died at

the hospital in Manama was brought back to his village by car. She was told that "the washing of the dead was never done at the hospital but took place in the village." It is likely that a similar system was in place in Eastern Province. Hansen, *Investigations in a Shī'a Village in Bahrain*, 130.

61. Interview with Julius W. Taylor, "Health and Disease in Saudi Arabia," 232.
62. Interview with Taylor, 233.
63. Interview with Taylor, 233.
64. Interview with Taylor, 216.
65. Interview with Taylor, 204, 205.
66. Interview with Taylor, 233.
67. Interview with Taylor, 233.
68. Interview with Taylor, 240.
69. Tom L. Beauchamp, "Informed Consent: Its History, Meaning, and Present Challenges," *Cambridge Quarterly of Healthcare Ethics* 20 (2011): 516.
70. Francis, "U.S. Hospital Oasis of Health for Arabs."
71. Parker, *Making the Desert Modern*, 55.
72. Daggy states, for example: "We had about 12,000 Saudi employees, and each one had one or two wives and a set of children." But then he continues, "We had 12–15,000 Saudi employees and 12–15,000 wives and kids." He later provides a more detailed set of numbers: "We had 10,000 employees and 9,000 wives, 29,000 kids in Saudi Arabia at that time." Interview with Richard Daggy, "Health and Disease in Saudi Arabia," 20–21, 25. Handschin reported, "During that time when I became medical director, we were caring for about 69,000 people. Thirteen thousand of them were employees. That constituted 19 percent of our people for whom we were responsible. Wives accounted for an additional 16 percent. Children accounted for 59 percent of the people we were responsible for. And the Saudi Arab parents, for whom we became responsible, accounted for 6 percent of the people that we had to care for." In sum, according to Handschin's figures, 19 percent of the local patients to whom Aramco was providing medical care were employees, but only 16 percent were employees' wives. Interview with Richard Handschin, "Health and Disease in Saudi Arabia," 139. Taylor, for his part, admits: "The number who had four wives was small; I think at one time it was like 10 or 12 percent of the employees had four wives. On the other end, there was 10 or 12 or 15 percent who had no wives: they weren't married at all. The biggest number of married Arabs had two wives; three wives was next; and then four wives was the least." Interview with Julius W. Taylor, "Health and Disease in Saudi Arabia," 182.
73. Interview with Robert and Patricia Oertley, "Health and Disease in Saudi Arabia," 362.

74. James R. McNiel, "Pediatric Practice in Eastern Saudi Arabia," *Clinical Pediatrics* 5, no. 6 (June 1966): 387.

75. Interview with Robert and Patricia Oertley, "Health and Disease in Saudi Arabia," 362.

76. Interview with Oertleys, 363.

77. Interview with Richard Handschin, "Health and Disease in Saudi Arabia," 156.

78. Interview with Handschin, 156.

79. Interview with Handschin, 155.

80. Interview with Handschin, 136.

81. Interview with Handschin, 137.

82. Interview with Handschin, 137.

83. Interview with Handschin, 149.

84. Interview with Handschin, 154.

85. Mahmood Mamdani, *The Myth of Population Control: Family, Caste, and Class in an Indian Village* (New York: Monthly Review Press, 1972), 149, 161–162. Thank you to Seçil Yılmaz for this reference.

86. Interview with Richard Handschin, "Health and Disease in Saudi Arabia," 151–152.

87. Interview with Handschin, 152.

88. Interview with Handschin, 141.

89. Interview with Handschin, 152.

90. Interview with Handschin, 140.

91. Interview with Ahmed Mustafa, "Health and Disease in Saudi Arabia," 554.

92. Interview with Richard Handschin, "Health and Disease in Saudi Arabia," 133.

93. Interview with Handschin, 130.

94. Interview with Handschin, 133.

95. Interview with Robert and Patricia Oertley, "Health and Disease in Saudi Arabia," 362.

96. Interview with Julius W. Taylor, "Health and Disease in Saudi Arabia," 227–228.

97. For a discussion of the global infrastructure that connected institutions in the Middle East to laboratories in Europe and North America, see Elise K. Burton, *Genetic Crossroads: The Middle East and the Science of Human Heredity* (Stanford, CA: Stanford University Press, 2021), ch. 3.

98. J. C. Snyder, R. C. Page, E. S. Murray, R. H. Daggy, S. D. Bell Jr., R. L. Nichols, N. A. Haddad, A. T. Hanna, and D. McComb, "Observations on the Etiology of Trachoma," *American Journal of Ophthalmology* 48, no. 3, pt. 2 (September 1959): 327.

99. Interview with Elinor Nichols, "Health and Disease in Saudi Arabia," 267.

100. Quoted in Vitalis, *America's Kingdom*, 34.

101. Arab Support Committee, "Struggle Oppression and Counter-Revolution in Saudi Arabia," translated from the original Arabic articles appearing in the 1972 issues of the Al Jazeerah Al-Jadeedah, the political organ of the People's Democratic Party of Al Jazeerah Al Arabiah—"Saudi Arabia" (Berkeley, CA, 1972), 14.

102. Vitalis, *America's Kingdom*, 27; Interview with Dorothy McComb, "Health and Disease in Saudi Arabia," 322.

103. Interview with McComb, 322.

104. E. S. Murray, S. D. Bell Jr., A. T. Hanna, R. L. Nichols, and J. C. Snyder, "Studies on Trachoma I. Isolation and Identification of Strains of Elementary Bodies from Saudi Arabia and Egypt," *American Journal of Tropical Medicine and Hygiene* 9, no. 2 (1960): 116. The Egyptian strains were taken from clinics at the Giza Memorial Ophthalmological Institute in Cairo.

105. Murray et al., 117.

106. Roger L. Nichols, D. E. McComb, N. Haddad, and E. S. Murray, "Studies on Trachoma. II. Comparison of Fluorescent Antibody, Gimesa and Egg Isolation Methods for Detection of Trachoma Viruses in Human Conjunctival Scrapings," *American Journal of Tropical Medicine and Hygiene* 12, no. 2 (1963): 223.

107. The Mayo Clinic's site on trachoma, for example, lists sex as a risk factor, and attributes the fact that "in some areas, women's rate of contracting the disease is two to six times higher than that of men" to women's greater contact with children, "who are the primary reservoir of infection." "Trachoma," Mayo Clinic, https://www.mayoclinic.org/diseases-conditions/trachoma/symptoms-causes/syc-20378505.

108. Interview with Dorothy McComb, "Health and Disease in Saudi Arabia," 303. One study references similar findings in the Punjab, where it was "suggested that the most important vehicle for the spread of eye infections is the village woman's shawl, a general purpose garment used for cleaning the faces of children." C. E. Taylor, P. V. Gulati, and J. Harinarain, "Eye Infections in a Punjab Village," *American Journal of Tropical Medicine and Hygiene* 7, no. 42 (1958), discussed in Arthur A. Bobb Jr. and Roger L. Nichols, "Influence of Environment on Clinical Trachoma in Saudi Arabia," *American Journal of Ophthalmology* 67, no. 2 (1969): 242.

109. Interview with Dorothy McComb, "Health and Disease in Saudi Arabia," 303.

110. Murray et al., "Studies on Trachoma I," 117.

111. Marie Feng, R. Shih-Man Chang, Taylor R. Smith, and John C. Snyder, "Adenoviruses Isolated from Saudi Arabia. II. Pathogenicity of Certain Strains for Man," *American Journal of Tropical Medicine and Hygiene* 8 (1959): 504.

112. Feng et al., 501.

113. "Aramco, Harvard Fight Trachoma in $500,000, Five-Year Program," *Arabian Sun and Flare* (Arabian American Oil Co, Dhahran, Saudi Arabia) 9, no. 44 (November 10, 1954), 6.

114. Parker, *Making the Desert Modern*, 7.

115. Samuel D. Bell Jr., Roger L. Nichols, and Nadim A. Haddad, "The Immunology of the Trachoma Agent with a Preliminary Report on Field Trials of Vaccine," *Investigative Ophthalmology & Visual Science* 2 (October 1963): 475.

116. Bell, Nichols, and Haddad, 475.

117. "Aramco, Harvard Fight Trachoma," 6. Jonas Salk began polio immunization research by immunizing monkeys in his University of Pittsburgh laboratory in the early 1950s. Brandt, "Polio, Politics, Publicity, and Duplicity," 259.

118. Interview with Elinor Nichols, "Health and Disease in Saudi Arabia," 269; Roger L. Nichols, Arthur A. Bobb, Nadim A. Haddad, and Dorothy E. McComb, "Immunofluorescent Studies of the Microbiologic Epidemiology of Trachoma in Saudi Arabia," *American Journal of Ophthalmology* 63 (1967): 1372.

119. Nichols et al., 1375–1376.

120. Interview with Dorothy McComb, "Health and Disease in Saudi Arabia," 305.

121. Interview with McComb, 306.

122. Murray et al., "Studies on Trachoma I," 117.

123. Interview with Dorothy McComb, "Health and Disease in Saudi Arabia," 308.

124. Interview with McComb, 307.

125. Interview with McComb, 321.

126. Interview with McComb, 316; "At War with Trachoma," *Aramco World* 11, no. 8 (October 1960): 6.

127. Interview with Dorothy McComb, "Health and Disease in Saudi Arabia," 309.

128. Interview with McComb, 306.

129. Burton, *Genetic Crossroads*, 21.

130. Interview with Elinor Nichols, "Health and Disease in Saudi Arabia," 270.

131. Interview with Nichols, 270–271.

132. Interview with Nichols, 271.

133. Dorothy E. McComb and Roger L. Nichols, "Antibodies to Trachoma in Eye Secretions of Saudi Arab Children," *American Journal of Epidemiology* 90, no. 4 (1969): 278.

134. Nichols et al., "Immunofluorescent Studies," 1406.

135. Nichols et al., 1373.

136. Nichols et al., 1373–1374.

137. Nichols et al., 1374.

138. Jones, *Desert Kingdom*, 136.

139. Nichols et al., "Immunofluorescent Studies," 1402.

140. Interview with Dorothy McComb, "Health and Disease in Saudi Arabia," 304.

141. Arthur A. Bobb Jr. and Roger L. Nichols, "Influence of Environment on Clinical Trachoma in Saudi Arabia," *American Journal of Ophthalmology* 67, no. 2 (1969): 242.

142. Interview with Elinor Nichols, "Health and Disease in Saudi Arabia," 272–273.

143. Bobb and Nichols, "Influence of Environment," 235.

144. Interview with Julius W. Taylor, "Health and Disease in Saudi Arabia," 225.

145. Interview with Dorothy McComb, "Health and Disease in Saudi Arabia," 314.

146. Interview with McComb, 314.

147. Interview with McComb, 302.

148. The Aramco-supported studies in *Trachoma and Related Disorders Caused by Chlamydial Agents: Proceedings of a Symposium Held in Boston, Massachusetts 17–20 August 1970*, ed. Roger L. Nichols (Amsterdam: Excerpta Medica, 1971), include the following: J. Dennis Mull and John H. Peters, "Lyzome (Muramidase) in Eye Secretions of Infants and Children in Regions with and without Endemic Trachoma," 211–216; A. Hathaway and J. H. Peters, "Characterization of Antibodies to Trachoma in Human Eye Secretions," 260–268; Roger L. Nichols, Karen von Fritzinger, and Dorothy E. McComb, "Epidemiological Data Derived from Immunotyping of 338 Trachoma Strains Isolated from Children in Saudi Arabia," 337–357; F. B. Gordon, R. L. Nichols and A. L. Quan, "Immunotyping of *Chlamydia trachomatis* with Fluorescent Antibody: Retention of Immunospecificity in Cell Culture Passage, and Typing with Infected Cell Monolayers," 358–362; E. S. Murray, C. E. O. Fraser, J. H. Peters, D. E. McComb, and R. L. Nichols, "The Owl Monkey as an Experimental Primate Model for Conjunctival Trachoma Infection," 386–395; Dorothy E. McComb, John H. Peters, C. E. Ovid Fraser, Edward S. Murray, A. Bruce MacDonald, and Roger L. Nichols, "Resistance to Trachoma Infection in Owl Monkeys Correlated with Antibody Status at the Outset in an Experiment to Test the Response to Topical Trachoma Antigens," 396–406; A. Bruce Macdonald and Joan Barenfanger, "A Quantitative Micromethod for Determining Antibody Concentrations in Antisera to Chlamydial Agents," 423–434; and Roger L. Nichols, Edward S. Murray, Pamela P. Scott, and Dorothy E. McComb, "Trachoma Isolation Studies in Saudi Arabia from 1957 through 1969," 517–528.

149. Mull and Peters, "Lyzome (Muramidase) in Eye Secretions," 215.

150. Armand P. Gelpi, "Introduction—Elinor Nichols," "Health and Disease in Saudi Arabia," 251.

151. Interview with Elinor Nichols, "Health and Disease in Saudi Arabia," 284–285.

152. Interview with Dorothy McComb, "Health and Disease in Saudi Arabia," 307.

Chapter 5

1. Amir A. Afkhami, *A Modern Contagion: Imperialism and Public Health in Iran's Age of Cholera* (Baltimore: Johns Hopkins University Press, 2019), 169.

2. World Health Organization, *Minutes of the First Meeting of the Fifteenth Session of the Regional Committee for the Eastern Mediterranean Held at the Africa Hall Addis-Ababa on Wednesday 22 September 1965*, EM/RC15A/Prog.min.1 (November 1965), 25–26, https://apps.who.int/iris/bitstream/handle/10665/124087/em_rc15_a_prog_min_1_en.pdf.

3. Laura Frances Goffman, "A Jar of Shaykhs' Teeth: Medicine, Politics, and the Fragments of History in Kuwait," *International Journal of Middle East Studies* 53, no. 4 (November 2021): 589–603.

4. "Al-Kulira," *Majallat al-Kuwayt*, 1 September 1965, 20/Ha/240, Kuwait University (hereafter KU).

5. "Ma'a Mala'ika al-Rahma fi al-Kuwayt," *Adwa' al-Kuwayt*, 13 September 1965, KU 20/dal/300.

6. "Ma'a Mala'ika al-Rahma fi al-Kuwayt."

7. "Ma'a Mala'ika al-Rahma fi al-Kuwayt."

8. This is not to suggest that Kuwait was a passive recipient of pan-Arab ideologies; as Talal Al-Rashoud has demonstrated, "Arab nationalist influence dominated" Kuwait's Education Department in the 1950s, and they offered their "Arab scholarships" to other Arab governments as well as nationalist activists, which "played a significant role in the region's cultural and political development." Talal Al-Rashoud, "From Muscat to the Maghreb: Pan-Arab Networks, Anti-Colonial Groups, and Kuwait's Arab Scholarships (1953–1961)," *Arabian Humanities* 12 (2019): https://doi.org/10.4000/cy.5004.

9. The Syrian Protestant College, later renamed American University of Beirut, opened the Nurses Training School in 1905. By 1952, 518 nurses and 59 midwives had graduated. Liat Kozma and Nicole Khayat, "Gendered Struggles over the Medical Profession in the Modern Middle East and North Africa," *Journal of Middle East Women's Studies* 18, no. 1 (2022): 4–5.

10. "5 Daqa'iq ma'a Ra'ida al-Tamrid fi al-Kuwayt," *Adwa' al-Kuwayt*, 12 August 1963, KU 20/dal/300.

11. From December 1947 and through the 1948 war, the Palestinian women's movement contributed to emergency medical services. Palestinian women, including those from the middle and upper classes, worked as nurses. Ellen L. Fleischmann,

The Nation and Its "New" Women: The Palestinian Women's Movement, 1920–1948 (Berkeley: University of California Press, 2003), 203; Shay Hazkani, *Dear Palestine: A Social History of the 1948 War* (Stanford, CA: Stanford University Press, 2021), 163.

12. Rosemarie Said Zahlan, "The Gulf States and the Palestine Problem, 1936–48," *Arab Studies Quarterly* 3, no. 1 (1981): 1–21.

13. "5 Daqa'iq ma'a Ra'ida al-Tamrid fi al-Kuwayt," *Adwa' al-Kuwayt*, 12 August 1963, KU 20/dal/300.

14. "5 Daqa'iq ma'a Ra'ida al-Tamrid fi al-Kuwayt."

15. Andrea Wright, *Between Dreams and Ghosts: Indian Migration and Middle Eastern Oil* (Stanford, CA: Stanford University Press, 2021), 5.

16. "5 Daqa'iq ma'a Ra'ida al-Tamrid fi al-Kuwayt," *Adwa' al-Kuwayt*, 12 August 1963, KU 20/dal/300.

17. Omar AlShehabi, "Histories of Migration to the Gulf," in *Transit States: Labour, Migration & Citizenship in the Gulf*, ed. Abdulhadi Khalaf, Omar AlShehabi, and Adam Hanieh (London: Pluto Press, 2015), 8.

18. Alex Cobb Boodrookas, "The Making of a Migrant Working Class: Contesting Citizenship in Kuwait and the Persian Gulf, 1925–1975" (PhD diss., New York University, 2020), 12.

19. IOR R/15/1/714, "Administration Reports 1925–1930," 1930, 54.

20. Khalid al-Jarallah, *Sihhat al-Kuwayt: Qira'a fi Watha'iq Kuwaytiyya wa Ajnabiyya* (Kuwait: Markaz al-Buhuth wa-l-Dirasat al-Kuwaytiyya, 2019), 143.

21. Farah Al-Nakib, *Kuwait Transformed: A History of Oil and Urban Life* (Stanford, CA: Stanford University Press, 2016), 61.

22. C. Stanley G. Mylrea, "Kuwait before Oil: Memoirs of Dr. C. Stanley G. Mylrea, Pioneer Medical Missionary of the Arabian Mission Reformed Church in America" (Center for Research and Studies on Kuwait, unpublished manuscript, written between 1945 and 1951), 27.

23. Abdulrahman Alebrahim, *Kuwait's Politics before Independence: The Role of the Balancing Powers* (Berlin, Germany: Gerlach Press, 2019), 53.

24. 'Abd Allah Khalid al-Hatim, *Min Huna Bada'at al-Kuwayt* (Damascus: al-Matba'a al-'Umumiyya, 1962), 149.

25. Boodrookas, "Making of a Migrant Working Class," 81.

26. H. R. P. Dickson, *Kuwait and Her Neighbours* (London: George Allen & Unwin, 1956), 370.

27. IOR R/15/1/715, "Administration Reports 1931–1935," 1935, 51. In Iran, Anglo-Iranian Oil Company (AIOC) recruited missionary nurses, offering them better pay and modern conveniences like air conditioning. Lydia Wytenbroek, "Nursing (Inter)nationalism in Iran, 1916–1947," *Journal of Middle East Women's Studies* 18, no. 1 (March 2022): 50.

28. Khalid al-Jarallah, *Tarikh al-Khadamat al-Sihhiyya fi al-Kuwayt* (Kuwait: Markaz al-Buhuth wa-l-Dirasat al-Kuwaytiyya, 1996), 102.

29. Dr. S. D. McClean, Chief Medical Officer, "Kuwait Oil Company—Medical Service. Recommendations," December 1952, ARC 59729, BP. Information and Images from the BP Archive. I am grateful to Joanne Burman, BP Archive assistant, for helping me to obtain these documents.

30. Medical care similarly emerged as a mark of royal privilege—and a point of contestation—in Saudi Arabia. See Laura Frances Goffman, "Popular Politics and Epidemics in Eastern Arabia," *Labor: Studies in Working-Class History* 20, no. 2 (May 2023): 74–94.

31. Jill Crystal, *Kuwait: The Transformation of an Oil State* (New York: Routledge, 1992), 17, 36.

32. Crystal, *Kuwait*, 18.

33. Jill Crystal, *Oil and Politics in the Gulf: Rulers and Merchants in Kuwait and Qatar* (Cambridge: Cambridge University Press, 1990), 47.

34. Crystal, *Oil and Politics in the Gulf*, 49.

35. Crystal, 49.

36. Talal Al-Rashoud, "Modern Education and Arab Nationalism in Kuwait, 1911–1961" (PhD diss., SOAS University of London, 2016), 125.

37. Al-Rashoud, "Modern Education and Arab Nationalism," 137.

38. Al-Rashoud, 151.

39. Crystal, *Oil and Politics in the Gulf*, 52.

40. IOR R/15/1/468, "File 45/23 (D 140) Kuwait Reforms," Enclosure in Bagdad Despatch No. 188 of 28.4.1938, "Al Istiqlal. The Movement in Koweit. Iraq's Sympathy," 26 April 1938.

41. IOR R/15/5/205, 'File 4/20 Koweit Situation,' Balance Sheet of the Kuwait Municipality for the Year 1356 (1937), "General Control."

42. IOR R/15/5/205, 'File 4/20 Koweit Situation,' Translation of the Law Governing the powers of the Kuwait Administrative Council as granted by H.M. the Ruler of Kuwait on 9 July 1938.

43. IOR R/15/5/205, 'File 4/20 Koweit Situation,' Appendix II. "Demands."

44. Sunil S. Amrith, *Decolonizing International Health: India and Southeast Asia, 1930–65* (New York: Palgrave Macmillan, 2006), 2.

45. Tony Judt, *Postwar: A History of Europe since 1945* (New York: Penguin Books, 2005), 74.

46. Al-Rashoud, "Modern Education and Arab Nationalism," 160.

47. Al-Nakib, *Kuwait Transformed*, 92.

48. Boodrookas, "Making of a Migrant Working Class," 338.

49. Talal Al-Rashoud, "Icon of Defiance and Hope: Gamal Abdel Nasser's Image in Gulf History," *Mada Masr*, November 28, 2020, https://www.madamasr.com/en/2020/11/28/opinion/u/icon-of-defiance-and-hope-gamal-abdel-nassers-image-in-gulf-history/.

50. Reem Alissa, "The Oil Town of Ahmadi since 1946: From Colonial Town to Nostalgic City," *Comparative Studies of South Asia, Africa and the Middle East* 33, no. 1 (2013): 48.

51. Farah Al-Nakib, "Public Space and Public Protest in Kuwait, 1938–2012," *City* 18, no. 6 (2014): 729.

52. Crystal, *Oil and Politics in the Gulf*, 79. For a detailed discussion of the 1959 Nationality Law, see Boodrookas, "Making of a Migrant Working Class," 179–186.

53. Al-Rashoud, "Modern Education and Arab Nationalism," 331.

54. KU: Department of Health Statistics and Statistical Research, "Annual Report 1958–1962" (Kuwait: Ministry of Public Health), 235.

55. "Kuwaiti Constitution," https://www.wipo.int/edocs/lexdocs/laws/en/kw/kw004en.pdf.

56. Crystal, *Oil and Politics in the Gulf*, 85.

57. Al-Nakib, *Kuwait Transformed*, 175.

58. Yusif al-Shihab, *Al-Kuwayt 'Abra al-Tarikh* (Kuwait: 1989), 290.

59. Samir Shamma, *Bitrul al-Kuwayt: Hadirhu wa Mustaqbalhu* (Damascus: Matabi' Ibn Zibdun, 1959), 79.

60. KU: Department of Health Statistics and Statistical Research, "Annual Report 1958–1962" (Kuwait: Ministry of Public Health), 115.

61. Roberto Fabbri, Sara Saragoça, and Ricardo Camacho, *Modern Architecture Kuwait 1949–1989* (Zurich, Switzerland: Niggli, 2016), 70; Crystal, *Oil and Politics in the Gulf*, 78.

62. "Jawla al-Iman fi Mu'assasat al-Sihha al-'Amma," *al-Iman* 12 (1954): 202, 204.

63. KU: Department of Health Statistics and Statistical Research, "Annual Report 1958–1962" (Kuwait: Ministry of Public Health), 38. Recorded deaths in 1962, for example, are broken down by age range, but also by the fact that 62.1 percent of the deceased were Kuwaiti, 37.4 percent were non-Kuwaiti, and 0.5 percent were of unknown nationality. The distribution of Kuwaiti and non-Kuwaiti deaths within the specific age ranges, however, is not provided. KU: Department of Health Statistics and Statistical Research, "Annual Report 1958–1962" (Kuwait: Ministry of Public Health), 34.

64. KU: Department of Health Statistics and Statistical Research, "Annual Report 1958–1962" (Kuwait: Ministry of Public Health), 152–153.

65. Julia R. Shatz observed a similar dynamic in Mandate Palestine. She argues that "it was through the organizations and practices of social welfare,

rather than formal politics that most Palestinians interacted with institutions of daily governance." Julia R. Shatz, "A Politics of Care: Local Nurses in Mandate Palestine," *International Journal of Middle East Studies* 50, no. 4 (2018): 670.

66. Susan L. Smith, *Sick and Tired of Being Sick and Tired: Black Women's Health Activism in America, 1890–1950* (Philadelphia: University of Pennsylvania Press, 1995), 148.

67. Sujani Reddy, *Nursing & Empire: Gendered Labor and Migration from India to the United States* (Chapel Hill: University of North Carolina Press, 2015), 12–13.

68. "Al-Ta'aqud ma'a 6 Atibba' wa 40 Mumarrida," *al-Ra'y al-'Am*, 26 April 1962, KU 20/dal/300; *Akhbar al-Kuwayt*, 24 March 1963, KU 20/dal/300; "Tashkil Lajnna min al-Sihha wa Diwan al-Muwazafin," *al-Ra'y al-'Am*, 4 July 1964, KU 20/dal/300; "Wizarat al-Sihha Tata'aqad ma'a 75 Mumarrid wa Mumarrida," *al-Ra'y al-'Am*, 20 July 1965 KU 20/dal/300; "Al-Sihha Tatlub 150 Mumarrida Qanuniyya min al-Muttahida," *Akhbar al-Kuwayt*, 2 January 1966, KU 20/dal/300; "'Adad Kabir min al-Mumarridat Tata'aqad Ma'ahunna Wizarat al-Sihha," *al-Siyasa*, 8 August 1967, KU 20/dal/300.

69. *Akhbar al-Kuwayt*, 24 March 1963, KU 20/dal/300.

70. "Ma'a Mala'ika al-Rahma fi al-Kuwayt," *Adwa' al-Kuwayt*, 13 September 1965, KU 20/dal/300.

71. Catherine Ceniza Choy, *Empire of Care: Nursing and Migration in Filipino American History* (Durham, NC: Duke University Press, 2003), 2.

72. Nurses' low pay and inferior professional and social status in the Middle East also was a legacy of the British empire. In Mandate Palestine, for example, "British nurses were paid the lowest salary among *all* officials in the Senior Division, locals included." Hagit Krik, "The Female Imperial Agent and the Intricacies of Power: British Nurses in Mandate Palestine," *Journal of Middle East Women's Studies* 18, no. 1 (March 2022): 25.

73. Boodrookas, "Making of a Migrant Working Class," 260.

74. There were also significant labor actions in 1963 at Shuwaikh Port and KOC. Boodrookas, "Making of a Migrant Working Class," 442–443; "Intaha Idrab Mumarridi Mustashfa al-'Azam," *al-Ra'y al-'Am*, 4 July 1963, KU 3/ha/040.

75. "Mumarridu wa Mumarridat al-Sihha," *al-Tali'a*, 3 July 1963, KU 20/dal/300.

76. "Intaha Idrab Mumarridi Mustashfa al-'Azam," *al-Ra'y al-'Am*, 4 July 1963, KU 3/ha/040.

77. "Mumarridu wa Mumarridat al-Sihha," *al-Tali'a*, 3 July 1963, KU 20/dal/300.

78. "Mumarridu wa Mumarridat al-Sihha."

79. "Mumarridu wa Mumarridat al-Sihha."

80. "Mumarridu wa Mumarridat al-Sihha."

81. "Mumarridu wa Mumarridat al-Sihha."

82. Elizabeth Faue and Josiah Rector, "The Precarious Work of Care: OSHA, AIDS, and Women Health-Care Workers, 1983–2000," *Labor: Studies in Working-Class History* 17, no. 4 (2020): 12.

83. Boodrookas, "Making of a Migrant Working Class," 280–281.

84. Mufida Hilmi, "Mala'ika al-Rahma fi Jahim!" *al-Nahda*, 20 November 1968, KU 20/dal/300.

85. Hilmi.

86. Faue and Rector, "The Precarious Work of Care," 14.

87. Hilmi, "Mala'ika al-Rahma fi Jahim!"

88. Hilmi.

89. Hilmi.

90. "Qanun Raqam 23," *al-Kuwayt al-Yawm*, 25 May 1964, KU 20/dal/300.

91. "Qanun Raqam 23."

92. Hilmi, "Mala'ika al-Rahma fi Jahim!" Barjas Hammud al-Barjas would go on to become the head of the Kuwaiti Red Crescent Society. See Nasr al-Majali, "Al-Kuwayt Tan'a Barjas Hammud al-Barjas, *Elaf*, 14 May 2014, https://elaph.com/Web/News/2014/5/904228.html.

93. Hilmi, "Mala'ika al-Rahma fi Jahim!"

94. K. A. Brent, "Are Nurses Getting Too Much Education?" *Hospital Management* 67 (April 1949): 68, quoted in Thetis M. Group and Joan I. Roberts, *Nursing, Physician Control, and the Medical Monopoly: Historical Perspectives on Gendered Inequality in Roles, Rights, and Range of Practice* (Bloomington: Indiana University Press, 2001), 182.

95. Hilmi, "Mala'ika al-Rahma fi Jahim!"

96. Hilmi.

97. Charlotte Dale, "The Social Exploits and Behaviour of Nurses during the Anglo-Boer War, 1899–1902," in *Colonial Caring: A History of Colonial and Post-Colonial Nursing*, ed. Helen Sweet and Sue Hawkins (Manchester, UK: Manchester University Press, 2015), 64.

98. Hilmi, "Mala'ika al-Rahma fi Jahim!"

99. "Mala'ika al-Rahma: Nawal al-Mir'ibi Namudhaj Ra'i'," *Adwa' al-Kuwayt*, 5 September 1966, KU 20/dal/300.

100. Hilmi, "Mala'ika al-Rahma fi Jahim!"

101. Hilmi.

102. Fabbri, Saragoça, and Camacho, *Modern Architecture Kuwait 1949–1989*, 70.

103. "Sakan la bal Sijn Mukayyaf bi-l-hawa," *al-Yaqiza*, 18 September 1968, KU 20/dal/300.

104. "Sakan la bal Sijn Mukayyaf bi-l-hawa."

105. Al-Nakib, *Kuwait Transformed*, 181.

106. "Ma'a Mala'ika al-Rahma fi al-Kuwayt," *Adwa' al-Kuwayt*, 13 September 1965, KU 20/dal/300.

107. "Sakan la bal Sijn Mukayyaf bi-l-hawa."

108. "Sakan la bal Sijn Mukayyaf bi-l-hawa."

109. Chris Rominger, "Nursing Transgressions, Exploring Difference: North Africans in French Medical Spaces during World War I," *International Journal of Middle East Studies* 50, no. 4 (2018): 698, 695.

110. Boodrookas, "Making of a Migrant Working Class," 192.

111. Boodrookas, 48. See also Mary Ann Tétreault and Haya al-Mughni, "Gender, Citizenship and Nationalism in Kuwait, *British Journal of Middle Eastern Studies* 22, nos. 1–2 (1995): 67.

112. Mary Ann Tétreault and Haya al-Mughni, "Modernization and Its Discontents: State and Gender in Kuwait, *Middle East Journal* 49, no. 3 (Summer 1995): 407.

113. Reddy, *Nursing & Empire*, 4.

114. "Madha Wara' Yad al-Ittiham?" *al-Risala*, 5 January 1964, KU 20/dal/300.

115. "Qalilan min al-Rahma..Ya Mala'ika al-Rahma," *Sawt al-Khalij*, 16 February 1967, KU 20/dal/300.

116. "Qalilan min al-Rahma."

117. Hilmi, "Mala'ika al-Rahma fi Jahim!"

118. Ahmadi Town was constructed as KOC headquarters in the late 1940s. See Alissa, "Oil Town of Ahmadi since 1946."

119. "Tawarra' qabl Tahkumi," *Usrati*, 23 December 1967, KU 20/dal/300.

120. "Ma'a Mala'ika al-Rahma fi al-Kuwayt," *Adwa' al-Kuwayt*, 13 September 1965, KU 20/dal/300.

121. "'Adad Kabir min al-Mumarridat tata'aqad Ma'ahunna Wizarat al-Sihha," *al-Siyasa*, 8 August 1967, KU 20/dal/300.

122. "'Adad Kabir min al-Mumarridat tata'aqad Ma'ahunna Wizarat al-Sihha."

123. Hilmi.

124. "Ma'a Mala'ika al-Rahma fi al-Kuwayt."

125. Hilmi, "Mala'ika fi al-Tariq ila Fawq," *al-Nahar*, 28 September 1968, KU 20/dal/300.

126. Hilmi.

127. Hilmi, "Mala'ika al-Rahma fi Jahim!"

128. On this "reverse migration," see Boodrookas, "Making of a Migrant Working Class," 527–528.

129. 'Abd al-Karim Beiruti, "Fi al-Kuwayt Azma Mumarridat," *al-Qabas*, 13 September 1973, KU 20/dal/300.

130. Smith, *Sick and Tired of Being Sick and Tired*, 134.

131. Such patterns continue in the twenty-first century. One study warns, for example, "In 2006, native nurses constituted only 6.6% of the nursing workforce; this affects the quality of provided health care owing to language, [religious] and socio-cultural barriers between foreign nurses and patients." K. F. Al-Jarallah, M. A. A. Moussa, S. K. Hakeem, and F. K. Al-Khanfar, "The Nursing Workforce in Kuwait to the Year 2020," *International Nursing Review* 56, no. 1 (March 2009): 65.

132. Beiruti, "Fi al-Kuwayt Azma Mumarridat." Tensions over the language used by citizen and noncitizen health-care workers in professional contexts persist in the region. In their study on nursing labor markets in Oman, for example, Crystal A. Ennis and Margaret Walton-Roberts describe how, on the one hand, "Omani nurses report feeling the need to fight for patient care to be discussed in English so all parties could participate, not just doctors and nurses from particular language groups," and on the other hand, some noncitizen nurses "report signing contracts or other documents in Arabic, without understanding the contents." Crystal A. Ennis and Margaret Walton-Roberts, "Labour Market Regulation as Global Social Policy: The Case of Nursing Labour Markets in Oman," *Global Social Policy* 18, no. 2 (2018): 179–180.

133. Reddy, *Nursing & Empire*, 15.

134. Reddy, 133.

135. "Ma'a Mala'ika al-Rahma fi al-Kuwayt."

136. "Sakan la bal Sijn Mukayyaf bi-l-hawa."

Chapter 6

1. Khalifa al-Sayyid Mohammad Salih al-Maliki, *Jawab Kull Sa'il 'ind Mu'alijin Qatar al-Awa'il* (Doha: Renoda Modern Printing Press, 2012), 36. Thank you to 'Isa al-Mulla for sharing this book with me.

2. Colleen Morgan, "Cures for Qataris: The First Hospital in Doha," *The Origins of Doha and Qatar Project*, March 10, 2015, https://originsofdoha.wordpress.com/2015/03/10/cures-for-qataris-the-first-hospital-in-doha/.

3. 'Abd Allah 'Ali al-Tabur, *Al-Tibb al-Sha'bi fi al-Imarat al-'Arabiyya al-Muttahida* (United Arab Emirates: Markaz al-Khalij li-l-Kutub, 1998).

4. Citizenship itself is a stratified and unstable category across the Gulf states. For an insightful discussion of Gulf populations who are permanently suspended in a temporary legal status, see Noora Lori, *Offshore Citizens: Permanent Temporary Status in the Gulf* (New York: Cambridge University Press, 2019). On Kuwait, see Anh Nga Longva, *Walls Built on Sand: Migration, Exclusion, and Society in Kuwait* (Boulder, CO: Westview Press, 1997).

5. Projit Bihari Mukharji, *Doctoring Traditions: Ayurveda, Small Technologies, and Braided Science* (Chicago: University of Chicago Press, 2016).

6. Richard S. Weiss, *Recipes for Immortality: Medicine, Religion, and Community in South India* (Oxford: Oxford University Press, 2009), 80. In practice, pluralities and hybridities persist despite this frame. See Projit Bihari Mukharji, "Symptoms of Dis-Ease: New Trends in the Histories of 'Indigenous' South Asian Medicines," *History Compass* 9, no. 12 (2011): 889.

7. "Doctors Prescribing Non-Ayurvedic Medicines Are Anti-national," *Times of India*, May 1, 2016, https://timesofindia.indiatimes.com/city/kolhapur/doctors-prescribing-non-ayurvedic-medicines-are-anti-national/articleshow/52058067.cms.

8. Banu Subramaniam, *Holy Science: The Biopolitics of Hindu Nationalism* (Seattle: University of Washington Press, 2019), 171–172.

9. Amal Sachedina, "Nizwa Fort: Transforming Ibadi Religion through Heritage Discourse in Oman," *Comparative Studies of South Asia, Africa and the Middle East* 39, no. 2 (August 2019): 328. There is a large and growing literature on heritage studies in the Gulf. See, e.g., Sulayman Khalaf, "Poetics and Politics of Newly Invented Traditions in the Gulf: Camel Racing in the United Arab Emirates," *Ethnology* 39, no. 3 (2000): 243–261; Erik Gilbert, "The Dhow as Cultural Icon: Heritage and Regional Identity in the Western Indian Ocean," *International Journal of Heritage Studies* 17, no. 1 (2011): 62–80; Karen Exell and Trinidad Rico, "'There Is No Heritage in Qatar': Orientalism, Colonialism and Other Problematic Histories," *World Archeology* 45, no. 4 (2013): 670–685; miriam cooke, *Tribal Modern: Branding New Nations in the Arab Gulf* (Berkeley: University of California Press, 2014); Ahmed al-Dailami, "'Purity and Confusion': The Hawala between Persians and Arabs in the Contemporary Gulf," in *The Persian Gulf in Modern Times: People, Ports, and History*, ed. Lawrence G. Potter (New York: Palgrave Macmillan, 2014), 299–326; Karen Exell and Trinidad Rico, eds., *Cultural Heritage in the Arabian Peninsula: Debates, Discourses and Practices* (Surrey, UK: Ashgate, 2014); Natalie Koch, "Gulf Nationalism and the Geopolitics of Constructing Falconry as a 'Heritage Sport,'" *Studies in Ethnicity and Nationalism* 15, no. 3 (2015): 522–539; Karen Exell, "Desiring the Past and Reimagining the Present: Contemporary Collecting in Qatar," *Museum & Society* 14, no. 2 (2016): 259–274; Elizabeth Derderian, "Authenticating an Emirati Art World: Claims of Tabula Rasa and Cultural Appropriation in the UAE," *Journal of Arabian Studies* 7 (2017): 12–27; Pamela Erskine-Loftus, Mariam Al-Mulla, and Victoria Hightower, eds., *Representing the Nation: Heritage, Museums, and Identity in the Arab Gulf States* (New York: Routledge, 2016); Farah Al-Nakib, "Modernity and the Arab Gulf States: The Politics of Heritage, Memory, and

Forgetting," in *Routledge Handbook of Persian Gulf Politics*, ed. Mehran Kamrava (New York: Routledge, 2020), 57–82; Fahad Ahmad Bishara, "The Fateh Al-Khayr," *Perspectives on History*, February 25, 2021, https://www.historians.org/publications-and-directories/perspectives-on-history/march-2021/the-emfateh-al-khayr/em; Amal Sachedina, *Cultivating the Past, Living the Modern: The Politics of Time in the Sultanate of Oman* (Ithaca, NY: Cornell University Press, 2021).

10. Ahmed Kanna, *Dubai: The City as Corporation* (Minneapolis: University of Minnesota Press, 2011), 27. The Arabic term is *khalal sukkānī*, or demographic distortion or imbalance. Kanna, 121.

11. Kanna, 26.

12. Al-Nakib, "Modernity and the Arab Gulf States," 58–59.

13. Al-Nakib, 75.

14. This section draws from my discussion of *al-ṭibb al-shaʿbī* in Laura Frances Goffman, "A Jar of Shaykhs' Teeth: Medicine, Politics, and the Fragments of History in Kuwait," *International Journal of Middle East Studies* 53, no. 4 (November 2021): 601–602.

15. A related and comparably complex term is *baladī*. As Janet Abu-Lughod writes, "This virtually untranslatable term, an adjective derived from the noun for community (country, city, town, village), now connoted native in contrast to Westernized; folk as contrasted with sophisticated; untutored and low class as opposed to refined; traditional as contrasted with modern." See Janet Abu-Lughod, *Cairo: 1001 Years of the City Victorious* (Princeton, NJ: Princeton University Press, 1971), 191. Cited in Nancy Y. Reynolds, *A City Consumed: Urban Commerce, the Cairo Fire, and the Politics of Decolonization in Egypt* (Stanford, CA: Stanford University Press, 2012), 243n69.

16. Orit Bashkin, "Hybrid Nationalisms: Waṭanī and Qawmī Visions of Iraq under ʿAbd Al-Karim Qasim, 1958–61," *International Journal of Middle East Studies* 31, no. 2 (2011): 296.

17. Ted Swedenburg, "Egypt's Music of Protest: From Sayyid Darwish to DJ Haha," *Middle East Report* 265 (Winter 2012): 42.

18. Swedenburg, 42.

19. Daniel J. Gilman, *Cairo Pop: Youth Music in Contemporary Egypt* (Minneapolis: University of Minnesota Press, 2014), 10.

20. Gilman, 11.

21. Mandana E. Limbert, "Caste, Ethnicity, and the Politics of Arabness in Southern Arabia," *Comparative Studies of South Asia, Africa and the Middle East* 34, no. 3 (2014): 592.

22. Limbert, 593.

23. Limbert, 590.

24. Mandana E. Limbert, *In the Time of Oil: Piety, Memory & Social Life in an Omani Town* (Stanford, CA: Stanford University Press, 2010), 9.

25. Dan Rabinowitz, *The Power of Deserts: Climate Change, the Middle East, and the Promise of a Post-Oil Era* (Stanford, CA: Stanford University Press, 2020), 14.

26. As Rachel Teskey and Norah Alkhamis point out, the perspectives gained from oral histories are particularly useful in constructing national narratives in the Gulf, where much written history is based on European sources. Rachel Teskey and Norah Alkhamis, "Oral History and National Stories: Theory and Practice in the Gulf Cooperation Council," in *Representing the Nation: Heritage, Museums, National Narratives, and Identity in the Arab Gulf States*, ed. Pamela Erskine-Loftus, Mariam Al-Mulla, and Victoria Hightower (New York: Routledge, 2016), 137.

27. His books address topics such as theater in the United Arab Emirates (1986), traditional games in the Emirates (1986), pottery in Wadi Hujail (1987), and traditional education in the Emirates (1992). "'Abd Allah 'Ali al-Tabur," *al-Tibrah*, http://altibrah.ae/author/281.

28. Al-Tabur, *Al-Tibb Al-Sha'bi*, 8.

29. Frauke Heard-Bey, *From Trucial States to United Arab Emirates: A Society in Transition* (London: Longman, 1982), 325–326.

30. Todd Reisz, *Showpiece City: How Architecture Made Dubai* (Stanford, CA: Stanford University Press, 2020), 138.

31. Al-Tabur, *Al-Tibb Al-Sha'bi*, 7.

32. Al-Tabur, 7. This is also one of Zayed's most frequently quoted lines in the contemporary United Arab Emirates.

33. Al-Tabur, 9.

34. Al-Tabur, 319–327.

35. Al-Tabur, 169.

36. Al-Tabur, 169.

37. Al-Tabur, 167.

38. Al-Tabur, 287–288.

39. Al-Tabur, 167.

40. Ana Vinea, "Possessed or Insane? Diagnostic Puzzles in Contemporary Egypt," *International Journal of Middle East Studies* (2023): 5, https://doi.org/10.1017/S0020743823000673.

41. Al-Tabur, *Al-Tibb Al-Sha'bi*, 167–168. Translation is from Sahih International.

42. Al-Tabur, 168.

43. Al-Tabur, 168.

44. Suzanne Miers, *Slavery in the Twentieth Century: The Evolution of a Global Problem* (Walnut Creek, CA: Alta Mira Press, 2003), 342. Slavery was officially

banned in Iran in 1929, Kuwait in 1949, Qatar in 1952, Saudi Arabia in 1962, and Oman in 1970. Behnaz Mirzai, *A History of Slavery and Emancipation in Iran, 1800–1929* (Austin: University of Texas Press, 2017), 158. See also Jerzy Zdanowski, *Speaking with Their Own Voices: The Stories of Slaves in the Persian Gulf in the 20th Century* (Cambridge: Cambridge Scholars Press, 2014); Hisham al-'Awadi, *Tarikh al-'Abid fi al-Khalij al-'Arabi* (Kuwait: Dar al-Tanweer, 2021)

45. Matthew S. Hopper, *Slaves of one Master: Globalization and Slavery in Arabia in the Age of Empire* (New Haven, CT: Yale University Press, 2015), 216.

46. Sachedina, *Cultivating the Past, Living the Modern*, 172–173.

47. Limbert, *In the Time of Oil*, 147–148; Sachedina, *Cultivating the Past, Living the Modern*, 188–196; Alice Wilson, *Afterlives of Revolution: Everyday Counterhistories in Southern Oman* (Stanford, CA: Stanford University Press, 2023), 25–26.

48. Al-Tabur, *Al-Tibb Al-Sha'bi*, 171.

49. Al-Tabur, 171.

50. British attempts to suppress trade in enslaved Africans, for example, paradoxically resulted in the expansion of other networks of exchange of enslaved people, particularly Baluchis. Mirzai, *Slavery and Emancipation in Iran*, 15.

51. Beatrice Nicolini, "Some Thoughts on the Magical Practice of *Zār* along the Red Sea in the Sudan," in *People of the Red Sea Project II, Held in the British Museum October 2004*, ed. Janet M. C. Starkey (Oxford, UK: Archeopress, 2005), 157.

52. Ehud Toledano, *As If Silent and Absent: Bonds of Enslavement in the Islamic Middle East* (New Haven, CT: Yale University Press, 2007), 220. Toledano, citing Fatima al-Misri, also makes the intriguing suggestion that *zār* entered Egypt in the 1820s in tandem with the Egyptian occupation of Sudan, but in the Arabian Peninsula, Reilly contends, "circumstantial evidence suggests that Khaybar's zar cult may have been of considerable antiquity." See Toledano, 220; Benjamin Reilly, *Slavery, Agriculture, and Malaria in the Arabian Peninsula* (Athens: Ohio University Press, 2015), 98.

53. Nicolini, "Magical Practice of *Zār* along the Red Sea," 159.

54. Reilly, *Slavery, Agriculture, and Malaria*, 97.

55. Toledano, *As If Silent and Absent*, 221; Reilly, *Slavery, Agriculture, and Malaria*, 155.

56. Taylor M. Moore, "Occult Epidemics," *History of the Present* 13, no. 1 (2023): 88.

57. On attacks on *zār* by early scripturalist reformers, or Salafis, in 1920s Aden, see Scott S. Reese, *Imperial Muslims: Islam, Community and Authority in the Indian Ocean, 1839–1937* (Edinburgh: Edinburgh University Press, 2018), 109–137. On how Salafi Qur'anic healers in contemporary Egypt reject what they perceive as unpermitted therapies such as *zār*, see Ana Vinea, "'What Is Your Evidence?'

A Salafi Therapy in Contemporary Egypt," *Comparative Studies of South Asia, Africa and the Middle East* 39, no. 3 (2019): 500–512.

58. Al-Tabur, *Al-Tibb Al-Sha'bi*, 171.
59. Al-Tabur, 174.
60. Al-Tabur, 175.
61. Al-Tabur, 175.
62. Al-Tabur, 175.
63. Al-Tabur, 171. Zubaydah Ashkanani has a similar explanation as to why women practiced *zār* in Kuwait in the late 1980s, writing, "The emotional distress and isolation which they feel in modern westernized Kuwait find expression and release in the world of *zar* with its caring rituals, consolation and mutually shared support, where their sense of identity, of self-worth, is assured and their sociocultural isolation and alienation is lessoned." Zubaydah Ashkanani, "*Zar* in a Changing World: Kuwait," in *Women's Medicine: The Zar-Bori Cult in Africa and Beyond*, ed. I. M. Lewis, Ahmed al-Safi, and Sayyid Hurreiz (Edinburgh: Edinburgh University Press, 1991), 220.
64. For scholarship on *zār* cults, see Nicolini, "Magical Practice of *Zār* along the Red Sea," 157; Toledano, *As If Silent and Absent*, 223. See also Al-Tabur, *Al-Tibb Al-Sha'bi*, 170–171.
65. Al-Tabur, 171.
66. Al-Tabur, 172.
67. Al-Maliki, *Jawab Kull Sa'il 'ind Mu'alijin Qatar al-Awa'il*, 6.
68. In addition to the book under consideration here, his publications cover topics such as *sha'bī* stories (2002), Qatari proverbs (2005), *sha'bī* markets in Qatar (2006), Proverbs in Qatar of Bedouin and townsfolk (2007), *sha'bī* trades (2008), Qatari Qur'an teachers (2009), and names of *sha'bī* diseases and treatments with herbs (2010). Al-Maliki, *Jawab Kull Sa'il 'ind Mu'alijin Qatar al-Awa'il*, back cover; "Khalifa al-Sayyid Mohammad Salih al-Maliki," *Good Reads*, https://www.goodreads.com/author/show/5075997._خليفة.
69. Al-Maliki, *Jawab Kull Sa'il 'ind Mu'alijin Qatar al-Awa'il*, 5.
70. Al-Maliki, 5.
71. Al-Maliki, 5.
72. Al-Maliki, 5.
73. Dwight F. Reynolds, ed., *Interpreting the Self: Autobiography in the Arabic Literary Tradition* (Berkeley: University of California Press, 2001), 41.
74. Al-Maliki, *Jawab Kull Sa'il 'ind Mu'alijin Qatar al-Awa'il*, 5.
75. Al-Maliki, 6.
76. Al-Maliki, 13.
77. Al-Maliki, 13.

78. Al-Maliki, 13.
79. Al-Maliki, 13.
80. Al-Maliki, 13.
81. Al-Maliki, 13–14.
82. David Commins, *The Gulf States: A Modern History* (London: I. B. Tauris, 2012), 150.
83. Al-Maliki, *Jawab Kull Sa'il 'ind Mu'alijin Qatar al-Awa'il*, 42.
84. Al-Maliki, 57.
85. Mirzai, *Slavery and Emancipation in Iran*, 129. In the early 1950s, a British political officer estimated that there were three thousand enslaved people in Qatar out of a population of around fifteen to twenty thousand people. Miers, *Slavery in the Twentieth Century*, 340.
86. Al-Maliki, *Jawab Kull Sa'il 'ind Mu'alijin Qatar al-Awa'il*, 32.
87. Maurice Halbwachs, *On Collective Memory*, trans. Lewis A. Coser (Chicago: University of Chicago Press, 1992).
88. "Oral History," Ministry of Presidential Affairs, National Archives, Official Portal of the United Arab Emirates, http://www.na.ae/en/archives/oralhistory/default.aspx
89. "Msheireb Museums showcase a new exhibition in collaboration with UCL Qatar's Masters Students titled 'Back to Msheireb: Shared Streets—Shared Stories,'" Msheireb Museums, https://msheirebmuseums.com/en/news/msheireb-museums-showcase-a-new-exhibition-in-collaboration-with-ucl-qatars-masters-students-titled-back-to-msheireb-shared-streets-shared-stories/.
90. "Steam Initiative: Oral History," Texas A&M University at Qatar, http://steam.qatar.tamu.edu/digital-narratives-2/oral-history/.
91. Goffman, "Jar of Shaykhs' Teeth."

Conclusion

1. Hissa 'Abd Allah al-Sharim, *Tarikh Ta'lim al-Tamrid bi Dawla Qatar, 1969–2008* (Doha: National Health Authority, 2007), 10.
2. Khalifa al-Sayyid Mohammad Salih al-Maliki, *Jawab Kull Sa'il 'ind Mu'alijin Qatar al-Awa'il* (Doha: Renoda Modern Printing Press, 2012), 160.
3. Al-Maliki, *Jawab Kull Sa'il 'ind Mu'alijin Qatar al-Awa'il*, 160.
4. Al-Maliki, 160.
5. See Laura Frances Goffman, "Malaria and Empire in Bahrain, 1931–1947," *Gulf Studies Monographic Series* 7 (2020): 1–30.

BIBLIOGRAPHY

Archival Collections
Arabian Gulf Digital Archives (AGDA), https://www.agda.ae/en
British Petroleum Archive (BP), University of Warwick, Coventry, UK
"Health and Disease in Saudi Arabia: Oral History Transcript: The Aramco Experience, 1940s–1990s/1998," Regional Oral History Office, Bancroft Library, University of California, Berkeley
India Office Records (IOR), British Library, London and Qatar Digital Library, https://www.qdl.qa/en
Kuwait University Archive (KU), Kuwait City, Kuwait
National Archives of India (NAI), New Delhi, India
National Archives of the United Kingdom (NAUK), Kew, United Kingdom
US National Archives at College Park, Maryland
William E. Mulligan Papers, Lauinger Library, Special Collections, Georgetown University, Washington, DC

Primary and Secondary Sources
"ʿAbd Allah ʿAli al-Tabur." *Al-Tibrah.* https://altibrah.ae/author/281.
Abi-Rached, Joelle M. *ʿAṣfūriyyeh: A History of Madness, Modernity, and War in the Middle East.* Cambridge: Massachusetts Institute of Technology Press, 2020.
Abugideiri, Hibba. "A Labor of Love: Making Space for Midwives in Gulf History." In *Gulf Women,* edited by Amira El-Azhary Sonbol, 167–200. Syracuse, NY: Syracuse University Press, 2012.
Abu-Hakima, Ahmad Mustafa. *Tarikh al-Kuwayt al-Hadith, 1750–1965* [Modern History of Kuwait, 1750–1965]. Kuwait: N.p., 1984.
Abu-Lughod, Janet. *Cairo: 1001 Years of the City Victorious.* Princeton, NJ: Princeton University Press, 1971.
Abu Saud, Abeer. *Qatari Women Past and Present.* Essex, UK: Longman Group, 1984.

Afkhami, Amir A. *A Modern Contagion: Imperialism and Public Health in Iran's Age of Cholera.* Baltimore, MD: Johns Hopkins University Press, 2019.

Albateni, Khaled. "The Arabian Mission's Effect on Kuwaiti Society, 1910–1967." PhD diss., Indiana University, 2014.

Alebrahim, Abdulrahman. *Kuwait's Politics before Independence: The Role of the Balancing Powers.* Berlin: Gerlach Press, 2019.

Alissa, Reem. "The Oil Town of Ahmadi since 1946: From Colonial Town to Nostalgic City." *Comparative Studies of South Asia, Africa and the Middle East* 33, no. 1 (2013): 41–58.

Allen, Calvin H., Jr. "The Indian Merchant Community of Masqat." *Bulletin of the School of Oriental and African Studies* 44, no. 1 (1981): 39–53.

Alsada, Maryam Mohamed Abdulla Ebrahim. "The Lives of Girls and Women in Bahrain and Qatar: Dress, Marriage, Health and Education in the Pearl Fishing and Early Oil Era." PhD diss., University College London, 2022.

AlShehabi, Omar. *Contested Modernity: Sectarianism, Nationalism, and Colonialism in Bahrain.* London: Oneworld Academic, 2019.

———. "Histories of Migration to the Gulf." In *Transit States: Labour, Migration & Citizenship in the Gulf,* edited by Abdulhadi Khalaf, Omar Alshehabi, and Adam Hanieh, 3–38. London: Pluto Press, 2015.

Amrith, Sunil S. *Decolonizing International Health: India and Southeast Asia, 1930–65.* New York: Palgrave Macmillan, 2006.

Anscombe, Frederick F. *The Ottoman Gulf: The Creation of Kuwait, Saudi Arabia, and Qatar.* New York: Columbia University Press, 1997.

Arab Support Committee. "Struggle Oppression and Counter-Revolution in Saudi Arabia." Translated from the original Arabic articles appearing in the 1972 issues of the Al Jazeerah Al-Jadeedah, the political organ of the People's Democratic Party of Al Jazeerah Al Arabiah—"Saudi Arabia." Berkeley, CA, 1972.

"Aramco, Harvard Fight Trachoma in $500,000, Five-Year Program." *Arabian Sun and Flare* (Arabian American Oil Co., Dhahran, Saudi Arabia) 9, no. 44 (1954).

Armerding, Paul L. *Doctors for the Kingdom: The Work of the American Mission Hospitals in the Kingdom of Saudi Arabia 1913–1955.* Grand Rapids, MI: William B. Eerdmans Publishing, 2003.

Arnold, David. "The Indian Ocean as a Disease Zone, 1500–1950. *South Asia: Journal of South Asian Studies* 14, no. 2 (1991): 1–21.

Arslan, Aytuğ, and Hasan Ali Polat. "Travel from Europe to Istanbul in the 19th Century and the Quarantine of Çanakkale. *Journal of Transport & Health* 4 (2017): 10–17.

Ashkanani, Zubaydah. "*Zar* in a Changing World: Kuwait." In *Women's Medicine: The Zar-Bori Cult in Africa and Beyond*, edited by I. M. Lewis, Ahmed al-Safi, and Sayyid Hurreiz, 219–229. Edinburgh: Edinburgh University Press, 1991.

"At War with Trachoma." *Aramco World* 11, no. 8 (October 1960): 3–6.

Ateş, Sabri. "Bones of Contention: Corpse Traffic and Ottoman-Iranian Rivalry in Nineteenth-Century Iraq." *Comparative Studies of South Asia, Africa, and the Middle East* 30, no. 3 (2010): 512–532.

Al-Atiqi, Suliman. "The Origins of Kuwaiti Nationalism: Rashid Rida's Influence on Kuwaiti National Identity." *Arab Studies Journal* 23, no. 1 (Fall 2015): 78–122.

Al-ʿAwadi, Hisham. *Tarikh al-ʿAbid fi al-Khalij al-ʿArabi* [The history of slaves in the Arab Gulf]. Kuwait: Dar al-Tanweer, 2021.

Al-Awaji, Ibrahim Mohamed. "Bureaucracy and Society in Saudi Arabia." PhD diss., University of Virginia, 1971.

Al-ʿAwwami, Hasan. "'Nuʿarkhum fi 'al-labbania' wa yarhhabun bina fi 'al-wadi'" [We fight them in al-Labbania and they welcome us in al-Wadi], *Sobra News*, 7 February 2021, https://www.sobranews.com/sobra/108836.

Al-ʿAwwami, Sayyid ʿAli al-Sayyid Baqir. "Al-Haraka al-Wataniyya Sharq al-Saʿudiyya 1373–1393 h/ 1953–1973 m" [The National Movement in eastern Saudi Arabia 1373–1392 h/1953–1973 m]. Unpublished, 2 vols., 2011.

Al-ʿAzmi, Mohammad Maʿyyid ʿAbd Allah. "Al-Maqabir wa-l-Shawahid al-Qabriyya fi al-Kuwayt: Masdar li-Darrasa baʿd Jawanib al-Tarikh al-Ijtimaʿiyy al-Kuwayti khilal al-Qarnayn" [Cemeteries and gravestones in Kuwait: A source for studying some aspects of Kuwaiti social history during two centuries]. Master's thesis, Al-Bayt University, 2016.

Al-Azri, Khalid M. *Social and Gender Inequality in Oman: The Power of Religious and Political Tradition*. New York: Routledge, 2013.

Al-Azri, Nasser Hammad. "Sent to Explore, Conquer and Heal: History of the Evolution of Biomedicine in Oman during the 19th Century." *SQU Medical Journal* 11, no. 2 (May 2011): 187–195.

Baldry, John. "The Ottoman Quarantine Station on Kamaran Island 1882–1914." *Studies in History of Medicine* 2, nos. 1–2 (March–June 1978): 3–138.

Baron, Beth. *The Orphan Scandal: Christian Missionaries and the Rise of the Muslim Brotherhood*. Stanford, CA: Stanford University Press, 2014.

Bashkin, Orit. "Hybrid Nationalisms: Waṭanī and Qawmī Visions of Iraq under ʿAbd Al-Karim Qasim, 1958–61." *International Journal of Middle East Studies* 31, no. 2 (2011): 293–312.

Bayat, Asef. *Life as Politics: How Ordinary People Change the Middle East*. 2nd ed. Stanford, CA: Stanford University Press, 2013.

Beauchamp, Tom L. "Informed Consent: Its History, Meaning, and Present Challenges." *Cambridge Quarterly of Healthcare Ethics* 20 (2011): 515–523.
Belgrave, Charles. *Personal Column*. London: Hutchinson & Co., 1960.
Bell, Samuel D., Jr., Roger L. Nichols, and Nadim A. Haddad. "The Immunology of the Trachoma Agent with a Preliminary Report on Field Trials of Vaccine." *Investigative Ophthalmology & Visual Science* 2 (October 1963): 471–481.
Benedict, Carol. *Bubonic Plague in Nineteenth-Century China*. Stanford, CA: Stanford University Press, 1996.
Bishara, Fahad Ahmad. "The Fateh Al-Khayr." *Perspectives on History*, February 25, 2021. https://www.historians.org/publications-and-directories/perspectives-on-history/march-2021/the-emfateh-al-khayr/em.
———. "The Many Voyages of *Fateh al-Khayr*: Unfurling the Gulf in the Age of Oceanic History." *International Journal of Middle East Studies* 52, no. 3 (2020): 397–412.
———. "'No Country but the Ocean': Reading International Law from the Deck of an Indian Ocean Dhow, ca. 1900." *Comparative Studies in Society and History* 60, no. 2 (2018): 338–366.
———. *A Sea of Debt: Law and Economic Life in the Western Indian Ocean, 1780–1950*. Cambridge: Cambridge University Press, 2017.
Al-Bishr, Ahmad. *Maqalat 'an al-Kuwayt* [Articles about Kuwait]. Kuwait: Maktabat al-Amal, 1966.
Bobb, Arthur A., and Roger L. Nichols. "Influence of Environment on Clinical Trachoma in Saudi Arabia." *American Journal of Ophthalmology* 67, no. 2 (1969): 235–243.
Bolaños, Isacar A. "The Ottomans during the Global Crises of Cholera and Plague: The View from Iraq and the Gulf." *International Journal of Middle East Studies* 51, no. 4 (2019): 603–620.
Boodrookas, Alex Cobb. "The Making of a Migrant Working Class: Contesting Citizenship in Kuwait and the Persian Gulf, 1925–1975." PhD diss., New York University, 2020.
Boodrookas, Alex, and Arang Keshavarzian. "The Forever Frontier of Urbanism: Historicizing Persian Gulf Cities." *International Journal of Urban and Regional Research* 43, no. 1 (2019): 14–29.
Borel, Frédéric. *Étude d'hygiene internationale: Choléra et peste dans le pèlerinage musulman, 1860–1903* [International hygiene study: Cholera and plague in the Muslim pilgrimage, 1860–1903]. Paris: Libraires de l'Académie de Médecine, 1904. https://archive.org/details/b21354315.

Brandt, Allan M. "Polio, Politics, Publicity, and Duplicity: Ethical Aspects in the Development of the Salk Vaccine." *International Journal of Health Services* 8, no. 2 (1978): 257–270.

———. "Racism and Research: The Case of the Tuskegee Syphilis Study." *Hastings Center Report* 6, no. 8 (1978): 21–29.

Bsheer, Rosie. "A Counter-Revolutionary State: Popular Movements and the Making of Saudi Arabia." *Past and Present* 238 (November 2018): 233–277.

Burton, Elise K. *Genetic Crossroads: The Middle East and the Science of Human Heredity.* Stanford, CA: Stanford University Press, 2021.

Busch, Briton Cooper. *Britain and the Persian Gulf, 1894–1914.* Berkeley: University of California Press, 1967.

Calverley, Edwin E. "Evangelistic Activities at Kuweit." *Neglected Arabia* 92 (January–March 1915): 8–10.

Calverley, Eleanor T. *My Arabian Days and Nights: A Medical Missionary in Old Kuwait.* New York: Thomas Y. Crowell Co., 1958.

Chalcraft, John. "Migration and Popular Protest in the Arabian Peninsula and the Gulf in the 1950s and 1960s." *International Labor and Working-Class History* 79, no. 1 (Spring 2011): 28–47.

"Cholera—*Vibrio cholerae* infection." Centers for Disease Control and Prevention. https://www.cdc.gov/cholera/general/index.html.

Choy, Catherine Ceniza. *Empire of Care: Nursing and Migration in Filipino American History.* Durham, NC: Duke University Press, 2003.

Commins, David. *The Gulf States: A Modern History.* London: I. B. Tauris, 2012.

———. *The Wahhabi Mission and Saudi Arabia.* London: I. B. Tauris, 2006.

cooke, miriam. *Tribal Modern: Branding New Nations in the Arab Gulf.* Berkeley: University of California Press, 2014.

Crouzet, Guillemette. *Inventing the Middle East: Britain and the Persian Gulf in the Age of Global Imperialism.* Montreal: McGill-Queen's University Press, 2022.

Crystal, Jill. *Kuwait: The Transformation of an Oil State.* New York: Routledge, 1992.

———. *Oil and Politics in the Gulf: Rulers and Merchants in Kuwait and Qatar.* Cambridge: Cambridge University Press, 1990.

Daggy, Richard H. "Malaria in Oases of Eastern Saudi Arabia." *American Journal of Tropical Medicine and Hygiene* 8 (1959): 223–291.

Daggy, Richard, and R. C. Page. "Aramco's Preventive Medicine Program." *Medical Bulletin* 16 (1956): 196–204.

Al-Dailami, Ahmed. "'Purity and Confusion': The Hawala between Persians and Arabs in the Contemporary Gulf." In *The Persian Gulf in Modern Times:*

People, Ports, and History, edited by Lawrence G. Potter, 299–326. New York: Palgrave Macmillan, 2014.

"Da'ira al-Sihha al-'Amma" [Public Health Department]. *Al-Kuwayt al-Yawm* 11 (February 1955): 6–7.

Dale, Charlotte. "The Social Exploits and Behaviour of Nurses during the Anglo-Boer War, 1899–1902." In *Colonial Caring: A history of Colonial and Post-Colonial Nursing*, edited by Helen Sweet and Sue Hawkins, 60–83. Manchester, UK: Manchester University Press, 2015.

Dalenberg, Cornelia. "From Shadowed Thresholds, Dark with Fear: A Village Woman's Story." *Arabia Calling* 225 (Autumn 1951): 12–14.

———. *Sharifa*. Grand Rapids, MI: Wm. B. Eerdmans Publishing Co., 1983.

———. "Unforgetable [sic] Patients." *Arabia Calling* 217 (Summer 1949): 12–13.

Department of Planning and Statistics, State of Kuwait. *Statistics Abstract in 25 Years*. Kuwait: Ministry of Planning Statistics & IT Sector, 1990.

Derderian, Elizabeth. "Authenticating an Emirati Art World: Claims of Tabula Rasa and Cultural Appropriation in the UAE." *Journal of Arabian Studies* 7 (2017): 12–27.

Dewachi, Omar. *Ungovernable Life: Mandatory Medicine and Statecraft in Iraq*. Stanford, CA: Stanford University Press, 2017.

Dickson, H. R. P. *Kuwait and Her Neighbours*. London: George Allen & Unwin, 1956.

"Doctors Prescribing Non-Ayurvedic Medicines Are Anti-National." *Times of India*, May 1, 2016. https://timesofindia.indiatimes.com/city/kolhapur/doctors-prescribing-non-ayurvedic-medicines-are-anti-national/articleshow/52058067.cms.

Dolbee, Samuel. "Borders, Disease, and Territoriality in the Post-Ottoman Middle East." In *Regimes of Mobility: Borders and State Formation in the Middle East, 1918–1946*, edited by Jordi Tejel and Ramazan Hakki Öztan, 205–227. Edinburgh: Edinburgh University Press, 2022.

Douglas, Mary. *Purity and Danger: An Analysis of Concepts of Pollution and Taboo*. 1966. Reprint, London: Routledge, 2000.

Doumato, Eleanor Abdella. *Getting God's Ear: Women, Islam, and Healing in Saudi Arabia and the Gulf*. New York: Columbia University Press, 2000.

Echenberg, Myron. *Plague Ports: The Global Urban Impact of Bubonic Plague*. New York: New York University Press, 2007.

El Guindi, Ismail. "Vaginal Atresia in Saudi Arabia." *BJOG: An International Journal of Obstetrics and Gynaecology* 69, no. 6 (December 1962): 996–998.

Ennis, Crystal A., and Margaret Walton-Roberts. "Labour Market Regulation as Global Social Policy: The Case of Nursing Labour Markets in Oman." *Global Social Policy* 18, no. 2 (2018):169–188.

Erskine-Loftus, Pamela, Mariam Al-Mulla, and Victoria Hightower, eds. *Representing the Nation: Heritage, Museums, National Narratives, and Identity in the Arab Gulf States*. New York: Routledge, 2016.

Exell, Karen. "Desiring the Past and Reimagining the Present: Contemporary Collecting in Qatar." *Museum & Society* 14, no. 2 (2016): 259–274.

Exell, Karen, and Trinidad Rico, eds. *Cultural Heritage in the Arabian Peninsula: Debates, Discourses and Practices*. Surrey, UK: Ashgate, 2014.

———. "'There Is No Heritage in Qatar': Orientalism, Colonialism and Other Problematic Histories." *World Archeology* 45, no. 4 (2013): 670–685.

Fabbri, Roberto, Sara Saragoça, and Ricardo Camacho. *Modern Architecture Kuwait 1949–1989*. Zurich, Switzerland: Niggli, 2016.

Fabian, Johannes. *Time and the Other: How Anthropology Makes Its Object*. New York: Columbia University Press, 1983.

Fahmy, Kamal. "Cervical and Vaginal Atresia due to Packing the Vagina with Salt after Labor." *American Journal of Obstetrics and Gynecology* 84, no. 11 (1962): 1466–1469.

———. "Salt Atresia in Arabia." *Australian and New Zealand Journal of Obstetrics and Gynaecology* 5, no. 2 (1965): 103–112.

Fahmy, Khaled. *In Quest of Justice: Islamic Law and Forensic Medicine in Modern Egypt*. Oakland: University of California Press, 2018.

Fattah, Hala. *The Politics of Regional Trade in Iraq, Arabia, and the Gulf 1745–1900*. Albany: State University of New York Press, 1997.

Faue, Elizabeth, and Josiah Rector. "The Precarious Work of Care: OSHA, AIDS, and Women Health-Care Workers, 1983–2000." *Labor: Studies in Working-Class History* 17, no. 4 (2020): 9–33.

Feng, Marie, R. Shih-Man Chang, Taylor R. Smith, and John C. Snyder. "Adenoviruses Isolated from Saudi Arabia. II. Pathogenicity of Certain Strains for Man." *American Journal of Tropical Medicine and Hygiene* 8 (1959): 501–504.

Fleischmann, Ellen L. *The Nation and Its "New" Women: The Palestinian Women's Movement, 1920–1948*. Berkeley: University of California Press, 2003.

Floor, Willem. *Muscat: City, Society & Trade*. Washington, DC: Mage Publishers, 2015.

———. *Public Health in Qajar Iran*. Odenton, MD: Mage Publishers, 2004.

———. "Qal'eh-ye Mehran Khan: The First Leprosarium in Iran." *Iranian Studies* 53, nos. 1–2 (2020): 9–41.

Foucault, Michel. *Security, Territory, Population: Lectures at the Collège de France, 1977–78*. Edited by Michel Senellart, François Ewald, and Alessandro Fontana. Translated by Graham Burchell. New York: Palgrave Macmillan, 2007.

Francis, Lorania K. "U.S. Hospital Oasis of Health for Arabs: Medical Science Defeats Tide of Ancient Diseases in Oil Area." *Los Angeles Times*, April 2, 1951.

Freitag, Ulrike. *A History of Jeddah: The Gate to Mecca in the Nineteenth and Twentieth Centuries*. New York: Cambridge University Press, 2020.

Frith, Kathleen. "Vaginal Atresia of Arabia: Four Cases." *BLOG: An International Journal of Obstetrics and Gynaecology* 67, no. 1 (February 1960): 82–85.

Fuccaro, Nelida. *Histories of City and State in the Persian Gulf: Manama since 1800*. Cambridge: Cambridge University Press, 2009.

———. "Knowledge at the Service of the British Empire: The Gazetteer of the Persian Gulf, Oman, and Central Arabia." In *Borders and the Changing Boundaries of Knowledge*, edited by Inga Brandell, Marie Carlson, and Önver Cetrez, 17–34. Istanbul: Swedish Research Institute in Istanbul, 2015.

Gamsa, Mark. "The Epidemic of Pneumonic Plague in Manchuria 1910–1911." *Past and Present* 190 (2006): 147–183.

Ghazal, Amal N. *Islamic Reform and Arab Nationalism: Expanding the Crescent from the Mediterranean to the Indian Ocean (1880s–1930s)*. London: Routledge, 2010.

Ghrawi, Claudia. "Structural and Physical Violence in Saudi Arabian Oil Towns, 1953–56." In *Urban Violence in the Middle East: Changing Cityscapes in the Transition from Empire to Nation State*, edited by Ulrike Freitag, Nelida Fuccaro, Claudia Ghrawi, and Nora Lafi, 243–264. New York: Berghahn Books, 2015.

———. "A Tamed Urban Revolution: Saudi Arabia's Oil Conurbation and the 1967 Riots." In *Violence and the City in the Modern Middle East*, edited by Nelida Fuccaro, 109–126. Stanford, CA: Stanford University Press, 2016.

Giladi, Avner. *Muslim Midwives: The Craft of Birthing in the Premodern Middle East*. Cambridge: Cambridge University Press, 2014.

Gilbert, Erik. "The Dhow as Cultural Icon: Heritage and Regional Identity in the Western Indian Ocean." *International Journal of Heritage Studies* 17, no. 1 (2011): 62–80.

Gilman, Daniel J. *Cairo Pop: Youth Music in Contemporary Egypt*. Minneapolis: University of Minnesota Press, 2014.

Goffman, Laura Frances. "A Jar of Shaykhs' Teeth: Medicine, Politics, and the Fragments of History in Kuwait." *International Journal of Middle East Studies* 53, no. 4 (November 2021): 589–603.

———. "Malaria and Empire in Bahrain, 1931–1947." *Gulf Studies Monographic Series* 7 (2020): 1–30.

———. "Medical Frontiers: Health, Empire, and Society in the Gulf and Arabian Peninsula, 1862–1959." PhD diss., Georgetown University, 2019.

———. "Popular Politics and Epidemics in Eastern Arabia." *Labor: Studies in Working-Class History* 20, no. 2 (May 2023): 74–94.

González, Alessandra L. *Islamic Feminism in Kuwait: The Politics and Paradoxes.* New York: Palgrave Macmillan, 2013.

Graboyes, Melissa. *The Experiment Must Continue: Medical Research and Ethics in East Africa, 1940–2014.* Athens: Ohio University Press, 2015.

Green, Monica H., and Lori Jones. "The Evolution and Spread of Major Human Diseases in the Indian Ocean World." In *Disease Dispersion and Impact in the Indian Ocean World*, edited by Gwyn Campbell and Eva-Maria Knoll, 25–57. London: Palgrave Macmillan, 2020.

Green, Nile. *Bombay Islam: The Religious Economy of the West Indian Ocean, 1840–1915.* Cambridge: Cambridge University Press, 2011.

Group, Thetis M., and Joan I. Roberts. *Nursing, Physician Control, and the Medical Monopoly: Historical Perspectives on Gendered Inequality in Roles, Rights, and Range of Practice.* Bloomington: Indiana University Press, 2001.

Al-Hajri, Hilal. "Through Evangelizing Eyes: American Missionaries to Oman." *Proceedings of the Seminar for Arabian Studies held at the British Museum, London 22 to 24 July 2010* 41 (2011): 121–131.

Halbwachs, Maurice. *On Collective Memory.* Translated by Lewis A. Cosger. Chicago: University of Chicago Press, 1992.

Halevi, Leor. *Modern Things on Trial: Islam's Global and Material Reformation in the Age of Rida, 1865–1935.* New York: Columbia University Press, 2019.

Halliday, Fred. *Arabia without Sultans.* Middlesex, UK: Penguin Books, 1974.

Hamed-Troyansky, Vladimir. "Ottoman and Egyptian Quarantines and European Debates on Plague in the 1830s–1840s." *Past and Present* 253, no. 1 (November 2021): 235–270.

Hamlin, Christopher. *Cholera: The Biography.* Oxford: Oxford University Press, 2009.

Hanna, Nabil Subhi. *Al-Tibb al-Sha'bi fi al-Khalij* [Folk medicine in the Gulf]. Doha: Markaz al-Turath al-Sha'bi li Majlis al-Ta'aun li Duwal al-Khalij al-'Arabi, 1998.

Hansen, Henny Harald. *Investigations in a Shī'a Village in Bahrain.* Copenhagen: National Museum of Denmark, 1967.

Harrison, Mark. *Contagion: How Commerce has Spread Disease.* New Haven, CT: Yale University Press, 2012.

Harrison, Paul. *The Arab at Home.* New York: Thomas Y. Cromwell Co., 1924.

Harvey, David. *Spaces of Hope.* Berkeley: University of California Press, 2000.

Al-Hatim, ʿAbd Allah Khalid. *Min Huna Badaʾat al-Kuwayt* [From here Kuwait began]. Damascus: Al-Matbaʿa al-ʿUmumiyya, 1962.

Hazkani, Shay. *Dear Palestine: A Social History of the 1948 War*. Stanford, CA: Stanford University Press, 2021.

Heard-Bey, Frauke. *From Trucial States to United Arab Emirates: A Society in Transition*. London: Longman, 1982.

Himes, Norman E. *Medical History of Contraception*. Baltimore: Williams and Wilkins Co., 1936. Reprint, New York: Schocken, 1970.

Hobbs, Mark. "A Polymath in Muscat." *Untold Lives* (blog), British Library, August 28, 2014. https://blogs.bl.uk/untoldlives/2014/08/a-polymath-in-muscat.html.

Hopper, Matthew S. "Imperialism and the Dilemma of Slavery in Eastern Arabia and the Gulf, 1873–1939." *Itinerario* 30, no. 3 (2006): 76–94.

———. *Slaves of One Master: Globalization and Slavery in Arabia in the Age of Empire*. New Haven, CT: Yale University Press, 2015.

Huber, Valeska. *Channelling Mobilities: Migration and Globalisation in the Suez Canal Region and Beyond, 1869–1914*. Cambridge: Cambridge University Press, 2013.

"Hygiene-Related Diseases: Trachoma." Centers for Disease Control and Prevention, US Department of Health and Human Services, August 2, 2016. https://www.cdc.gov/healthywater/hygiene/disease/trachoma.html.

Inhorn, Marcia C. *Quest for Conception: Gender, Infertility, and Egyptian Medical Traditions*. Philadelphia: University of Pennsylvania Press, 1994.

Al-Jarallah, Khalid. *Dawakhana: Dirasa Tawthiqiyya fi Tarikh al-Kuwayt al-Sihhi min Khilal Dafatir ʿAbd al-Ilah al-Qinaʿi* [Dawakhana: A documentary study in the history of Kuwait through the notebooks of ʿAbd al-Ilah al-Qinaʿi]. Kuwait: Markaz al-Buhuth wa-l-Dirasat al-Kuwaytiyya, 2005.

———. *Sihhat al-Kuwayt: Qiraʾa fi Wathaʾiq Kuwaytiyya wa Ajnabiyya* [Kuwait's health: Reading in Kuwaiti and foreign documents]. Kuwait: Markaz al-Buhuth wa-l-Dirasat al-Kuwaytiyya, 2019.

———. *Tarikh al-Khadamat al-Sihhiyya fi al-Kuwayt* [History of health services in Kuwait]. Kuwait: Markaz al-Buhuth wa-l-Dirasat al-Kuwaytiyya, 1996.

Al-Jarallah, K. F., M. A. A. Moussa, S. K. Hakeem, and F. K. Al-Khanfar. "The Nursing Workforce in Kuwait to the Year 2020." *International Nursing Review* 56, no. 1 (March 2009): 65–72.

Jones, James H. *Bad Blood: The Tuskegee Syphilis Experiment*. New and expanded ed. New York: Free Press, 1993.

Jones, Marc Owen. *Political Repression in Bahrain*. New York: Cambridge University Press, 2020.

Jones, Stephanie. "British India Steamers and the Trade of the Persian Gulf, 1862–1914." *The Great Circle* 7, no. 1 (1985): 23–44.
Jones, Toby Craig. *Desert Kingdom: How Oil and Water Forged Modern Saudi Arabia*. Cambridge, MA: Harvard University Press, 2010.
Judt, Tony. *The Memory Chalet*. New York: Penguin Books, 2010.
———. *Postwar: A History of Europe since 1945*. New York: Penguin Books, 2005.
Kanna, Ahmed. *Dubai: The City as Corporation*. Minneapolis: University of Minnesota Press, 2011.
Kanna, Ahmed, Amélie Le Renard, and Neha Vora. *Beyond Exception: New Interpretations of the Arabian Peninsula*. Ithaca, NY: Cornell University Press, 2020.
Khalaf, Sulayman. "Poetics and Politics of Newly Invented Traditions in the Gulf: Camel Racing in the United Arab Emirates." *Ethnology* 39, no. 3 (2000): 243–261.
"Khalifa al-Sayyid Mohammad Salih al-Maliki." *Good Reads*, https://www.goodreads.com/author/show/5075997.
Khalili, Laleh. *Sinews of War and Trade: Shipping and Capitalism in the Arabian Peninsula*. London: Verso, 2020.
Al-Khalili, Saʿid bin Khalfan. *Ajwibat Al-Muhaqqiq al-Khalili* [The investigator al-Khalili's answers]. Vol. 6. Muscat, Oman: Maktabat Al-Jil Al-Waʿid, 2010.
Kingston, A. E. "The Vaginal Atresia of Arabia." *BJOG: An International Journal of Obstetrics and Gynaevology* 64, no. 6 (December 1957): 836–839.
Koch, Natalie. "Gulf Nationalism and the Geopolitics of Constructing Falconry as a 'Heritage Sport,'" *Studies in Ethnicity and Nationalism* 15, no. 3 (2015): 522–539.
Kozma, Liat, and Nicole Khayat. "Gendered Struggles over the Medical Profession in the Modern Middle East and North Africa." *Journal of Middle East Women's Studies* 18, no. 1 (2022): 1–11.
Kozma, Liat, and Diane Samuels. "Beyond Borders: The Egyptian 1947 Epidemic as a Regional and International Crisis." *British Journal of Middle Eastern Studies* (2017): 1–18. https://doi.org/10.1080/13530194.2017.1370999.
Krik, Hagit. "The Female Imperial Agent and the Intricacies of Power: British Nurses in Mandate Palestine." *Journal of Middle East Women's Studies* 18, no. 1 (March 2022): 12–35.
"Kuwaiti Constitution." https://www.wipo.int/edocs/lexdocs/laws/en/kw/kw004en.pdf.
Lackner, Helen. *A House Built on Sand: A Political Economy of Saudi Arabia*. London: Ithaca Press, 1978.
Landen, Robert Geran. *Oman since 1856: Disruptive Modernization in a Traditional Arab Society*. Princeton, NJ: Princeton University Press, 1967.

Lang, John G. "The Quarantine Camp at El Tor." *Public Health Reports (1896–1970)* 17, no. 20 (1902): 1156–1159.

Laskow, Sarah. "How the Plastic Bag Became So Popular." *The Atlantic*, October 10, 2014. https://www.theatlantic.com/technology/archive/2014/10/how-the-plastic-bag-became-so-popular/381065/.

Leak, W. Norman. "Medicine and the Traditions." *Neglected Arabia*, no. 125 (April–June 1923): 3–5.

Lefebvre, Henri. *The Production of Space*. Translated by Donald Nicholson-Smith. Oxford: Blackwell, 1991.

Lei, Sean Hsiang-lin. *Neither Donkey nor Horse: Medicine in the Struggle over China's Modernity*. Chicago: University of Chicago Press, 2014.

Lerner, Barron H. *The Breast Cancer Wars: Hope, Fear, and the Pursuit of a Cure in Twentieth-Century America*. Oxford: Oxford University Press, 2003.

Limbert, Madana E. "Caste, Ethnicity, and the Politics of Arabness in Southern Arabia." *Comparative Studies of South Asia, Africa and the Middle East* 34, no. 3 (2014): 590–598.

———. *In the Time of Oil: Piety, Memory & Social Life in an Omani Town*. Stanford, CA: Stanford University Press, 2010.

Longva, Anh Nga. *Walls Built on Sand: Migration, Exclusion, and Society in Kuwait*. Boulder, CO: Westview Press, 1997.

Lori, Noora. *Offshore Citizens: Permanent Temporary Status in the Gulf*. New York: Cambridge University Press, 2019.

Lorimer, J. G. *The Gazetteer of the Persian Gulf, Oman and Central Arabia*. Farnborough, UK: Gregg International, 1970.

Low, Michael Christopher. "Empire and the Hajj: Pilgrims, Plagues, and Pan-Islam under British Surveillance, 1865–1908." *International Journal of Middle East Studies* 40, no. 2 (2008): 269–290.

———. *Imperial Mecca: Ottoman Arabia and the Indian Ocean Hajj*. New York: Columbia University Press, 2020.

Lynteris, Christos. "Skilled Natives, Inept Coolies: Marmot Hunting and the Great Manchurian Pneumonic Plague (1910–1911)." *History and Anthropology* 24, no. 3 (2013): 303–321.

Al-Majali, Nasr. "Al-Kuwayt Tan'a Barjas Hammud al-Barjas" [Kuwait mourns Barjas Hammud al-Barjas], *Elaf*, May 14, 2014, https://elaph.com/Web/News/2014/5/904228.html.

Al-Maliki, Khalifa al-Sayyid Mohammad Salih. *Jawab Kull Sa'il 'ind Mu'alijin Qatar al-Awa'il* [Answer for every questioner from the early healers of Qatar]. Doha: Renoda Modern Printing Press, 2012.

Mamdani, Mahmood. *The Myth of Population Control: Family, Caste, and Class in an Indian Village*. New York: Monthly Review Press, 1972.

Mathew, Johan. *Margins of the Market: Trafficking and Capitalism across the Arabian Sea*. Oakland: University of California Press, 2016.

Matthiesen, Toby. "The Cold War and the Communist Party of Saudi Arabia, 1975–1991." *Journal of Cold War Studies* 22, no. 3 (Summer 2020): 32–62.

———. "Migration, Minorities, and Radical Networks: Labour Movements and Opposition Groups in Saudi Arabia, 1950–1975." *International Review of Social History* 59, no. 3 (Autumn 2014): 473–504.

———. *The Other Saudis: Shiism, Dissent and Sectarianism*. Cambridge: Cambridge University Press, 2015.

McComb, Dorothy E., and Roger L. Nichols. "Antibodies to Trachoma in Eye Secretions of Saudi Arab Children." *American Journal of Epidemiology* 90, no. 4 (1969): 278–284.

McDow, Thomas F. *Buying Time: Debt and Mobility in the Western Indian Ocean*. Athens: Ohio University Press, 2018.

McNiel, James R. "Pediatric Practice in Eastern Saudi Arabia." *Clinical Pediatrics* 5, no. 6 (June 1966): 385–390.

Megill, Allan. "The Reception of Foucault by Historians." *Journal of the History of Ideas* 48, no. 1 (1987): 117–141.

Meier, Paul. "The Biggest Public Health Experiment Ever: The 1954 Field Trial of the Salk Poliomyelitis Vaccine." In *Statistics: A Guide to the Unknown*, edited by Judith M. Tanur, Frederick Mosteller, William H. Kruskal, Richard F. Link, Richard S. Peters, and Gerald R. Rising, 2–13. San Francisco, CA: Holden-Day, 1972.

Ménoret, Pascal. *The Saudi Enigma: A History*. London: Zed Books, 2005.

Miers, Suzanne. *Slavery in the Twentieth Century: The Evolution of a Global Problem*. Walnut Creek, CA: Alta Mira Press, 2003.

Mirzai, Behnaz A. *A History of Slavery and Emancipation in Iran, 1800–1929*. Austin: University of Texas Press, 2017.

Mishra, Saurabh. "Incarceration and Resistance in a Red Sea Lazaretto, 1880–1930." In *Quarantine: Local & Global Histories*, edited by Alison Bashford, 54–65. London: Palgrave, 2016.

Moore, Taylor M. "Occult Epidemics." *History of the Present* 13, no. 1 (2023): 87–100.

Morgan, Colleen. "Cures for Qataris: The First Hospital in Doha." *The Origins of Doha and Qatar Project*, March 10, 2015. https://originsofdoha.wordpress.com/2015/03/10/cures-for-qataris-the-first-hospital-in-doha/.

"Msheireb Museums Showcase a New Exhibition in Collaboration with UCL Qatar's Masters Students Titled 'Back to Msheireb: Shared Streets—Shared Stories." https://msheirebmuseums.com/en/news/msheireb-museums-showcase-a-new-exhibition-in-collaboration-with-ucl-qatars-masters-students-titled-back-to-msheireb-shared-streets-shared-stories/.

Al-Mughni, Haya. *Women in Kuwait: The Politics of Gender.* Rev. ed. London: Saqi Books, 2001.

Mukharji, Projit Bihari. *Doctoring Traditions: Ayurveda, Small Technologies, and Braided Sciences.* Chicago: University of Chicago Press, 2016.

———. "Symptoms of Dis-Ease: New Trends in the Histories of 'Indigenous' South Asian Medicines." *History Compass* 9, no. 12 (2011): 887–899.

Murray, E. S., S. D. Bell Jr., A. T. Hanna, R. L. Nichols, and J. C. Snyder. "Studies on Trachoma 1. Isolation and Identification of Strains of Elementary Bodies from Saudi Arabia and Egypt." *American Journal of Tropical Medicine and Hygiene* 9, no. 2 (1960): 116–124.

Mylrea, C. Stanley G. "A Case of Snake Bite in Kuwait, Arabia." *Transactions of the Royal Society of Tropical Medicine and Hygiene* 21, no. 5 (February 1928): 426.

———. "The Enemy at the Gates." *Neglected Arabia* 117 (April–June 1921): 3–7.

———. "Kuwait before Oil." Unpublished ms., written between 1945 and 1951. Kuwait: Center for Research and Studies on Kuwait.

Al Najjar, Sabika, and Fawzeya Matar. *Al-Mar'a al-Bahrayniyya fi al-Qarn al-'Ishrin: Marhalat ma Qabl al-Istiqlal 1900–1970* [Bahraini women in the twentieth century: Pre-independence period 1900–1970]. Ottawa: Masaa Publishing and Distribution, 2017.

Najmabadi, Afsaneh. *Professing Selves: Transsexuality and Same-Sex Desire in Contemporary Iran.* Durham, NC: Duke University Press, 2014.

Al-Nakib, Farah. *Kuwait Transformed: A History of Oil and Urban Life.* Stanford, CA: Stanford University Press, 2016.

———. "Modernity and the Arab Gulf States: The Politics of Heritage, Memory, and Forgetting." In *Routledge Handbook of Persian Gulf Politics,* edited by Mehran Kamrava, 57–82. New York: Routledge, 2020.

———. "Public Space and Public Protest in Kuwait, 1938–2012." *City* 18, no. 6. (2014): 723–734.

Nichols, Roger L., ed. *Trachoma and Related Disorders caused by Chlamydial Agents: Proceedings of a Symposium held in Boston, Massachusetts 17–20 August 1970.* Amsterdam: Excerpta Medica, 1971.

Nichols, Roger L., Arthur A. Bobb, Nadim A. Haddad, and Dorothy E. McComb. "Immunofluorescent Studies of the Microbiologic Epidemiology of

Trachoma in Saudi Arabia." *American Journal of Ophthalmology* 63 (1967): 1372–1408.

Nichols, Roger L., D. E. McComb, N. Haddad, and E. S. Murray. "Studies on Trachoma. II. Comparison of Fluorescent Antibody, Gimesa and Egg Isolation Methods for Detection of Trachoma Viruses in Human Conjunctival Scrapings." *American Journal of Tropical Medicine and Hygiene* 12, no. 2 (1963): 223–229.

Nicolini, Beatrice. "Some Thoughts on the Magical Practice of *Zār* along the Red Sea in the Sudan." In *People of the Red Sea Project II, Held in the British Museum October 2004*, edited by Janet M. C. Starkey, 157–162. Oxford, UK: Archeopress, 2005.

Nutton, Vivian. "The Seeds of Disease: An Explanation of Contagion and Infection from the Greeks to the Renaissance." *Medical History* 27 (1983): 1–24.

Onley, James. *The Arabian Frontier of the British Raj: Merchants, Rulers, and the British in the Nineteenth-Century Gulf*. Oxford: Oxford University Press, 2007.

———. "Indian Communities in the Persian Gulf, c. 1500–1947." In *The Persian Gulf in Modern Times: People, Ports, and History*, edited by Lawrence G. Potter, 231–266. New York: Palgrave Macmillan, 2014.

"Oral History." Ministry of Presidential Affairs, National Archives, Official Portal of the United Arab Emirates. https://www.na.ae/en/archives/oralhistory/default.aspx.

Parker, Chad H. *Making the Desert Modern: Americans, Arabs, and Oil on the Saudi Frontier, 1933–1973*. Amherst: University of Massachusetts Press, 2015.

Patterson, Lucy M. "Nine Months Medical Work at Bahrein." *Neglected Arabia* 52 (October–December 1904): 7–10.

———. "Two Weeks at the Hospital." *Neglected Arabia* 50 (April–June 1904): 10–11.

Porter, Roy. *The Greatest Benefit to Mankind: A Medical History of Humanity from Antiquity to the Present*. London: Fontana Press, 1999.

Potter, Lawrence G. Introduction to *The Persian Gulf in History*, edited by Lawrence G. Potter, 1–26. New York: Palgrave Macmillan, 2009.

———, ed. *The Persian Gulf in Modern Times: People, Ports, and History*. New York: Palgrave Macmillan, 2014.

———. *Society in the Persian Gulf: Before and after Oil*. Doha: Georgetown University in Qatar, Center for International and Regional Studies, 2017.

Al-Qinaʻi, Yusif. *Safahat min Tarikh al-Kuwayt* [Pages from the history of Kuwait]. Kuwait: Matbaʻat Hukumat al-Kuwayt, 1968.

Rabinowitz, Dan. *The Power of Deserts: Climate Change, the Middle East, and the Promise of a Post-Oil Era*. Stanford, CA: Stanford University Press, 2020.
Al-Rasheed, Madawi. *A History of Saudi Arabia*. 2nd ed. Cambridge: Cambridge University Press, 2010.
———. *A Most Masculine State: Gender, Politics, and Religion in Saudi Arabia*. Cambridge: Cambridge University Press, 2013.
Al-Rashoud, Talal. "From Muscat to the Maghreb: Pan-Arab Networks, Anti-Colonial Groups, and Kuwait's Arab Scholarships (1953–1961)." *Arabian Humanities* 12 (2019): https://doi.org/10.4000/cy.5004.
———. "Icon of Defiance and Hope: Gamal Abdel Nasser's Image in Gulf History." *Mada Masr*, November 28, 2020. https://www.madamasr.com/en/2020/11/28/opinion/u/icon-of-defiance-and-hope-gamal-abdel-nassers-image-in-gulf-history/.
———. Modern Education and Arab Nationalism in Kuwait, 1911–1961." PhD diss., SOAS University of London, 2016.
Reddy, Sujani. *Nursing & Empire: Gendered Labor and Migration from India to the United States*. Chapel Hill: University of North Carolina Press, 2015.
Reese, Scott S. *Imperial Muslims: Islam, Community and Authority in the Indian Ocean, 1839–1937*. Edinburgh: Edinburgh University Press, 2018.
———. "The Myth of Immobility: Women and Travel in the British Imperial Indian Ocean" *Journal of World History* 33, no. 2 (June 2022): 301–320.
Reilly, Benjamin. *Slavery, Agriculture, and Malaria in the Arabian Peninsula*. Athens: Ohio University Press, 2015.
Reinhart, A. Kevin. "Impurity/No Danger." *History of Religions* 30, no. 1 (August 1990): 1–24.
Reisz, Todd. *Showpiece City: How Architecture Made Dubai*. Stanford, CA: Stanford University Press, 2020.
Reverby, Susan M. *Examining Tuskegee: The Infamous Syphilis Study and its Legacy*. Chapel Hill: University of North Carolina Press, 2009.
———, ed. *Tuskegee's Truths: Rethinking the Tuskegee Syphilis Study*. Chapel Hill: University of North Carolina Press, 2012.
Reynolds, Dwight F., ed. *Interpreting the Self: Autobiography in the Arabic Literary Tradition*. Berkeley: University of California Press, 2001.
Reynolds, Nancy Y. *A City Consumed: Urban Commerce, the Cairo Fire, and the Politics of Decolonization in Egypt*. Stanford, CA: Stanford University Press, 2012.
Rifa'i, 'Abd al-'Aziz and Sayyid Ahmad Yunis. *Bina' al-Dawla al-'Arabiyya al-Sa'udiyya fi al-'Asr al-Hadith wa-l-Mu'asir 1902–1953* [Building the Saudi Arabian state in the modern and contemporary era]. Cairo: Al-Maktaba al-'Alamiyya, 1978.

Rizzo, Helen Mary. *Islam, Democracy, and the Status of Women: The Case of Kuwait*. New York: Routledge, 2005.
Rominger, Chris. "Nursing Transgressions, Exploring Difference: North Africans in French Medical Spaces during World War I." *International Journal of Middle East Studies* 50, no. 4 (2018): 691–713.
Al-Rumaydi, Talal Saʿd. *al-Kuwayt wa-l-Khalij al-ʿArabi fi al-Salnama al-ʿUthmaniyya* [Kuwait and the Arab Gulf in the Ottoman salname]. Kuwait: N.p., 2009.
Al-Sabah, Meshal. *Gender and Politics in Kuwait: Women and Political Participation in the Gulf*. London: I. B. Tauris, 2013.
Sachedina, Amal. *Cultivating the Past, Living the Modern: The Politics of Time in the Sultanate of Oman*. Ithaca, NY: Cornell University Press, 2021.
———. "Nizwa Fort: Transforming Ibadi Religion through Heritage Discourse in Oman." *Comparative Studies of South Asia, Africa and the Middle East* 39, no. 2 (August 2019): 328–343.
Al-Saliʿ, ʿAbd Allah. *Al-Khadamat al-Sihhiyya bi Madinat Mecca al-Mukarrama* [Health services in Mecca]. Mecca, Saudi Arabia: Umm Al-Qura University, 1983.
Al-Salimi, ʿAbdullah bin Humayd. *Jawabat al-Imam al-Salimi* [Imam al-Salimi's responses]. Vol. 2. Edited by ʿAbdullah bin Muhammad bin ʿAbdullah al-Salimi and ʿAbd al-Sattar Abu Ghuddah. Muscat: Maktabat al-Imam al-Salimi, 2010.
Samin, Nadav. *Of Sand or Soil: Genealogy & Tribal Belonging in Saudi Arabia*. Princeton, NJ: Princeton University Press, 2015.
Sammut, Charlie. "The Life of Dr Jayakar. A British Agency Surgeon in Muscat." Transcript. *BOS Podcasts*. British Omani Society, May 12, 2020. https://www.ao-soc.org/news/aos/podcast-transcript-cs.
———. "Medicine and Politics at the Edge of Empire: Surgeon Lt Col Atmaram Sadashiva Grandin Jayakar." YouTube video, Anglo-Omani Society, May 18, 2022. https://www.youtube.com/watch?v=YRC8-j_MjWk.
Sariyildiz, Gülden, and Oya Dağlar Macar. "Cholera, Pilgrimage, and International Politics of Sanitation: The Quarantine Station on the Island of Kamaran." In *Plague and Contagion in the Islamic Mediterranean*, edited by Nükhet Varlık, 243–273. Kalamazoo, MI: Arc Humanities Press, 2017.
Al-Sayegh, Fatma Hassan. "American Women Missionaries in the Gulf: Agents for Cultural Change." *Islam and Christian-Muslim Relations* 9, no. 3 (1998): 339–356.
Scalenghe, Sara. *Disability in the Ottoman Arab World, 1500–1800*. New York: Cambridge University Press, 2014.

Schotthoefer, Anna M., Scott W. Bearden, Jennifer L. Holmes, Sara M. Vetter, John A. Montenieri, Shanna K. Williams, Christine B. Graham, Michael E. Woods, Rebecca J. Eisen, and Kenneth L. Gage. "Effects of Temperature on the Transmission of *Yersinia Pestis* by the Flea, *Xenopsylla Cheopis*, in the Late Phase Period." *Parasites & Vectors* 4, 191 (2011). https://doi.org/10.1186/1756-3305-4-191.

Scott, David. "Colonial Governmentality." *Social Text*, no. 43 (1995): 191–220.

Shamma, Samir. *Bitrul al-Kuwayt: Hadiruhu wa Mustaqbaluhu* [Kuwait petroleum: Its present and future]. Damascus: Matabi' Ibn Zibdun, 1959.

Al-Sharim, Hissa 'Abd Allah. *Tarikh Ta'lim al-Tamrid bi Dawla Qatar, 1969–2008* [History of nursing education in Qatar, 1969–2008]. Doha: National Health Authority, 2007.

Shatz, Julia R. "A Politics of Care: Local Nurses in Mandate Palestine." *International Journal of Middle East Studies* 50, no. 4 (2018): 669–689.

Al-Shaybani, Muhammad bin Ibrahim. *Al-Amrad al-Fattaka fi Tarikh al-Kuwayt: al-Ta'un, al-Judariyy, al-Influwanza* [Fatal diseases in Kuwait's history: Plague, smallpox, influenza]. Kuwait: Markaz al-Makhtutat wa-l-Turath wa-l-Watha'iq, 2017.

Al-Shaybani, Sultan bin Mubarak bin Hamad. *Al-Tawa'in fi al-Dhakira al-'Umaniyya* [Plagues in Omani memory]. Muscat: Mahboub, 2021.

Shihab, Yusif. *Al-Kuwayt 'Abra al-Tarikh* [Kuwait throughout history]. Kuwait: N.p., 1989.

Sinan, Mahmoud. *Tarikh Qatar al-'Amm* [General history of Qatar]. Baghdad: Al-Ma'aref Press, 1966.

Singha, Radhika. "Passport, Ticket, and India-Rubber Stamp: 'The Problem of the Pauper Pilgrim' in Colonial India c. 1882–1925." In *The Limits of British Colonial Control in South Asia: Spaces of Disorder in the Indian Ocean Region*, edited by Ashwini Tambe and Harald Fischer-Tiné, 49–78. New York: Routledge, 2009.

Smith, Susan L. *Sick and Tired of Being Sick and Tired: Black Women's Health Activism in America, 1890–1950*. Philadelphia: University of Pennsylvania Press, 1995.

Snyder, J. C., R. C. Page, E. S. Murray, R. H. Daggy, S. D. Bell Jr., R. L. Nichols, N. A. Haddad, A. T. Hanna, and D. McComb. "Observations on the Etiology of Trachoma." *American Journal of Ophthalmology* 48, no. 3, pt. 2 (September 1959): 325–329.

"Steam Initiative: Oral History." Texas A&M University at Qatar. http://steam.qatar.tamu.edu/digital-narratives-2/oral-history/.

Steinberg, Guido. "Ecology, Knowledge, and Trade in Central Arabia (*Najd*) during the Nineteenth and Early Twentieth Centuries." In *Counter-Narratives:*

History, Contemporary Society, and Politics in Saudi Arabia and Yemen, edited by Madawi Al-Rasheed and Robert Vitalis, 77–102. New York: Palgrave Macmillan, 2004.

Stolz, Daniel A. "The Voyage of the *Samannud*: Pilgrimage, Cholera, and Empire on an Ottoman-Egyptian Steamship Journey in 1865–66." *International Journal of Turkish Studies* 23, nos. 1–2 (2017): 1–18.

Storm, Ida Paterson. "Touring Troubles." *Arabia Calling* 218 (Autumn–Winter 1949–1950): 3–12.

Subramaniam, Banu. *Holy Science: The Biopolitics of Hindu Nationalism*. Seattle: University of Washington Press, 2019.

Suzuki, Hideaki. *Slave Trade Profiteers in the Western Indian Ocean: Suppression and Resistance in the Nineteenth Century*. Cham, Switzerland: Palgrave Macmillan, 2017.

Swedenburg, Ted. "Egypt's Music of Protest: From Sayyid Darwish to DJ Haha." *Middle East Report* 265 (Winter 2012): 39–43.

Al-Tabur, ʿAbd Allah ʿAli. *Al-Tibb al-Shaʿbi fi al-Imarat al-ʿArabiyya al-Muttahida* [Folk medicine in the United Arab Emirates]. Dubai: Markaz al-Khalij li-l-Kutub, 1998.

Tagliacozzo, Eric. "Hajj in the Time of Cholera: Pilgrim Ships and Contagion from Southeast Asia to the Red Sea." In *Global Muslims in the Age of Steam and Print*, edited by James L. Gelvin and Nile Green, 103–120. Berkeley: University of California Press, 2013.

Takriti, Abdel Razzaq. *Monsoon Revolution: Republicans, Sultans, and Empires in Oman, 1965–1976*. Oxford: Oxford University Press, 2013.

Tang, F. F., H. Chang, Y. Huang, and K. Wang, "Studies on the Etiology of Trachoma with Special Reference to Isolation of the Virus in Chick Embryo." *Chinese Medical Journal* 75 (1957): 429–447.

Teskey, Rachel, and Norah Alkhamis, "Oral History and National Stories: Theory and Practice in the Gulf Cooperation Council." In *Representing the Nation: Heritage, Museums, National Narratives, and Identity in the Arab Gulf States*, edited by Pamela Erskine-Loftus, Mariam Al-Mulla, and Victoria Hightower, 133–147. New York: Routledge, 2016.

Tétreault, Mary Ann, and Haya al-Mughni. "Gender, Citizenship and Nationalism in Kuwait." *British Journal of Middle Eastern Studies* 22, nos. 1–2 (1995): 64–80.

———. "Modernization and Its Discontents: State and Gender in Kuwait." *Middle East Journal* 49, no. 3 (Summer 1995): 403–417.

Thoms, Marion Wells. "Bahrein Station." *Neglected Arabia* 36 (October–December 1900): 7–11.

———. "Women Patients." *Neglected Arabia* 44 (October–December 1902): 17–20.

Thoms, S. J. "Bahrein." *Neglected Arabia* 37 (January–March 1901): 6–8.

———. "The Hospital at Bahrein." *Neglected Arabia* 44 (October–December 1902): 12–16.

———. "Opening Work at Bahrein: A Shark Bite." *Neglected Arabia* 35 (July–September 1900): 6.

Thomson, Theodore. *Report by Dr. Theodore Thomson on the Sanitary Requirements of Certain Places in or near the Persian Gulf, &.*, Printed for the use of the Foreign Office, October 1906. London School of Hygiene & Tropical Medicine Library & Archives Service. https://archive.org/details/b21359118.

Tiffany, M. N. "Women's Medical Work in Bahrain." *Neglected Arabia* 154 (July–September 1930): 7–10.

Tilley, Helen. "Medical Cultures, Therapeutic Properties, and Laws in Global History." In "Therapeutic Properties: Global Medical Cultures, Knowledge, and Law," edited by Helen Tilley. Special Issue, *Osiris* 36 (2021): 1–24.

Toledano, Ehud. *As If Silent and Absent: Bonds of Enslavement in the Islamic Middle East*. New Haven, CT: Yale University Press, 2007.

"Trachoma." Mayo Clinic. https://www.mayoclinic.org/diseases-conditions/trachoma/symptoms-causes/syc-20378505.

"Trachoma." World Health Organization, May 9, 2021. https://www.who.int/news-room/fact-sheets/detail/trachoma.

Underhill, Betty M. L. "Salt-Induced Vaginal Stenosis of Arabia." *BJOG: An International Journal of Obstetrics and Gynaecology* 71, no. 2 (1964): 293–298.

Valeri, Marc. "High Visibility, Low Profile: The Shi'a in Oman under Sultan Qaboos." *International Journal of Middle East Studies* 42, no. 2 (2010): 251–268.

Van Ess, John. "The Annual Meeting." *Neglected Arabia* 45 (January–March 1903): 3–5.

Varlık, Nükhet. *Plague and Empire in the Early Modern Mediterranean World: The Ottoman Experience, 1347–1600*. New York: Cambridge University Press, 2015.

Vassiliev, Alexei. *The History of Saudi Arabia*. London: Saqi Books, 2000.

Vinea, Ana. "Possessed or Insane? Diagnostic Puzzles in Contemporary Egypt." *International Journal of Middle East Studies* (2023): 1–15. https://doi.org/10.1017/S0020743823000673.

———. "'What Is Your Evidence?' A Salafi Therapy in Contemporary Egypt." *Comparative Studies of South Asia, Africa and the Middle East* 39, no. 3 (2019): 500–512.

Visser, Reidar. *Basra, the Failed Gulf State: Separatism and Nationalism in Southern Iraq*. London: Global Book Marketing, 2005.

Vitalis, Robert. *America's Kingdom: Mythmaking on the Saudi Oil Frontier.* Stanford, CA: Stanford University Press, 2007.
Watson, Janet C. E. "Travel to Mecca from Southern Oman in the Pre-Motorized Period." In *The Hajj: Collected Essays*, edited by Venetia Porter and Liana Saif, 96–99. London: British Museum Press, 2013.
Watts, S. J. "From Rapid Change to Stasis: Official Responses to Cholera in British-Ruled India and Egypt: 1860 to C. 1921." *Journal of World History* 12, no. 2 (Fall 2001): 321–374.
Webb, James L. A., Jr. *Humanity's Burden: A Global History of Malaria.* Cambridge: Cambridge University Press, 2009.
Weiss, Richard S. *Recipes for Immortality: Medicine, Religion, and Community in South India.* Oxford: Oxford University Press, 2009.
Wellsted, J. R. *Travels to the City of the Caliphs along the Shores of the Persian Gulf and the Mediterranean.* 2 vols. London: Henry Colburn, 1840.
Wilkinson, J. C. *The Imamate Tradition of Oman.* Cambridge: Cambridge University Press, 1987.
———. *Water and Tribal Settlement in South-East Arabia: A Study of the Aflāj of Oman.* Oxford: Oxford University Press, 1977.
Wilson, Alice. *Afterlives of Revolution: Everyday Counterhistories in Southern Oman.* Stanford, CA: Stanford University Press, 2023.
Woodward, Catherine S. "The Discourse and Experience of the Arabian Mission's Medical Missionaries: Part I 1920–39." *Middle Eastern Studies* 47, no. 5 (2011): 779–805.
———. "The Discourse and Experiences of the Arabian Mission's Medical Missionaries: Part II 1939–1960." *Middle Eastern Studies* 47, no. 6 (2011): 885–910.
World Health Organization. Minutes of the First Meeting of the Fifteenth Session of the Regional Committee for the Eastern Mediterranean Held at the Africa Hall Addis-Ababa on Wednesday 22 September 1965. Doc. No. EM/RC15A/Prog.min.1, November 1965. https://apps.who.int/iris/bitstream/handle/10665/124087/em_rcl5_a_prog_min_1_en.pdf.
Wright, Andrea. *Between Dreams and Ghosts: Indian Migration and Middle Eastern Oil.* Stanford, CA: Stanford University Press, 2021.
Wytenbroek, Lydia. "Nursing (Inter)nationalism in Iran, 1916–1947." *Journal of Middle East Women's Studies* 18, no. 1 (March 2022): 36–58.
Yamani, Mai Ahmad Zaki. "Birth and Behaviour in a Hospital in Saudi Arabia." *Bulletin (British Society for Middle Eastern Studies)* 13, no. 2 (1986): 169–176.
Zahlan, Rosemarie Said. "The Gulf States and the Palestine Problem, 1936–48." *Arab Studies Quarterly* 3, no. 1 (1981): 19.

Zdanowski, Jerzy. *Speaking with Their Own Voices: The Stories of Slaves in the Persian Gulf in the 20th Century.* Cambridge: Cambridge Scholars Press, 2014.

Zwemer, Amy E. "Lay-Preaching in the Women's Dispensary." *Neglected Arabia* 43 (July–September 1902): 8–10.

———. "The Ups and Downs of Work for the Women." *Neglected Arabia* 47 (July–September 1903): 7–10.

———. "Work for Women." *Neglected Arabia* 37 (January–March 1901): 9–10.

Zwemer, S. M. "Bahrein." *Neglected Arabia* 35 (July–September 1900): 3–5.

INDEX

Page numbers in *italic* refer to images or tables.

'Abd Allah bin Salih al-Yaf i, 187–88
Abdalla Salim, 138
'Abd al-'Aziz bin Ahmad Al Ahmad Al Thani, Shaykh, 184–86
'Abd al-'Aziz Ibn Sa'ud, 101, 224n25
'Abd al-Malik, Maryam, 191–92
Abdullah al-Salem, Shaykh, 140, 141
Abdulla bin Khamis, 19, 20
Abdul Rahman, Ali, 123
abortion, 91
Abugideiri, Hibba, 220n59
Abu-Hakima, Ahmad Mustafa, 26–27
Abu-Lughod, Janet, 241n15
Abu Saud, Abeer, 93
al-Afghani, Sara, 147–48
Agha Khani community, 49, 52, 212n9
Ahmadi Town, 158, 238n118
Ahmad al-Jabir, Shaykh, 137, 138, 140
Alexandria, cholera epidemic, 208n55
'Ali, Layla, 161
'Ali ibn 'Abbas Majusi, 82
Ali Salman, 19
Alkhamis, Norah, 242n26
Alsada, Maryam, 201n30, 217n2
American University of Beirut, 132, 232n9
Al-Amiri Hospital (Kuwait), 142
Amrith, Sunil, 140
Anglo-Boer War, 149–50

Anglo-Iranian Oil Company (AIOC), 233n27
Anglo-Persian Oil Company, 138
animals, contagion of, 27
anthrax, 27
Arab Charitable Association, 68
Arabian Mission: competition with government medical services, 77–78; and medical institutional change, 55; recruitment of women doctors and nurses, 60–61; resistance to, 56–58, 59–60. *See also* hospitals; missionaries
Arab nationalism, 138–39, 141, 145, 232n8
Arabness, 171–72
Arab Support Committee, 117
Aramco (Arabian American Oil Company): accountability of employees, 108–9; corporate colonialism and state building, 14–15, 97, 100–105, 224n18; employee living conditions, 96, 124–27, *125*, *126*; hierarchical medical interventions, 106–10; politics of health, 99–100; trachoma vaccine tests (overview), 14–15. *See also* experiments
Aramco-Harvard research. *See* experiments

architecture of hospitals: and gendered medicine, 51, 53, 62–63; and local climate, 56
Ashkanani, Zubaydah, 244n63
al-'Awwami, 'Ali al-Sayyid Baqir, 79–80, 90, 105
Al-'Azam Hospital (Kuwait), 145
Al-Azri, Nasser Hammad, 213n18

Bahrain: childbirth, 76–77, 85; corpses, handling of, 226n60; dispensaries, 65–67; epidemic mortalities, 34; eye disease, 104–5; hospitals, 53, 55–56, 63–65, 70–71, 187, 213n23; hospitals, government–missionary competition, 77–78; immigration to, 187; missionaries, 55–56, 63–67, 75, 76–78; oil discovery date, 172; plague, 34, 65–67, 216n82; quarantine, 33, 45
Barghash bin Sa'id (Sultan of Zanzibar), 208n62
al-Barjas, Barjas Hammud, 148–49, 153, 237n92
Basra: Arabian Mission in, 55; plague, 26, 40; quarantine measures by Ottomans, 40–42; quarantine stations, 24, 43, 44, 45, 46
Bediyyu bin Farhan, 188
Bedouins, 58–59, 85–86, 101
Belgrave, Charles, 81, 104
Bhatia community, 49, 51, 53
biomedicine: definition, 202n41; and folk medicine, 170, 173, 188–89; and state power (overview), 191–96; as Trojan Horse, 54, 213n18. *See also* folk medicine (*al-ṭibb al-sha'bī*); health and power; local health practices
Boodrookas, Alex, 135
Borel, Frédéric, 25–26
British Agency medical dispensaries, 49, 57–58

British imperialism. *See* Government of India; Great Britain
British India Steam Navigation Company, 24
British Petroleum, 140
Burton, Elise, 123
Bushire: cholera, 28; epidemics, 37–39; political and economic importance, 36–37; quarantine, 25; quarantine stations, *40, 41, 42*

Calverley, Edwin, 67–68
Calverley, Eleanor, 62, 75–76
cataract treatment, 61, 64, 215n71
cauterization (*al-kayy*), 31–32, 185–87, 209n71
childbirth: overview, 14, 72–74, 94–95; in Aramco hospitals, 111; in folk medicine, 86–94, 221n73; vaginal packing, 72–74, 78–86, 94, 217n2; women missionaries and medical conversion, 74–78, 217n6; women navigating medicalization, 94–95. *See also* hospitals
Childs, J. Rives, 117
China and plague, 47–48, 209n78, 211n106
cholera: Alexandria, 208n55; Bushire, 28; Hijaz, 22–23; introduced from India, 28; Iran, 131; Kuwait, 131–32; Oman, 30–31; Oman and Muscat, 1–4, 6, 199n20, 205n30; and Ottoman expansionism, 40–41; pandemics, 197n5; Qatif, 28; vaccinations in Kuwait, 131–32; and water systems, 2–3, 199n20, 209n66
Choy, Catherine Ceniza, 144–45
citizen-noncitizen binaries: in Gulf region, 239n132; and health care, 167; in Kuwait, 15, 141–46, 157–62, 239n131; and medical nostalgia, 15–16, 169–70, 173, 175, 241n10; in Oman, 239n132; in Saudi Arabia,

96, 99–103, 106–11, 225n40, 227n72; in United States, 144. *See also* Aramco (Arabian American Oil Company); gendered medicine; hierarchies of race and/or class; nurses

citizenship: nationality law (Kuwait), 141, 155; as unstable, 239n4

class distinctions. *See* hierarchies of race and/or class

clinical misogyny, 110–16, 227n72. *See also* gendered medicine

colonialism and medical interventions. *See* health and power

Commins, David, 207n46

contagion: overview, 13, 19–22; globalization of disease, 22–26; and imperialism, British, 32–40, 45–47; and imperialism, Ottoman, 40–47; in pre-imperial Gulf communities, 26–32; public health as coercion, 47–48

contagion of animals, 27

contraception, 82, 91, 112, 115–16, 220n37

corporate colonialism: overview, 14–15, 97; and state building, 14–15, 97, 100–105, 224n18. *See also* Aramco (Arabian American Oil Company); experiments

corpses, handling of, 30–31, 108, 226n60

Crystal, Jill, 138

Curzon, Lord George (Viceroy of India), 24–25

Daggy, Richard, 102, 103, 227n72
Dale, Charlotte, 149–50
Dalenberg, Cornelia, 36, 76–77, 103–4
Dammam, development in, 100
Davies, Fred, 97
Dawud, Fawziyya, 147
Dewachi, Omar, 202n37

Dhahran, development in, 100
Dhahran Health Center, 96
Dhahran Hospital (Saudi Arabia), 111
Dhahran laboratory, 97, 117. *See also* experiments
Dickson, H. R. P., 137
disabilities, 88, 220n56
Doha, hospitals in, 164–65
Doumato, Eleanor Abdella, 209n71
Dubai, epidemic mortalities, 34

Eastern Province, Saudi Arabia: clinical and epidemiological studies, 118; preventive medicine, 102–3; underdevelopment, 100, 224n19. *See also* experiments

Educational Council (Kuwait), 138–39

Egypt: medicine and policy, 202n37; missionaries in, 55, 78; *sha'bī* music, 170–71; trachoma studies, 229n104; *zār* in, 243n52

El Guindi, Ismail, 79

El Tor lazaretto, 23–24, 205n17

Emirates: demographic imbalance, 169, 241n10; hospitals, 174–75; isolation of patients, 28; magical medicine, enslaved people, and women, 177–81; magical medicine and Islamic tradition, 173–77; National Archives oral history initiative, 189; oil discovery date, 172; smallpox vaccinations, 174

Ennis, Crystal A., 239n132

enslaved people: contagion among, 27; and magical medicine practice, 172, 179–81; manumission of, 70–71; numbers of, 177, 245n85; trade in, 19, 20, 177–78, 203n2, 203n6, 243n50. *See also* slavery

epidemics: British records of mortalities, 34; Bushire, 37–39; and mobility of pearl divers, 26,

epidemics (*continued*)
29–30; smallpox, 136–37. *See also* cholera; immunizations; plague
experiments: overview, 14–15, 96–100, 128–30; clinical misogyny, 110–16, 227n72; corporate colonialism and state building, 14–15, 97, 100–105, 224n18; hierarchical medical interventions, 106–10
—, TRACHOMA PROJECT: environmental differences, 96, 124–27, *125, 126*; identification of pathogen, 98, 116–19, 229n104; state knowledge of, 123–24; symptoms and treatment, 103–5; transmission, 118–19, 225n45, 229nn107–108; vaccine development, 98–99, 119–23, *122*
eye diseases, 103–5, 118–19, 225n45, 226n48, 229nn107–108. *See also* experiments, trachoma project

Fahmy, Kamal, 59, 80, 82, 85
Fahmy, Khaled, 202n37
Faisal bin ʿAbd al-ʿAziz Al Saʿud, 224n21
Faysal bin Turki, Sultan of Muscat and Oman: cholera epidemic, 1–2, 4, 6; hospital construction, 49–53, 59–60; quarantine enforcement, 19–21, 33
folk medicine (*al-ṭibb al-shaʿbī*): overview, 15–16, 164–67, 189–90; childbirth in, 86–94, 221n73; magical medicine, enslaved people, and women, 177–81; magical medicine and Islamic tradition, 173–77; as national heritage of Qatar, 181–89; and politics of heritage, 167–73, 241n15, 242n26. *See also* childbirth; local health practices
Foucault, Michel, 10–11
French flagging of ships, 20
Frith, Kathleen, 81, 83–85, 86

gender: and hardships of work, 146–47; and Indian Ocean mobilities, 9, 201n30; in Kuwait nationality law, 155; and morbidity, 4; tensions surrounding methods of healing, 175–76, 179. *See also* gendered medicine; nurses
gendered medicine: cauterization by opposite sex, 31–32; and citizen-noncitizen binaries for nurses, 160–61; clinical misogyny, 110–16, 227n72; hospital architecture, 51, 53, 62–63; and hospitals (overview), 13–14; male role in childbirth, 74–78, 92, 217n6, 221n76; and missionaries, 60–62, 69–70; and misunderstandings, 63–66; sexualization of patients' body parts, 80–81, 219n29; trachoma project, 110–16, 227n72; trachoma transmission, 118–19, 229nn107–108. *See also* childbirth; hierarchies of race and/or class; hospitals; nurses
Giladi, Avner, 74, 217n6
Gilman, Daniel J., 171
Giza Memorial Ophthalmological Institute (Egypt), 229n104
global influenza pandemic, 101, 224n25
globalization of disease, 22–26
Government of India: hospital funding in Muscat, 49, 50; hospitals in Bahrain, 56; oversight of Muscat's foreign affairs, 36; and politics of contagion, 34. *See also* Indians
Great Britain: competition with Ottomans, 45–46, 57; institutionalized health care, 49–50, 52; protection of Kuwait, 43–44, 57; quarantine stations, 19–20, 24–25; separation of Zanzibar from Muscat, 198n12;

slave trade, 19, 20, 243n50; support of coastal rulers, 21, 198n7; welfare state, 140
Great Manchurian Plague, 47–48, 209n78
Great War: effects on missionary–British dynamics, 68; racism during, 155
Gulf Oil, 138

Hadad, Regina, 156
Haddad, Nadim, 123
al-Hadidi, Yahiya, 142
al-Hajiri, Yusuf Ya'qub, 101–2
hajj (pilgrimage): quarantine measures, 22–23, 204n16; steamship transportation, 208n62
Hamad 'Abd Allah al-Saqr, 69
Hamad ibn Isa Al Khalifa, Shaykh of Bahrain, 69
Hamud bin Mohammad, Sultan of Zanzibar, 3
Handschin, Richard, 112–14, 115, 227n72
Hanna, Nabil Subhi, 86–94
Hansen, Henny Harold, 104–5, 226n60
Harb, Wadi'a, 151–52
Harrison, Paul, 27, 31–32, 101
al-Harthi, Saleh bin 'Ali, 208n62
Harvard School of Public Health (HSPH). *See* experiments
Harvard University. *See* experiments
al-Hasa, Saudi Arabia, 100, 101, 103, 222n4
al-Hatim, 'Abd Allah Khalid, 29–30, 70
health and power: overview, 1–7, 191–96; beyond national borders and chronologies, 7–10; methods of study, 16–17, 199n22, 202n37, 202n41; between politics of health and theories of power, 10–12. *See also* childbirth; contagion; experiments; folk medicine (*al-ṭibb al-sha'bī*); hospitals; nurses; state building
health and religious and cultural norms. *See* religious and cultural norms
health care and state building. *See* state building
hierarchical medical interventions, 106–10. *See also* citizen-noncitizen binaries
hierarchies of race and/or class: American lens of, 64–65; antagonism toward *zār*, 179–81; in Aramco practices, 96, 99–101, 106–10; in Kuwait medical institutions, 58–59, 157–58; and morbidity, 3–4; and quarantine infrastructure, 21–22, 35–36, 39, 47; in travel, 32–33. *See also* citizen-noncitizen binaries; gender; gendered medicine
hierarchies of religion, 51–52, 53
Hilmi, Mufida, 151–52, 158, 160
Himes, Norman E., 220n37
Holland, R. E., 60
Hopper, Matthew, 31, 177–78
hospitals: overview, 6–7, 13–14, 70–71; architecture of, 51–52, 53, 56, 62–63; in Bahrain, 63–65, 187, 213n23; competition among, 54–60; in Emirates, 174–75; gendered medicine and missionaries, 60–62, 69–70; gendered medicine and misunderstandings, 63–66; in Kuwait, 137–38, 142, 151–52, 156–58; local treatments and hospitals, 63–64, 66–67; in Muscat, 49–53, 59–60, 62–63, 212nn9–10; non-Christian alternatives to, 56, 67–69; and patients, 70–71; in Qatar, 164–65; vs. quarantine system, 53–54; sanatoriums, 156–57. *See also* childbirth; folk medicine (*al-ṭibb al-sha'bī*); local health practices; nurses

HSPH (Harvard School of Public Health). *See* experiments
Hussa Ahmad bin Sayf, 72–73

Ibadi Imamate, 208n62
Ibn Saʿud. *See* ʿAbd al-ʿAziz Ibn Saʿud
Ibn Sina, 215n71
Ibrahim Bey, 43–44
Ikhwan, 68, 101, 207n46
immunizations: of Aramco employees' dependents, 115, 130; cholera, 131–32; polio, 97, 120, 230n117; of sheep against anthrax, 27; smallpox, 120, 136–37, 174. *See also* epidemics; experiments; experiments, trachoma project
imperialism. *See* contagion; Great Britain; health and power; hospitals; Ottomans; state building
India, politics of heritage, 168, 240n6
Indian Medical Service (IMS), 25
Indians: in Kuwait, 161–62; in Muscat, 199n18; in Oman, 199n17; in quarantine stations, 204n16; in United States, 144. *See also* Government of India
infertility, 89–91
influenza pandemic, global, 101, 224n25
informed consent, 110, 128. *See also* experiments
Inhorn, Marcia, 89–90
insecticide use, 103
Iran: cholera, 131; missionary nurses, 233n27; Qajar state, 24, 36–39; slavery, 242n44
Iranians in Kuwait, 136
Iraq, 141, 202n37
Iraqi press, 139
Isa bin Ali Al Khalifa, Shaykh, 33
Islamic tradition: healers in Qatar, 183–85; and magical medicine, 173–77, 187–88. *See also* gendered medicine; religious and cultural norms
Al Istiqlal (Iraqi newspaper), 139

al-Jasir, Hamad, 226n48
Jawab Kull Saʾil ʿind Muʿalijin Qatar al-Awaʾil (al-Maliki), 166–67, 181–84
Jayakar, Atmaram Sadashiva Grandin: career, 10, 197n1; cholera epidemic, 1–4, 6, 199n18, 205n30
jinn, 176–78, 179–81, 188
Juraj, Michael, 108–9

Kamaran Island, 23–24, 204n16
Kanna, Ahmed, 169
al-Karani, Ibrahim, 164–65
al-Khal, Farhan, 68
Khalfan bin Hamad bin Mahomed, 21
al-Khalili, Saʿid bin Khalfan, 31, 208n62, 208n63
al-Khatib, Ahmad, 139
Khaybar, 179
Khobar, 100
Al-Khobar Pediatric and Maternity Hospital (Saudi Arabia), 111
Khojas, 49, 212nn9–10
Khoury, Jamila Fadil, 131–33, 144, 154, 159–60, 161–62
King ʿAbd al-ʿAziz Hospital (Saudi Arabia), 102
Kingston, A. E., 81
Kutchi, Memon Abdul Latif Isani, 52
Kuwait: attack by Ikhwan, 68; British dispensary, 57, 214n40; childbirth, 75–76, 85–86; cholera, 131–32; citizen-noncitizen binaries, 15, 141–46, 157–62, 239n131; hospitals, 53, 62, 142, 151–52, 156–58; hospitals, missionary–government competition in, 77–78; hospitals, resistance to missionary institu-

tions, 57–58, 67–68; ideological quarantine, 207n46; labor disputes, 145, 236n74; medical care as royal privilege, 137; missionaries in, 62, 75–78; nationality law, 141, 155; oil discovery date, 172; pan-Arabism, 132, 133, 232n8; plague, 26, 29–30; population, 141, 214n34; population, medical staff, and beds, 1965–1970, *143*; quarantine and sanitation measures, 42–47, 57, 207n46; recorded deaths, 235n63; slavery, 242n44; smallpox epidemic, 136–37; state building in post-oil era, 137–43; state building in pre-oil era, 134–37; *zār*, 244n63. *See also* Kuwait Municipality; nurses

Kuwaiti merchant class, 67–68, 69, 135–37, 138–40

Kuwaiti press, 155–57, 162

Kuwait Municipality, 135–40. *See also* Kuwait

Kuwait Oil Company (KOC), 137–42, 238n118

labor disputes: Kuwait, 145, 236n74; Saudi Arabia, 96

leprosy, 28

Lerner, Barron H., 219n29

Limbert, Mandana E., 171–72

Lister Institute (London), 117

livestock, contagion in, 27

local health practices: cauterization (*al-kayy*), 31–32, 185–87, 209n71; contagion in pre-imperial Gulf communities, 26–32; eye disease, 104; foreign attitudes toward, 80–81; and interactions with foreign doctors, 82–84; isolation of patients, 28; odors and disease, 58–59; persistence of, 86; for shark injuries, 63. *See also* childbirth; folk medicine (*al-ṭibb al-shaʿbī*)

magical medicine: and enslaved people and women, 177–81; and Islamic tradition, 173–77, 187–88

Majlis movement (Kuwait), 138–40

Al Maktum Hospital (Dubai), 174–75

malaria, 101, 102–3, 105, 113, 221n73, 225n34

al-Maliki, Khalifa al-Sayyid Mohammad Salih: career, 182, 244n68; as source, 164–65, 166–67, 181–85

Mamdani, Mahmood, 113

Manama, hospitals in, 63–64

Mandate Palestine, 235n65, 236n72. *See also* Palestine war (1948); Palestinians

maps, *5, 35*

mashmashi (disease of mules), 27

Mason Memorial Hospital (Bahrain), 55–56, 213n23

Mazmun, ʿAbd al-Rahman, 164, 165

McComb, Dorothy, 118–19, 120, 121–23, 126, 130

McVean, N. N. G. C., 62–63

measles, 28

Mecca, health services in, 102

medical care as royal privilege, 137, 140, 234n30

medical experiments. *See* experiments

medical infrastructure. *See* hospitals; quarantine stations

medical materialism, 30

medical nostalgia: and citizen-noncitizen binaries, 15–16, 169–70, 173, 175, 241n10; in India, 168, 240n6. *See also* folk medicine (*al-ṭibb al-shaʿbī*); local health practices

Memon community, 52, 212n10

methods of study, 16–17, 199n22, 202n37, 202n41

midwives: hiring and paying of, 217n6; and nurse training, 191–92; in opposition to missionary doctors, 74–76; postpartum practices,

midwives (*continued*)
72–74, 78–86, 94, 217n2; training of, 220n59. *See also* childbirth
al-Mir'ibi, Nawal, 150–51
missionaries: access of to privileged spaces, 54, 213n18; in Bahrain, 55–56, 63–67, 75, 76–78; childbirth and medical conversion, 74–78, 217n6; in competition with state health care, 77–78; in Egypt, 78; and hospitals, 13–14, 49–50, 54–58, 60–66, 69–70, 187; in Iran, 233n27; in Kuwait, 46, 57–58, 62, 67–68, 75–78; misunderstandings with locals, 63–65; in Oman, 59–60; and "progress" of local peoples, 8, 61, 71; recruitment of women doctors and nurses, 60–61; relationship with British agencies, 55, 68; resistance to in Kuwait, 57–58, 67–68
Mission Medical Service, 77
modern medicine. *See* biomedicine
Modi, Narendra, 168
Moore, Taylor M., 179
morbidity, 3–4
Movement of Arab Nationalists, 145–46
Msheireb Museums, 189
Mubarak al-Sabah, Shaykh, 43–47, 57, 58, 101
Mukharji, Projit Bihari, 168
Mull, J. Dennis, 129
Muscat, 2; cholera, 1–4, 6; hospitals, 49–53, 59–60, 62–63, 212nn9–10; Indian presence, 49, 199n18, 212nn9–10; oversight of foreign affairs, 36; population, 199n15; quarantine stations, 19–21, 36, *37*, *38*, *39*; separation from Zanzibar, 198n12
Muttrah: cholera, 1–2; plague, 4; population, 199n15; quarantine stations, 36, 205n30
Mylrea, Stanley, 59, 68–69, 101, 137

Najmabadi, Afsaneh, 202n37
Al-Nakib, Farah, 169
Nasser, Gamal Abdel, 141
National Archives of the United Arab Emirates, 189
National Foundation for Infantile Paralysis, 97
nationality law (Kuwait), 141, 155
Neglected Arabia (magazine), 61
New State Hospital (Kuwait), 77
New York, quarantines in, 47
New York Neurological Center, 106–7
Nichols, Elinor, 98–99, 117, 123–24, 129–30
Nichols, Roger, 98–99, 121, *122*, 123–24, 127, 129, 225n45
non-Christian alternatives to hospitals, 56, 67–69
noncitizen workers. *See* citizen-noncitizen binaries; nurses
North Africans, racism against, 155
nurses: overview, 15, 131–34, 162–63; deportment at work, 149–52; deportment outside work, 152–55; health care and state building, post-oil, 137–43; health care and state building, pre-oil, 134–37; Kuwaitization of nursing, 157, 159–62; misconduct implications and accusations, 155–59; training of, 148–49, 159–60, 191–92, 232n9; working conditions, 143–49, 236n72

Oertley, Bob, 111, 112, 115–16
oil industry, discovery dates, 172. *See also* experiments; state building
Oman: cholera, 1–4, 6, 30–31, 205n30; citizen-noncitizen binaries, 239n132; enslaved people and slavery, 19, 20, 178, 203n2, 203n6; historical name, 198nn6–7; Indian presence, 199n17, 212n9; missionary medical practice, 59–60;

noncitizen nurses, 239n132; oil discovery date, 172; population, 198n14, 199n15; separation from Zanzibar, 198n12; water system, 2–3, 199n20, 209n66
oral histories, 173, 174, 189–90, 242n26
Ottomans: in Kuwait, 42–47, 57; medicine and policy in Egypt, 202n37; plague, 200n23; quarantine and sanitation, 40–47, 57; quarantine stations, 24, *43*, *44*, *45*, *46*, 204n16; *zār*, 179

Page, R. C., 102
Palestine, Mandate, 235n65, 236n72
Palestine war (1948), 132–33
Palestinians: interactions with daily governance, 235n65; as medical service providers, 232n11; as teachers, 139
pan-Arabism, 132–33, 141, 232n8
pandemics: cholera, 197n5; global influenza pandemic, 101, 224n25; third global plague pandemic, 44–45, 65–67, 211n106. *See also* cholera; contagion; epidemics; plague
Parker, Chad R., 111
Paterson Storm, Ida, 79, 90
pearl divers: jurisdiction over, 32; mobility and epidemics, 26, 29–30; as patients, 63, 70–71; proposed hospital care for, 69; wives of, 91
Peters, John H., 129
pilgrimage (hajj): quarantine measures, 22–23, 204n16; steamship transportation, 208n62
pilgrims, Shi'i, 41
placentas, disposal of, 93–94
plague: Bahrain, 34, 65–67, 216n82; Basra, 26, 40; deaths from, 210n82; Dubai, 34; epidemic of 1831, 29–30, 207n52; Great Manchurian Plague, 47–48, 209n78; and handling corpses, 30–31; Kuwait, 26; Muscat, 4; Muttrah, 4; Oman, 199n20; Ottoman experience, 200n23; Qatif, 26; Sharjah, 34; temperature and transmission, 66, 216n82; terms for, 207n50, 209n65; third global pandemic, 44–45, 65–67, 211n106. *See also* contagion; quarantine; quarantine stations
polio vaccine, 97, 120, 230n117
politics of contagion. *See* contagion
politics of heritage, 167–73, 240n6, 241n15, 242n26. *See also* folk medicine (*al-ṭibb al-shaʿbī*)
Potter, Lawrence G., 199n22
public health and medicine: communication with locals, 20, 21–22, 48; and governance, 4, 6, 32–33, 59–60, 135–37. *See also* health and power
Punjab, 229n108

Qajar state, 24, 36–39. *See also* Iran
Qatar: childbirth, 93; enslaved people and slavery, 242n44, 245n85; folk healers, 164–65; malaria control, 221n73; national heritage of folk medicine, 181–89; nurses training, 191–92; oil discovery date, 172; quarantine stations, 45
Qatif: cholera, 28; conquest of, 101; disease prevalence, 105; health care facilities, 101; malaria control, 103; plague, 26; quarantine stations, 45; underdevelopment, 100
al-Qattan, ʿAwataf, 161
quarantine: ideological, 207n46; and imperialism, British, 32–40, 45–47; and imperialism, Ottoman, 40–47; isolation of patients

quarantine (*continued*)
in pre-imperial Gulf, 28; motivations for, 33–34, 53–54. *See also* local health practices; quarantine stations
quarantine stations: overview, 6–7, 13; El Tor lazaretto, 23–24, 205n17; escapes from, 19–22; Kamaran Island, 23–24, 204n16; Muscat, *37*, *38*, *39*; race and class hierarchies in, 21–22, 35–36, 39, *40*, *41*, *42*, *43*, *44*, *45*, *46*, 47; and regional trade, 210n84. *See also* quarantine

Rahman, Daudur, 57, 58, 214n40
ranj (disease of mules), 27
Ras Al Khaimah, 28
al-Rashid, ʿAbd al-ʿAziz, 30
Rashid Rida, Muhammad, 67–68
Al-Rashoud, Talal, 139, 141
Reddy, Sujani, 155
Red Sea, sanitation and quarantine measures, 22–23
Reformed Church in America, 53, 55
Reilly, Benjamin, 179, 243n52
religious and cultural norms, 30–32, 108, 116, 226n60. *See also* folk medicine (*al-ṭibb al-shaʿbī*); gendered medicine; local health practices
Rominger, Chris, 155
al-Rumaydi, Talal Saʿd, 43–44
Rushdi, Rasim, 58–59
Russia: international rivalries, 22, 38–39; quarantine stations, 25, 37
Russian doctors, 47–48

Al-Sabah, ʿAbd Allah al-Jabir, Shaykh, 136
Al-Sabah, Fahad al-Salem, Shaykh, 133
Al-Sabah Hospital (Kuwait), 142, 151–52
Sachedina, Amal, 168–69, 178
Salih, ʿAʾisha, 160, 161
al-Salimi, ʿAbdullah bin Humayd, 30, 31, 208n62

Salk, Jonas, 97, 230n117
sanatoriums, 156–57
Saʿud bin ʿAbd al-ʿAziz Al Saʿud, 101, 224n21
Saudi Arabia: citizen-noncitizen binaries, 96, 99–103, 106–11, 225n40, 227n72; contraception in, 112, 115–16; global influenza pandemic, 101, 224n25; medical care as royal privilege, 234n30; oil discovery date, 172; public health care expansion, 105; slavery, 242n44; state building, 14–15, 97, 100–105, 224n18. *See also* Aramco (Arabian American Oil Company)
Sayyid Saʿid al Bu-Saʿidi, Sultan of Muscat and Oman, 198n12
Scalenghe, Sara, 220n56, 226n48
scientific medicine. *See* biomedicine
Scott, Norman, 53
sexualization of patients' body parts, 80–81, 219n29
Sharjah, epidemic mortalities, 34
Shatz, Julia R., 235n65
Shiʿi pilgrims, 41
slavery: banning of, 242n44; contagion control, 27. *See also* enslaved people
smallpox, 28, 120, 136–37, 174
Snyder, John C., 96–97, 99
social boundaries. *See* citizen-noncitizen binaries; hierarchies of race and/or class; hierarchies of religion
Standard Oil, 100
state building: and corporate colonialism, 14–15, 97, 100–105, 224n18; and national heritage, 169–70; in post-oil Kuwait, 137–43; in pre-oil Kuwait, 134–37
Suez Canal, 22–23, 24, 141
Sur, slavery in, 19, 203n2
Suwailim bin Faraj, 70–71
al-Suwaydi, ʿAbd al-Rahman bin ʿAbd Allah, 26

Swedenburg, Ted, 170–71
syphilis, 90
Syrian Protestant College, 232n9

al-Tabur, 'Abd Allah 'Ali, 28, 166–67, 173–80, 242n27
Tahiya bint Hemd, 123
al-Tali'a (pro-labor mouthpiece), 145–46, 147
Tang, F. F., 98, 116–17
Taylor, Julius W., 106, 107–8, 109, 110, 116, 127, 227n72
Teskey, Rachel, 242n26
Thoms, Marion, 64–65
Thoms, Sharon, 56, 61, 63
Thomson, Theodore, 34–36, 38–39, 42, 46–47
al-ṭibb al-sha'bī (folk medicine). *See* folk medicine (*al-ṭibb al-sha'bī*); local health practices
Al-Tibb al-Sha'bi fi al-Imarat al-'Arabiyya al-Muttahida (al-Tabur), 166–67
Tiffany, M. N., 76
Toledano, Ehud, 179, 243n52
trachoma: symptoms and treatment, 103–5; transmission, 118–19, 225n45, 229nn107–108. *See also* experiments, trachoma project
traditional medicine. *See* folk medicine (*al-ṭibb al-sha'bī*); local health practices
tuberculosis, 142

Underhill, Betty, 81–82, 84, 85
United States: citizen-noncitizen binaries, 144; gendered hardships of work, 146; health care workers, 161; sexualization of patients' body parts, 219n29; treaty with Oman, 59–60
Usrati (Kuwaiti women's publication), 158
'Uthman bin Bashr, 28, 29

vaccines. *See* experiments; immunizations
vaginal packing and atresia, 72–74, 78–86, 94, 217n2. *See also* childbirth
Van Ess, John, 56
Varlık, Nükhet, 200n23
venereal disease, 90
Victoria Memorial Hospital (Bahrain), 56
Vinea, Ana, 176–77
Vitalis, Robert, 100, 224n18

Wahhabi clerics, 101
Wahhabi movement, 179
Walton-Roberts, Margaret, 239n132
water access, 92, 191, 221n73
water infrastructure in Oman, 2–3, 199n20, 209n66
Weiss, Richard, 168
Wellsted, James Raymond, 29
women: as healers, 172, 174, 176; practice of *zār*, 179, 180, 244n63. *See also* childbirth; gender; gendered medicine; nurses
Woodward, Catherine S., 74–75
World Health Organization (WHO), 191
World War I: missionary–British dynamics, 68; racism, 155
Wright, Andrea, 134

Yamani, Mai Ahmad Zaki, 93

Zanzibar, 198n12
zār, 176–81, 188, 243n52, 244n63. *See also* folk medicine (*al-ṭibb al-sha'bī*)
Zayed bin Sultan Al Nahyan, Shaykh, 174
Zwemer, Amy, 62, 66, 216n82
Zwemer, Samuel, 67